CMC Vellore Handbook of
EMERGENCY MEDICINE

CMC Vellore Handbook of
EMERGENCY MEDICINE

THIRD EDITION

Editor

KPP Abhilash

MBBS MD PDF (Emergency Medicine)

Professor and Head
Department of Emergency Medicine
Christian Medical College Hospital
Vellore, Tamil Nadu, India

Foreword

K Prasad Mathews

MD FRACP (Geriatrics)
Medical Superintendent, CMC

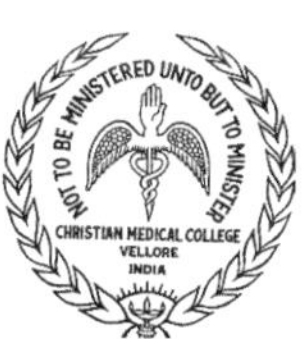

**CMC Vellore Handbook of Emergency Medicine, previously called
Emergency Medicine at CMC (EMAC)**

A Compendium for
Emergency Department Registrars

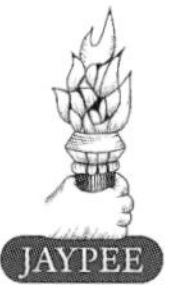

JAYPEE BROTHERS MEDICAL PUBLISHERS
The Health Sciences Publisher
New Delhi | London

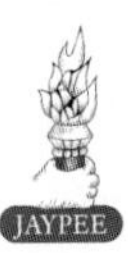 **Jaypee Brothers Medical Publishers (P) Ltd**

Headquarters
EMCA House
23/23-B, Ansari Road, Daryaganj
New Delhi 110 002, India
Landline: +91-11-23272143, +91-11-23272703
+91-11-23282021, +91-11-23245672
E-mail: jaypee@jaypeebrothers.com

Corporate Office
Jaypee Brothers Medical Publishers (P) Ltd.
4838/24, Ansari Road, Daryaganj
New Delhi 110 002, India
Phone: +91-11-43574357
Fax: +91-11-43574314
E-mail: jaypee@jaypeebrothers.com

Overseas Office
JP Medical Ltd.
83, Victoria Street, London
SW1H 0HW (UK)
Phone: +44-20 3170 8910
Fax: +44(0)20 3008 6180
E-mail: info@jpmedpub.com

Website: www.jaypeebrothers.com
Website: www.jaypeedigital.com

© 2022, Jaypee Brothers Medical Publishers

CMC Vellore Handbook of Emergency Medicine/KPP Abhilash

First Edition: 2016

Third Edition: 2022

Reprint: 2023, 2024, **2025**

ISBN: 978-93-5465-132-8

Printed at: Samrat Offset Pvt. Ltd.

Dedicated to

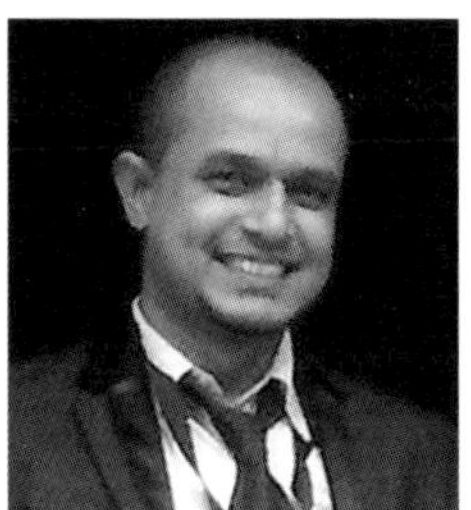

Dr Shubhanker Mitra (1981–2016) who was a fantastic colleague and friend, an outstanding clinician and researcher. Born on January 16, 1981, he joined Christian Medical College, Vellore, Tamil Nadu, India in the year 2000. He completed MD in General Medicine in 2010 and joined the department of General medicine and later Emergency department as a faculty. He lived his life with joyful exuberance, reckless investigation, legendary neologisms, irrepressible mischief, a penchant for drama and touching mindfulness for those around him.

Many will vouch for his diligence in the process of diagnosis, commitment to true hands-on personal care, and willingness to teach others as he learnt. His work ethic, devotion to his patients, and drive toward self-improvement, was exemplary and an example to all his colleagues. As a teacher, he was instrumental in spurring many into research fields, if not into plain pure inquisitiveness.

Over the last 5 years, he had been instrumental in resurrecting the culture of undergraduate research. He was the force behind Cognitio: CMC's Undergraduate Research Conference. Our undergraduates have since gone on to be regular features in conferences, winning awards at several conferences.
He would certainly be missed by all those who had the privilege to know and work with him.

Contributors

Priya G MD (Anesthesiology)
Department of Emergency Medicine
Christian Medical College
Vellore, Tamil Nadu, India

Surendra Kumar FAEM, D Ortho
Department of Emergency Medicine
Christian Medical College
Vellore, Tamil Nadu, India

Debasis Das Adhikari DCh DNB (Pediatrics)
FAEM FAPEM
Department of Pediatric Emergency
Christian Medical College
Vellore, Tamil Nadu, India

David Vincent FAEM
Department of Emergency Medicine
Christian Medical College
Vellore, Tamil Nadu, India

Ashwin Rajanesh MD (General Medicine)
Department of Emergency Medicine
Christian Medical College
Vellore, Tamil Nadu, India

Vineet Subodh FAEM
Department of Emergency Medicine
Christian Medical College
Vellore, Tamil Nadu, India

TS Ravi Kumar MSc (Nursing)
Department of Emergency Medicine
Christian Medical College
Vellore, Tamil Nadu, India

Esther Paul BSc (Nursing)
Department of Emergency Medicine
Christian Medical College
Vellore, Tamil Nadu, India

Sisha Liz Abraham MS DipNB
(Otorhinolaryngology) FHNS
Department of ENT
Christian Medical College
Vellore, Tamil Nadu, India

Roshna Rose Paul MS (Otorhinolaryngology)
Department of ENT
Christian Medical College
Vellore, Tamil Nadu, India

Sandeep David MD (Anesthesiology)
Department of Emergency Medicine
Christian Medical College
Vellore, Tamil Nadu, India

Sivanandan MD Anesthesiology
Department of Emergency Medicine
Christian Medical College
Vellore, Tamil Nadu, India

John Jesudasan FAEM
Department of Emergency Medicine
Christian Medical College
Vellore, Tamil Nadu, India

Gautham Raja FAEM MRCEM
Department of Emergency Medicine
Christian Medical College
Vellore, Tamil Nadu, India

Anne George MD O(bstetrics and Gynecology)
Department of Community Medicine
Christian Medical College
Vellore, Tamil Nadu, India

Moses Kirubairaj DipNB (Family Medicine)
FAEM
Department of Emergency Medicine
Christian Medical College
Vellore, Tamil Nadu, India

Jeyalinda Christopher MSc (Nursing)
Department of Emergency Medicine
Christian Medical College,
Vellore, Tamil Nadu, India

Sri Ranjani BSc (Nursing)
Department of Emergency Medicine
Christian Medical College
Vellore, Tamil Nadu, India

Suma Mary Thampi MD (Anesthesiology)
Department of Anesthesia
Christian Medical College
Vellore, Tamil Nadu, India

Deepu David MD DM (Gastroenterology)
Department of Gastroenterology Christian
Medical College
Vellore, Tamil Nadu, India

Foreword

I am very happy to write the foreword for the 3rd Edition of the *Handbook of Emergency Medicine.* "Emergency Medicine" is an emerging specialty in India. Christian Medical College, Vellore, Tamil Nadu has been at the forefront of Emergency Medicine in India and has been conducting the course on "Early management of Trauma" from 1998. 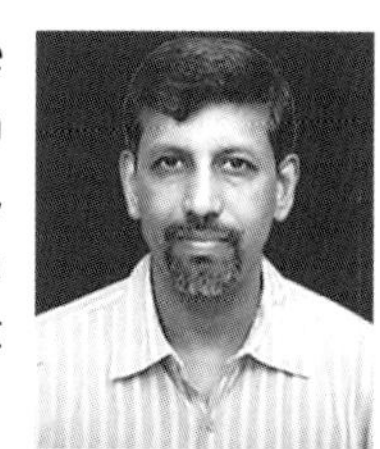

The Department of Emergency Medicine has grown exponentially over the years. The volume and variety of patients managed has increased dramatically. The number of faculty and staff has increased accordingly. Training for all doctors in emergency medicine through standardized protocols written in this book has greatly helped in improving the quality of patient care. Early trauma management and the art of making a quick diagnosis are essential for the quick recovery of the patient. This manual provides a valuable resource in emergency medicine for doctors working in all settings.

I wish the Emergency Medical team all the very best in their efforts to educate more doctors and paramedical workers in this important specialty.

K Prasad Mathews
MD FRACP (Geriatrics)
Medical Superintendent
CMC Medical Superintendent
Christian Medical College
Vellore, Tamil Nadu, India

Preface to the Third Edition

There has been a perceived need to have comprehensive guidelines for all acute medical and surgical emergencies presenting to the emergency department (ED) of Christian Medical College (CMC), Vellore, Tamil Nadu, India. This book is a compilation of all management guidelines and protocols followed in our ED. Since the ED of CMC was formed 22 years ago, there have been various changes in the structure and concept of emergency care.

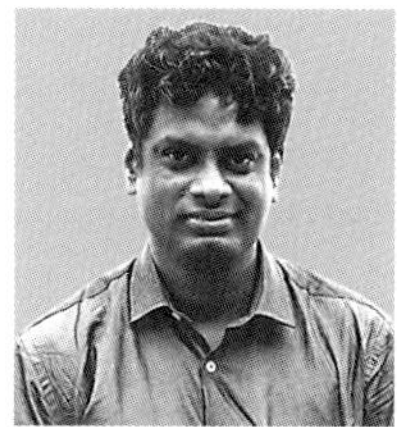

Our adult ED is one of the largest in the country with 100 beds and an annual patient load of more than 80,000 patients. The ED registrars are exposed to a wide spectrum of disease conditions. The COVID-19 pandemic thrust the emergency department to the forefront and all emergency physicians rose up to the challenge and weathered the storm. Through this book an attempt has been made to cover the basics of all the commonly seen medical and surgical conditions in our ED and the emergency management principles in a simplified manner. Many newer concepts have replaced the traditional management practices. Every effort has been taken to incorporate the latest evidence-based recommendations in the *CMC Handbook of Emergency Medicine*.

I hope that this book would serve the purpose of achieving the goal of protocol-based evaluation and evidence-based management of the common emergencies. If this book helps to provide better patient care and stimulates interest in emergency medicine among medical, nursing, and paramedic students, our efforts will indeed have been worthwhile.

All comments and constructive suggestions are welcome for further editions of the *Handbook of Emergency Medicine*.

Wishing all the readers the very best!

KPP Abhilash

MBBS MD PDF (Emergency Medicine)

Professor and Head

Emergency Department

Christian Medical College

Vellore, Tamil Nadu, India

Acknowledgments

- I acknowledge all the contributions who helped to prepare the 1st, 2nd, and 3rd editions of this handbook of emergency medicine. The final product is the result of intensive work put in by these contributors.
- Mr Senthil, Ms Bagyalakshmi, and Mr Sathish Kumar for their assistance in putting it all together.
- Dr Latif Rajesh Johnson for the photoshoot of the cover picture.
- The "emergency department" registrars, consultants, nurses and paramedics for all their suggestions and comments.
- The patients in the emergency department who teach us something new every day.
- To my parents, Dr KPA Chandrasekhar and Mrs KLT Priyadarshini, brother, sister-in-law, my niece, and friends for their everlasting support.
- We especially appreciate the constant support and encouragement of Shri Jitendar P Vij (Group Chairman), Mr Ankit Vij (Managing Director), Mr MS Mani (Group President), Jaypee Brothers Medical Publishers (P) Ltd, New Delhi, India in publishing this handbook and also their associates particularly Dr Richa Saxena (Associate Director-Professional Publishing), and Ms Prerna Bajaj (Development Editor) who have been prompt, efficient, and most helpful.

- Treat the patient's symptoms. Do not treat the monitors or laboratory investigations.
- *Do not* start your workup by looking at outside investigations. Your diagnosis will be totally biased.
- History is the most vital component needed to make a diagnosis. A wrong history will always lead you to the wrong diagnosis.
- *Never ignore* abnormal vital signs. They are more accurate in assessing the severity of the illness than your visual assessment of the patient.
- Develop your clinical skills. Never depend on the laboratory to make a clinical diagnosis. Train your brain to be better than a machine.
- History, examination findings, clinical diagnosis, and the laboratory investigations should be internally consistent. Otherwise, something is wrong somewhere. It is most probably a laboratory error (if your brain is smart enough).
- It is good to follow guidelines, but that should not limit your thinking process.
- Learn to make a list of differential diagnoses after history taking and clinical examination, *not* after viewing the results of blood investigations or imaging.
- Change is the only permanent thing in life. Be rational, question existing protocols, and try to improve yourself, patient care, and the department.
- Strive for academic excellence through research. The ED is an untapped goldmine for research.

Contents

Section 1: Basic Life Support and Management of Cardiac Arrest

1. Basic Life Support — 3
2. Management of Cardiac Arrest — 14

Section 2: Anaphylaxis, Shock and Airway

3. Anaphylaxis — 29
4. Overview of Shock — 32
5. Septic Shock — 35
6. Airway Management — 40
7. Respiratory Support — 44

Section 3: Fluid and Electrolytes

8. Fluid Therapy — 51
9. Sodium — 53
10. Potassium — 56
11. Calcium — 59
12. Magnesium — 62
13. Acid-base Abnormalities — 64

Section 4: Infectious Diseases

14. Antibiotic Protocol for Common Conditions — 71
15. Dengue — 75
16. Scrub Typhus — 78
17. Malaria — 80
18. Community-acquired Pneumonia — 82
19. Influenza and H1N1 — 84
20. COVID-19 — 86
21. Rabies — 90
22. Food Poisoning and Acute Gastroenteritis — 93
23. Urinary Tract Infections — 95
24. Acute Central Nervous System Infections — 98
25. Tetanus — 101
26. Antibiotic Doses and Spectrum — 103

Section 5: Toxicology

27.	General Measures	109
28.	Drug Overdose	111
29.	Insecticide Poisoning	116
30.	Rodenticides	121
31.	Plant Poisons	124
32.	Snake Bites	128
33.	Insect Envenomation	131
34.	Substance Abuse	134
35.	Miscellaneous	137

Section 6: Cardiac Emergencies

36.	Acute Coronary Syndrome	147
37.	Hypertensive Emergencies	154
38.	Pulmonary Edema	157
39.	Atrial Fibrillation	159
40.	Atrial Flutter	162
41.	Paroxysmal Supraventricular Tachycardia	164
42.	Wide Complex Tachycardias	166
43.	Valvular Emergencies	169
44.	Basics of Electrocardiogram	171

Section 7: Respiratory Emergencies

45.	Bronchial Asthma	179
46.	Chronic Obstructive Pulmonary Disease	183
47.	Pulmonary Embolism	186
48.	Pneumothorax	188
49.	Hemoptysis	190

Section 8: Neurological Emergencies

50.	Cerebrovascular Accidents	195
51.	Cerebral Venous Thrombosis	199
52.	Intracranial Hemorrhage	202
53.	Guillain–Barré Syndrome	205
54.	Hanging	207
55.	Seizures	209
56.	Headache	213

57. Bell's Palsy 216
58. Acute Dystonia 218
59. MRI Stroke Protocol 219

Section 9: Gastrointestinal and Hepatic Emergencies

60. Gastrointestinal Bleeding 225
61. Acute Pancreatitis 227
62. Spontaneous Bacterial Peritonitis 229
63. Hepatic Encephalopathy 231
64. Acute Cholangitis 233

Section 10: Hematological Emergencies

65. Anemia 237
66. Febrile Neutropenia 240
67. Acute Leukemia 241
68. Tumor Lysis Syndrome 243
69. Sickle Cell Crisis 245
70. Anticoagulants 247
71. Bleeding and Clotting Disorders 250
72. Hemophilia and von Willebrand Disease 253
73. Blood Products and Transfusion 255

Section 11: Endocrine Emergencies

74. Thyrotoxic Crisis 259
75. Myxedema Coma 261
76. Adrenal Insufficiency 263
77. Diabetic Emergencies 265
78. Pheochromocytoma 270

Section 12: Obstetric and Gynecological Emergencies

79. Ectopic Pregnancy 273
80. Bleeding Per Vagina 275
81. Hyperemesis Gravidarum 278
82. Pelvic Inflammatory Disease 279
83. Ovarian Torsion 280
84. Pregnancy Induced Hypertension (Preeclampsia and Eclampsia) 282
85. Postpartum Hemorrhage 284

Section 13: ENT Emergencies

86.	Epistaxis	289
87.	Stridor	291
88.	Vertigo and Benign Paroxysmal Positional Vertigo	292
89.	Deep Neck Space Infections	297

Section 14: Urological Emergencies

90.	Nephrolithiasis	301
91.	Torsion Testis	303
92.	Epididymo-orchitis	305
93.	Penile Emergencies	307

Section 15: Surgical Emergencies

94.	Skin and Soft Tissue Infections	313
95.	Duodenal Ulcer Perforation	315
96.	Acute Appendicitis	317
97.	Acute Cholecystitis	320
98.	Intestinal Obstruction	322
99.	Mesenteric Ischemia	324
100.	Gas Gangrene	326
101.	Nail Bed Emergencies	327
102.	Anorectal Emergencies	331
103.	Vascular Emergencies	334
104.	Breast Disorders	338

Section 16: Trauma

105.	Early Management of Trauma	341
106.	Hemorrhagic Shock	345
107.	Head Injury	348
108.	Cervical Spine	350
109.	Maxillofacial Trauma	355
110.	Thoracic Injuries	358
111.	Abdominal Injuries	361
112.	Extremity Injuries	364
113.	Wound Management	379
114.	Scalp Laceration	381
115.	Compartment Syndrome	383

116.	Trauma in Pregnancy	385
117.	Pediatric Trauma	388
118.	Geriatric Trauma	392
119.	X-rays in Trauma	394
120.	Eponyms in Trauma	396

Section 17: Pediatric Emergencies

121.	Assessment of a Sick Child in the Emergency Department	405
122.	Febrile Seizures	412
123.	Acute Asthma and Status Asthmaticus	414
124.	Acute Stridor and Epiglottitis	417
125.	Pneumonia and Bronchiolitis	420
126.	Acute Otitis Media and Otitis Externa	423
127.	Acute Gastroenteritis	424
128.	Drugs and Dosages in Pediatric Emergencies	426

Section 18: Disaster Management

129.	Mass Casualty Incidents	435

Section 19: Medicolegal Cases

130.	Medicolegal Cases	441

Section 20: Triage

131.	Triage Priorities	445

Section 21: Miscellaneous

132.	Heat-related Illnesses	451
133.	Malignant Hyperthermia	453
134.	Neuroleptic Malignant Syndrome	455
135.	Electrical Injuries	457
136.	Burns	459
137.	Drowning or Submersion Injuries	462
138.	Alcohol-related Emergencies	464
139.	Sudden Visual Loss	466
140.	Acute Red Eye	469
141.	Dermatological Emergencies	471
142.	Needle-stick Injuries	473

143.	Drugs in Pregnancy	476
144.	Acute Arthritis	479
145.	Procedural Sedation	481

Section 22: Procedures

146.	Nerve Blocks	485
147.	Central Venous Access	493
148.	Chest Tube Insertion	495
149.	Intraosseous Line	497
150.	Cricothyroidotomy	499
151.	Pericardiocentesis	502
152.	Pleural Tap	504
153.	Ascitic Tap (Paracentesis)	505

Section 23: Protocols

154.	Intubation Protocol	509
155.	Investigations Protocol	511
156.	Pain Protocol in the Emergency Department	513
157.	Polytrauma/Trauma Team Activation Protocol	515
158.	Prophylactic Antibiotic Protocol for Trauma Patients in the Emergency Department	517

Index	521

PLATE

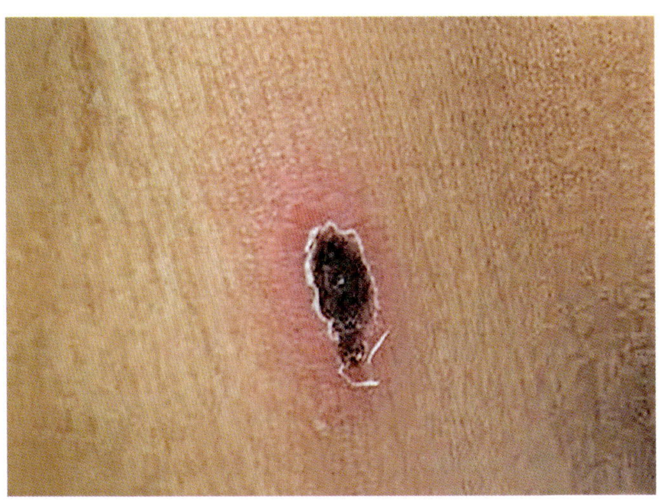

FIG. 1: Eschar of scrub typhus. *(Chapter 16)*

Basic Life Support and Management of Cardiac Arrest

Basic Life Support

CHAPTER 1

INTRODUCTION

Basic life support (BLS) is the component of the immediate care provided for the victims of life-threatening conditions, leading to cardiac arrest, and injuries till the patient can be shifted to a hospital. It can be given by doctors, nurses, paramedics, or even by a trained bystander.

The brain is very sensitive to hypoperfusion. Therefore, the main objective of BLS is to restore cerebral perfusion at the earliest.

The American Heart Association (AHA) periodically revises the guidelines for BLS and Advanced Cardiac Life Support (ACLS). The 2020 AHA guidelines laid emphasis on the following:

- *Sequence of BLS*: Circulation–Airway–Breathing (C–A–B)
- High-quality cardiopulmonary resuscitation (CPR)
- Use of naloxone (intramuscular or intranasal) in suspected opioid overdose
- Use of defibrillator for witnessed cardiac arrests as soon as possible
- Early epinephrine as soon as possible
- Monitoring arterial waveform with $ETCO_2$
- Real-time audio–visual feedback to improve team performance.

BASIC LIFE SUPPORT/CARDIOPULMONARY RESUSCITATION FOR ADULTS

Basic life support consists of the following main parts:

- Chest compressions
- Airway
- Breathing
- Defibrillation

Overview of Initial Basic Life Support Steps (Table 1)

- Assessment and scene safety.
- Remove victim from the hazardous environment to a place where care may be provided without putting the victim or BLS provider at a risk of harm.
- Look for response and breathing pattern. If there is no response and the victim is not breathing or is gasping, shout for help.
- Check the victim's carotid pulse (take at least 5 seconds but no more than 10 seconds) (**Fig. 1**).

TABLE 1: Steps of basic life support.		
Step 1	Assessment and scene safety	• Make sure that the scene of the incident is safe for you and for the victim • Relocate victim from hazardous environment
Step 2	Recognize the cardiac arrest	
	Look for response and breathing	• Tap the victim's shoulder and shout, "Are you all right?" • If there is no response, no breathing or gasping, shout for help
	Check the victim's pulse	• Take at least 5 seconds but no more than 10 seconds to check for pulse • Locate the trachea using two or three fingers • Feel the carotid pulse between trachea and the muscles of the neck (lateral to the thyroid cartilage). If no pulse is felt, activate the emergency response system
Step 3	Activate the emergency response system	• If you are alone with an unresponsive victim and do not have a mobile phone: Activate the emergency response system, get an AED, if available and then begin the CPR • If you have help at hand: Send them to get the AED and begin CPR
Step 4	Start CPR with 30 chest compressions and 2 breaths	
	Chest compressions	• Position yourself beside the victim • Keep the victim in supine position and on a firm surface • Place the heel of one hand on the lower half of the victim's sternum • Place the heel of the other hand on the top of the first hand and interlock your fingers • Straighten your elbows and position your shoulders directly over your hands • Push hard and fast • Allow for complete chest recoil • Minimize interruptions
	Rescue breaths	• Head tilt, chin lift to open the airway • In case of suspected cervical spine injury, use only jaw thrust. Avoid head tilt and chin lift • Provide two rescue breaths keeping the nose pinched after every 30 compressions • Use an improvised mask device, if available • Look for a chest rise with each rescue breath • If unable to provide breaths, continue with chest compressions

(AED: automated external defibrillator; CPR: cardiopulmonary resuscitation)

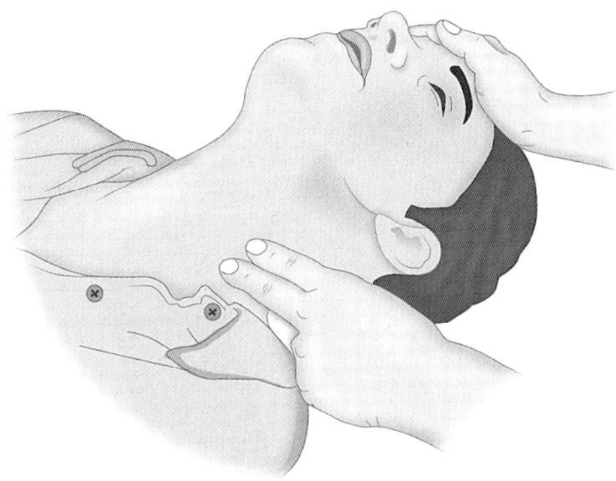

FIG. 1: Carotid pulse check.

- Activate the emergency response system and get an automatic external defibrillator (AED), if available and return to the patient.
- Start CPR. Perform five cycles of chest compressions and breaths (30:2), starting with compressions (C–A–B sequence).

Chest Compressions

High-quality CPR improves a victim's chance of survival. The BLS provider should follow these critical characteristics of chest compressions while providing high-quality CPR (**Fig. 2**).

- *Start compressions within 10 seconds* of recognition of cardiac arrest.
- *Push hard, push fast*: Compress at a rate of at least 100–120/min with a depth of at least 5 cm (2 inches) for adults, approximately 5 cm (2 inches) for children, and approximately 4 cm (1½ inches) for infants.
- *Allow complete chest recoil* after each compression.
- *Minimize interruptions* in compressions (try to limit interruptions to <10 s).
- In case of lay rescuer or sole rescuer present, compression only CPR is sufficient.
- *Give effective* breaths that make the chest rise. With an advanced airway in place, deliver 10 breaths/min or 1 breathe every 6 seconds.

Airway Maneuvers

In an unresponsive patient, the airway may be occluded due to decreased tone of the tongue and pharyngeal muscles. There are two methods of opening the airway to provide rescue breaths (**Table 2** and **Figs. 3A** and **B**).

Use only jaw thrust in cases of suspected head injury or cervical spine injury. Avoid head tilt–chin lift maneuver in these circumstances.

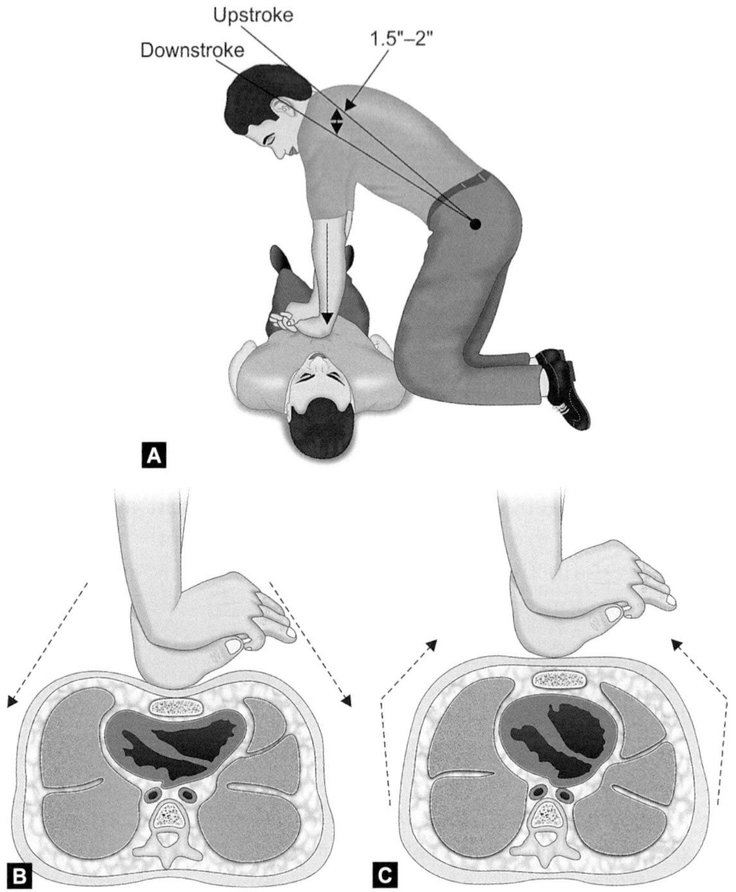

FIGS. 2A TO C: Technique of chest compressions.

TABLE 2: Two methods of opening the airway.	
Method	*Description*
Head tilt–chin lift	This maneuver lifts the tongue off the posterior pharynx thus opening up the airway. Avoid in cases of suspected cervical injury • Place your palm on the victim's forehead and apply downward pressure thus, tilting the head backward • Place the tips of the index and middle fingers at the mentum of the mandible and lift the chin upward
Jaw thrust	Jaw thrust is indicated if the victim has a head or neck injury • Place one hand on each side of the victim's head, resting the elbows on the surface on which the victim is lying • Place the fingers under the angles of the victim's mandible and lift with both the hands, displacing the jaw forward The jaw thrust displaces the mandible and tongue anteriorly, thus preventing the lax tongue from occluding the airway

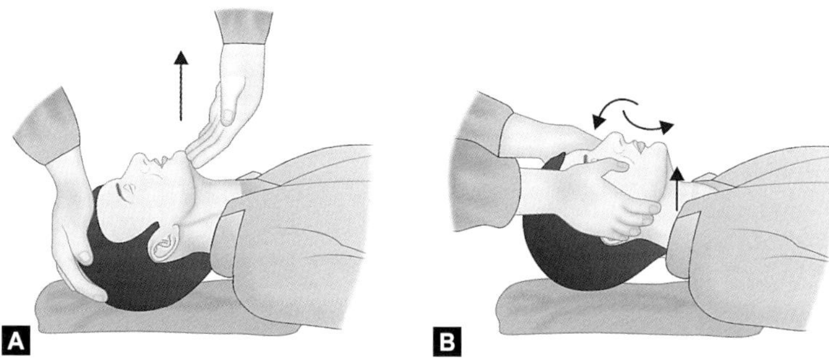

FIGS. 3A AND B: (A) Head tilt–chin lift; and (B) Jaw thrust.

Caution

- Avoid pressing deeply into the soft tissue under the chin as this may block the airway.
- Avoid using the thumb to lift the chin.
- Do not close the victim's mouth completely.

Ventilation

Respiratory arrest is a condition where the patient's respiratory efforts are either inadequate to maintain oxygenation or completely absent.

Management of a respiratory arrest includes the following components:
- Administering oxygen
- Keeping the airway open using basic airway adjuncts
- Suctioning if necessary, to clear secretions
- Providing basic ventilation using bag mask equipment
- Securing an advanced airway
- Identifying the cause.

Basic Airway Adjuncts

In unresponsive patients, the tongue can fall back and obstruct the airway due to loss of tone of the throat muscles. This can be prevented by the basic airway opening techniques (head tilt-chin lift or jaw thrust). In addition to this, two basic airway adjuncts (oropharyngeal airway or nasopharyngeal airway) can be used to facilitate ventilation during resuscitation (**Fig. 4**). These are indicated only in unconscious patients and come in various sizes. The correct size should be chosen for each patient for maximum benefit and to minimize complications such as oral trauma.

Oropharyngeal Airway

- *Choose the correct size*: It should be the distance between the first incisor and the angle of the mandible.
- If it is too large, it may close the glottis and block the airway.

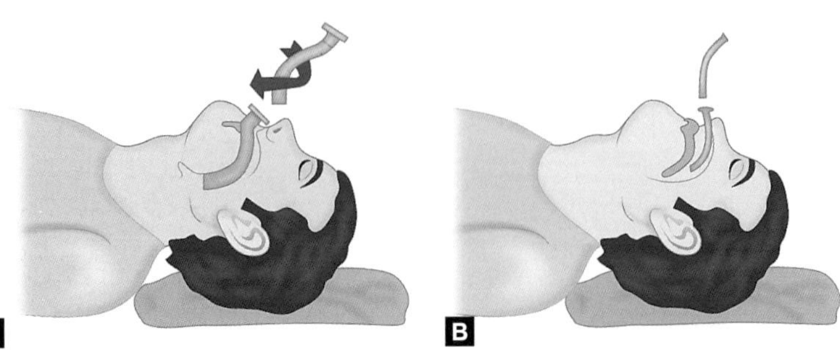

FIGS. 4A AND B: Basic airway adjuncts: Oropharyngeal airway and nasopharyngeal airway.

- *In adults*: Insert the tube with the concavity upward and then rotate it to 180 degree, when it touches the back of the throat.
- *In children and infants*: Insert the tube with the concavity downward while using a tongue depressor to hold the tongue forward.
- It is contraindicated in conscious patients as it can induce a gag resulting in vomiting.

Nasopharyngeal Airway

- *Choose the correct size*: It should be the distance between the tip of the nose and the earlobe.
- It is inserted through one of the nostrils after lubricating it with an anesthetic jelly. Push it till the flared end is at the nostril.
- It can be inserted in semiconscious patients.
- It is contraindicated in patients with base of skull fractures and nasal bleeds.

Rescue Breaths

- Ventilation may be provided mouth-to-mouth or mouth-to-nose.
- A mask or an improvised device (such as a rolled-up board) may be used.
- Give two rescue breaths after every 30 compressions.
- Give sharp rescue breaths, each over not more than 1 second.
- Provide enough tidal volume to see the chest rise, but avoid excessive ventilation.
- In an in-hospital setting, get a bag-mask for ventilation, if available.

Bag-mask Ventilation

Bag-mask ventilation (BMV) is a very efficient method of temporarily providing positive pressure ventilation.

The BMV device consists of:
- Self-inflating reservoir bag along with a mask
- A one-way valve which prevents rebreathing the exhaled air
- Oxygen port for supplying supplemental oxygen.

Use the E–C clamp technique to bag-mask a patient (**Table 3**). If done properly, it is as effective as a secured airway. Bag-mask ventilation can be done by one or two people (**Fig. 5**).

TABLE 3: E–C clamp technique.

Single rescuer	Use your thumb and first finger to form a C around the mask and place your third, fourth, and fifth finger under the bony part of the mandible forming an E to lift the jaw. Use the other hand to bag-mask
Two rescuers bag mask	One person stands at the headend of the patient and holds the mask firmly with both hands over the patient's face using the E–C technique. The other rescuer slowly squeezes the bag over for 1 s to provide an effective chest rise

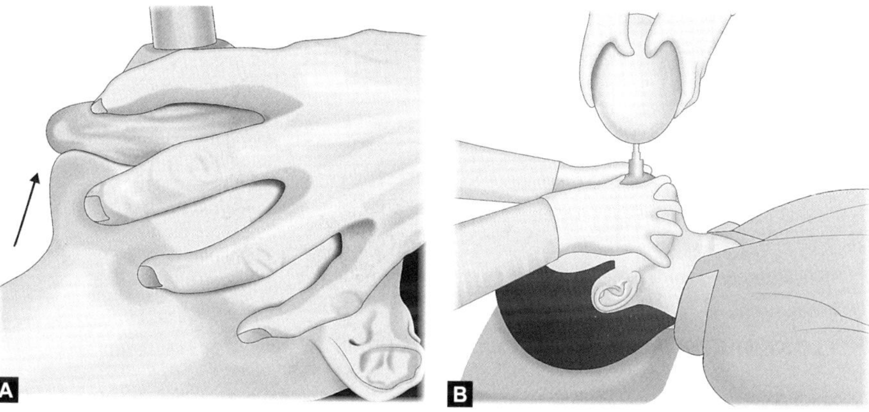

FIGS. 5A AND B: E–C clamp technique: Single rescuer and double rescuer.

The following are the steps involved in bag-mask ventilation:
1. Place mask on the victim's face. Use an airway adjunct if available.
2. The nasal end of the mask should cover the bridge of the nose, not extending over the eyes; the body of the mask should cover the nose and mouth, and the other end not extending beyond the chin.
3. Hold the mask using a single hand E-C technique or with both the hands (preferred) if an additional rescuer is present.
4. Apply firm pressure, forming a good mask seal.
5. Ventilate using a volume just sufficient to cause chest rise (not more than 8–10 mL/kg).
6. Squeeze the bag steadily over a second. Avoid explosive squeezing.
7. Connect bag-mask device to reservoir bag with O_2 supply, if available.
8. Give two ventilations after every 30 compressions for patients without an advanced airway.
9. Give asynchronous ventilation every 8–10 seconds (6–8/min) to patients with an advanced airway in place.
   Basic life support for adults is explained in **Flowchart 1**.

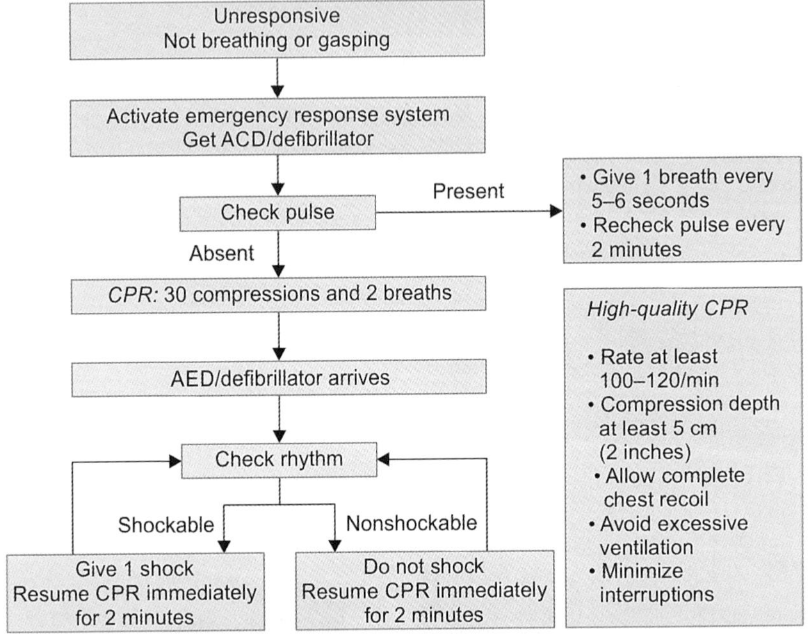

FLOWCHART 1: Adult basic life support algorithm.

BASIC LIFE SUPPORT/CARDIOPULMONARY RESUSCITATION FOR CHILDREN (CHILDREN FROM 1 YEAR OF AGE TO PUBERTY)

The child BLS sequence is similar to the sequence in adults. Following are the key differences:

- Compression–ventilation ratio for two rescuer CPR is 15:2 and for lone rescuer is 30:2
- *Compression depth*: Compress at least one-third of the depth of the chest, approximately 5 cm (2 inches).
- *Compression technique*: Can use one- or two-handed chest compressions for very small children.
- *Defibrillation dose*: First shock: 2 J/kg, second shock: 4 J/kg, subsequent shocks >4 J/kg, and maximum dose 10 J/kg or adult dose.
- To activate the emergency response system, following points are to be considered:
  - In case of unwitnessed arrest and if the rescuer is alone, provide 2 minutes of CPR before leaving the child to activate the emergency response system and get the defibrillator.
  - In case of sudden and witnessed arrest, leave the child to activate the emergency response system and get the defibrillator.

BASIC LIFE SUPPORT/CARDIOPULMONARY RESUSCITATION FOR INFANTS

The key points for infant BLS are:
- *Pulse check*: Feel the brachial artery in infants to check pulse.
- *Technique of chest compressions*: Two fingers for single rescuer and two thumb encircling hand technique for two rescuers (**Fig. 6**).
- *Compression depth*: At least one-third the chest depth, approximately 4 cm (1½ inches).
- Compression–ventilation ratio for two rescuers CPR is 15:2 and for lone rescuer, 30:2.
- *Defibrillation dose*: First shock: 2 J/kg, second shock: 4 J/kg, subsequent shocks >4 J/kg, and maximum dose 10 J/kg.
- To activate the emergency response system, follow the same steps as followed for children.
  Basic life support for children and infants is explained in **Flowchart 2**.

Defibrillation and Cardioversion

- Defibrillation is the nonsynchronized delivery of a shock that depolarizes the entire cardiac tissue into a refractory period, making it unable to sustain or propagate an aberrant circuit. It is performed during a cardiac arrest in a pulseless patient.
- Cardioversion is the delivery of energy that is synchronized to the QRS complex, thus only depolarizing the active circuit causing arrhythmia. It is used to revert arrhythmias in awake patients (**Table 4**).

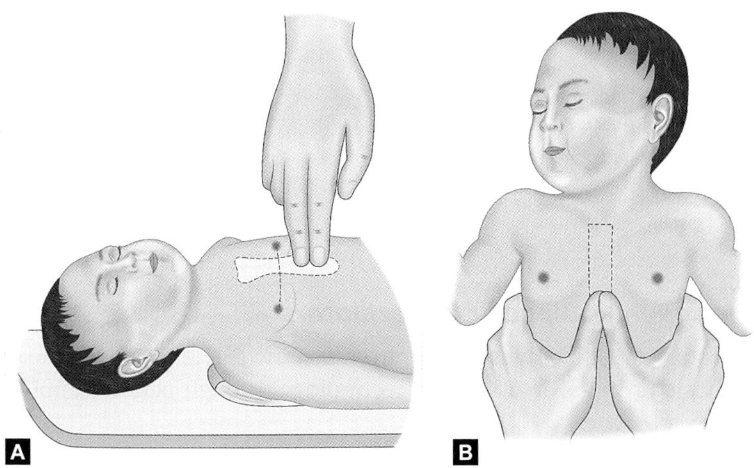

FIGS. 6A AND B: Technique of chest compression in children.

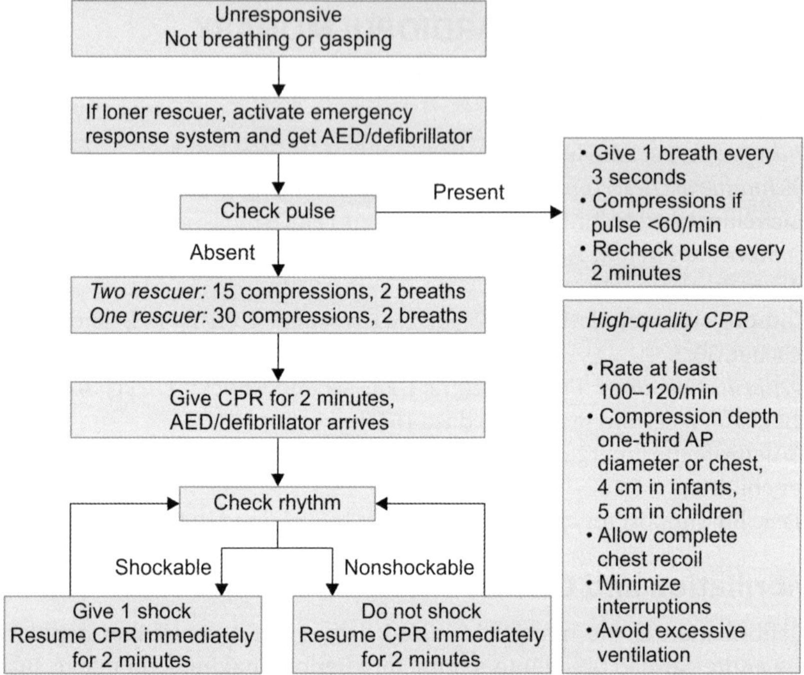

FLOWCHART 2: Pediatric basic life support algorithm.

TABLE 4: Differences between cardioversion and defibrillation.

Cardioversion	Defibrillation
Elective procedure	Emergency procedure
Victim is awake but frequently sedated	Victim is unconscious
Shock is synchronized with QRS	Shock is not synchronized
Indications	*Indications*
• Refractory supraventricular tachycardia	Pulseless ventricular tachycardia
• Unstable atrial fibrillation/flutter	Ventricular fibrillation
• Unstable ventricular tachycardia with pulse	
50–200 J (biphasic)	• 200 J (biphasic)
	• 360 J (monophasic)

Monophasic versus Biphasic Defibrillators

- Defibrillators are machines that deliver electrical energy to the heart by monophasic or biphasic waveform technology through paddles applied on the chest wall.
- Monophasic defibrillators deliver the charge in only one direction, from one electrode to the other. They use higher energy, typically 360 J and have many disadvantages. They are no longer used in most emergency departments (EDs).

- Biphasic defibrillators use lesser energy, are more efficient and cause lesser damage to the heart. They deliver a charge in one direction in the first half and the direction is reversed in the second half; hence a biphasic waveform.
- Currently, almost all the AEDs, manual and implantable defibrillators use the biphasic waveform technology.

Using an Automatic External Defibrillator

- Read the instructions on the AED.
- Stick the pads on the chest wall.
- Place the right pad (white) below the right clavicle and the left pad (red) on the left inferior-lateral chest, lateral to the apex.
- If the patient has an open thorax injury, respective pads may be placed on the left and right axilla.
- Turn on the AED and follow the voice prompts.
- The AED will analyze the cardiac rhythm and will deliver defibrillation if a shockable rhythm is present.

Using a Biphasic Defibrillator

- Turn on the defibrillator to the manual mode.
- Select the desired dose of energy (200 J in adults and 2 J/kg in children).
- Remove paddles, apply gel on the paddles.
- Charge paddles using the charge button on the paddles or on the device.
- Place paddles over the chest wall (Sternal paddle below the right clavicle and apex paddle on left lateral chest wall).
- Resuscitation team should stay clear of contact, oxygen circuit should be disconnected.
- Deliver shock by using the discharge button on the paddles or on the device.
- Resume CPR immediately; do not pause to check pulse/electrical rhythm soon after the shock.

Cardioversion Using a Biphasic Defibrillator

- Obtain consent from the patient and administer sedation with ketamine 1 mg/kg or midazolam 2 mg plus fentanyl 50 µg.
- Turn on the defibrillator to the manual mode.
- Select the desired dose of energy (50–200 J).
- Remove paddles, apply gel on the paddles. Pads may also be used, if available.
- Place paddles/pads over the chest wall. (Sternal paddle below the right clavicle and apex paddle on left lateral chest wall).
- Turn on the synchronized mode.
- Resuscitation team should stay clear of contact and oxygen circuit should be disconnected.
- Keep paddles on contact for at least 5 seconds while holding discharge till shock is delivered.
- Check pulse and electrical activity immediately after the shock.
- If arrhythmia persists, repeat the cardioversion with higher doses.

CHAPTER 2

Management of Cardiac Arrest

INTRODUCTION

To revive a victim of a cardiac arrest successfully, advanced technology and equipment like defibrillator, intubation facilities, oxygen, and drugs are required in most cases. Advanced life support can be effectively performed in a well-equipped emergency department (ED). The ED team may include doctors, nurses, and paramedics, who work together as a team with each member performing their role seamlessly. The team leader should take charge of the resuscitation team and assign roles to team members, make treatment decisions but respect and give constructive criticism to the team members.

As soon as a cardiac arrest is identified, the emergency response system should be activated as per basic life support (BLS) protocol and follows the following steps (**Flowchart 1**):

1. Connect the patient to the monitor to determine the cardiac rhythm and take necessary action.
2. Establish peripheral venous access. If two attempts fail, start an intraosseous line. Endotracheal tube (ET) may also be used to administer drugs, if the patient is already intubated.
3. If the patient is not already intubated, insert an oropharyngeal or nasopharyngeal airway to maintain airway patency by keeping the tongue out of the way, till intubation can be performed.
4. Remember the 5Hs and the 5Ts that are the reversible causes of a cardiac arrest (**Table 1**).

The overview of drugs used in cardiac arrest and the drugs that can be given through the ET tube are shown in **Tables 2** and **3**, respectively.

BRADYARRHYTHMIAS

Bradyarrhythmia is defined as a rhythm disorder in which the heart rate (HR) is less than 60 per minute, e.g., third-degree atrioventricular (AV) block or sinus bradycardia (**Table 4; Figs. 1** to **3**).

Symptomatic Bradycardia

Intervention is required when patients develop features of inadequate tissue perfusion as a result of bradycardia. The HR is generally <50 per minute. The signs and symptoms of unstable bradyarrhythmia are:

- Hypotension or other signs of shock
- Altered sensorium

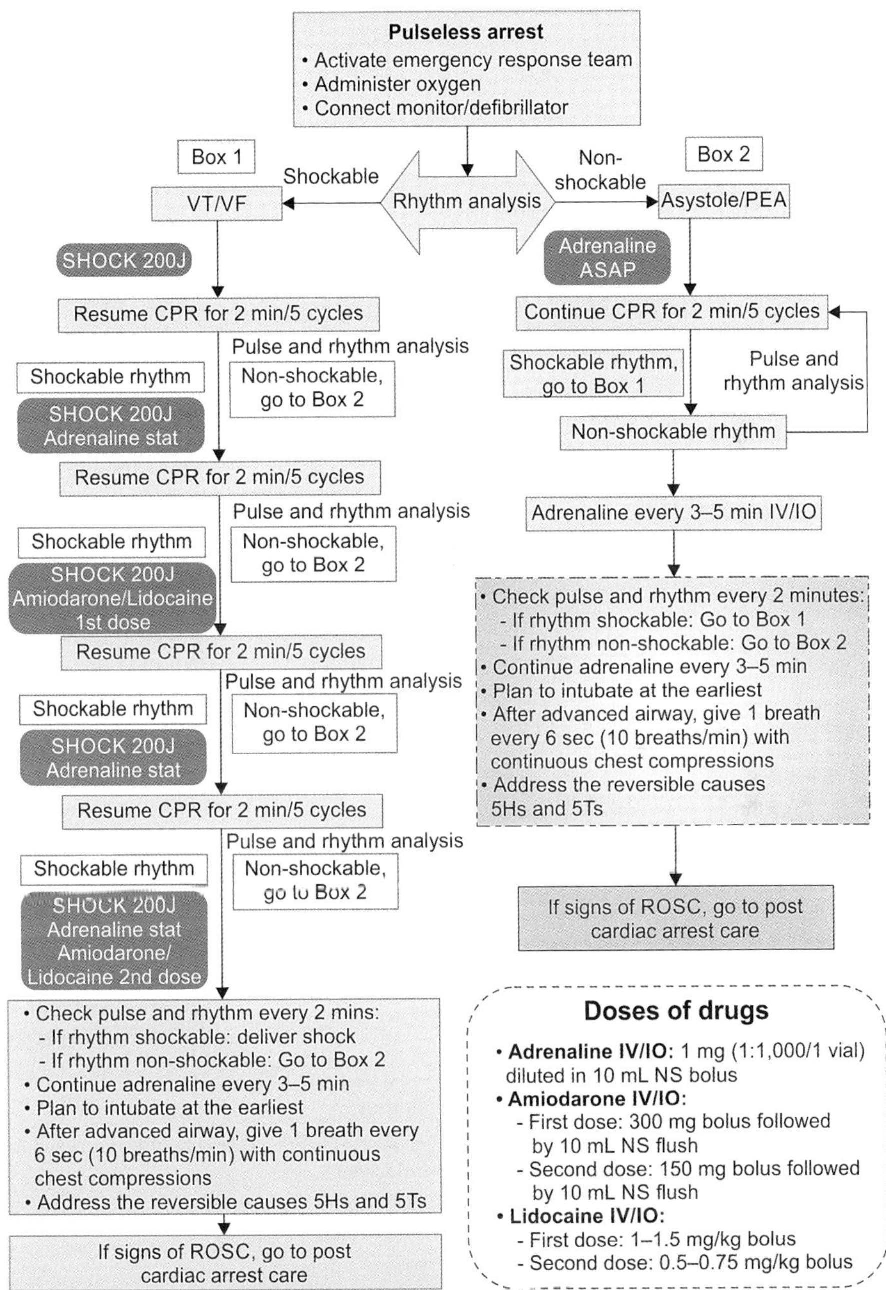

FLOWCHART 1: Adult cardiac arrest algorithm.

TABLE 1: Reversible causes: 5Hs and 5Ts.

• Hypoxia	• Tension pneumothorax
• Hypovolemia	• Tamponade cardiac
• Hydrogen ion (acidosis)	• Toxins
• Hypo/hyperkalemia	• Thrombosis, pulmonary
• Hypothermia	• Thrombosis, coronary

TABLE 2: Overview of drugs used in cardiac arrest.

Drugs	Indications	Dosage
Adrenaline	• VF • Pulseless VT • PEA • Asystole	• 1 mg (1:1000) IV/IO diluted in 10 mL NS every 3–5 minutes • 0.1–0.5 µg/kg/min continuous infusion
Amiodarone	• Refractory VF and VT • Stable VT • Polymorphic VT • WCT of unknown origin	• During cardiac arrest: 300 mg IV/IO first dose. If VT persists 150 mg IV/IO push second dose • In case of arrhythmias: 150 mg over 10 minutes followed by 1 mg/min infusion for 6 hours
Lignocaine/lidocaine	• Refractory VF and VT • Stable VT • Polymorphic VT • WCT of unknown origin	• First dose: 1–1.5 mg/kg • Second dose: 0.5–0.75 mg/kg
Atropine	• Symptomatic bradycardia	1 mg IV every 3–5 minutes, maximum dose: 3 mg
Dopamine	• Symptomatic bradycardia (refractory to atropine) • Hypotension with signs and symptoms of shock	5–20 µg/kg/min IV infusion
Magnesium sulfate	Torsades de pointes	1–2 g diluted in 5% dextrose over 20 minutes

(VF: ventricular fibrillation; VE: ventricular ectopics; PEA: pulseless electrical activity; IV/IO: intravenous/intraosseous; WCT: wide complex tachycardia; NS: normal saline)

- Active ischemic chest pain
- Acute pulmonary edema.

The following drugs may be given via ET tube in case of difficult IV/IO access. The dose required to be administered via ET tube is typically 2–3 times the usual IV dose (**Table 3**).

TABLE 3: Drugs that can be given through the ET tube.

Drugs	Dosage (triple the recommended IV dose)	When to administer?
Adrenaline	2–3 mg	If you fail to secure an IV access in two attempts during a cardiac arrest, proceed with IO/ET route
Atropine	2–3 mg	
Vasopressin	80–120 mg	
Naloxone	800 µg	
Lignocaine	3 mg/kg	

(ET: endotracheal; IO: intraosseous; IV: intravenous)

TABLE 4: Bradycardia rhythms (HR <60/min).

	Rhythm	P-wave	P-R interval	QRS
Sinus bradycardia	Regular	Before each QRS, identical	0.12–0.2 ms	<0.12 ms
First-degree AV block	Regular	Before each QRS, identical	>0.20 ms	<0.12 ms
Second-degree Mobitz type 1 AV block (Wenckebach)	Irregular	Present	Progressive prolongation	Dropped in a repeating pattern
Second-degree Mobitz type 2 AV block	Irregular	Present	Constant	Intermittent dropping of QRS complexes
Third-degree AV block (complete heart block)	Regular	Present, regular P-P interval	Variable	No relation with P-wave. Regular R-R intervals

(HR: heart rate; AV: atrioventricular)

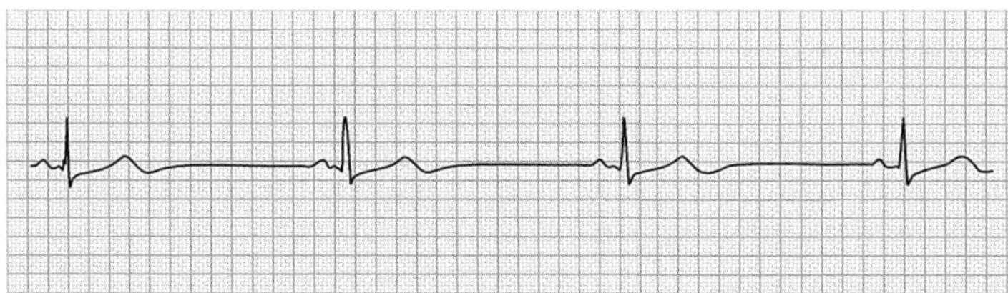

FIG. 1: Sinus bradycardia.

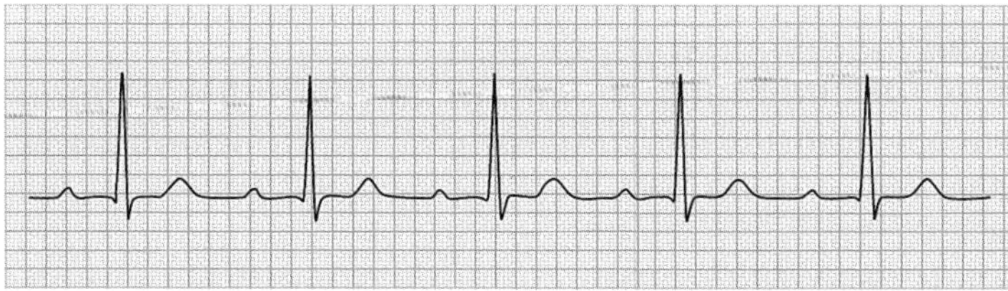

FIG. 2: First-degree AV block.

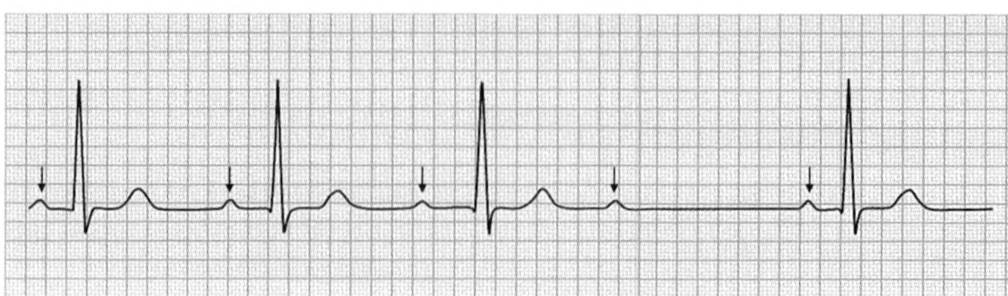

FIG. 3: Second-degree Mobitz type 1 AV block (Wenckebach).

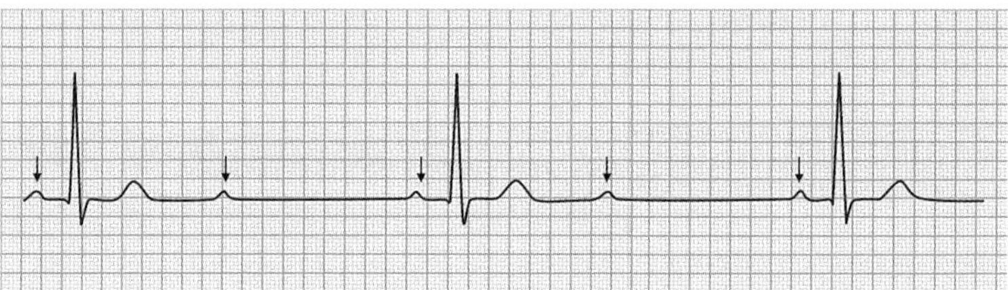

FIG. 4: Second-degree Mobitz type 2 AV block.

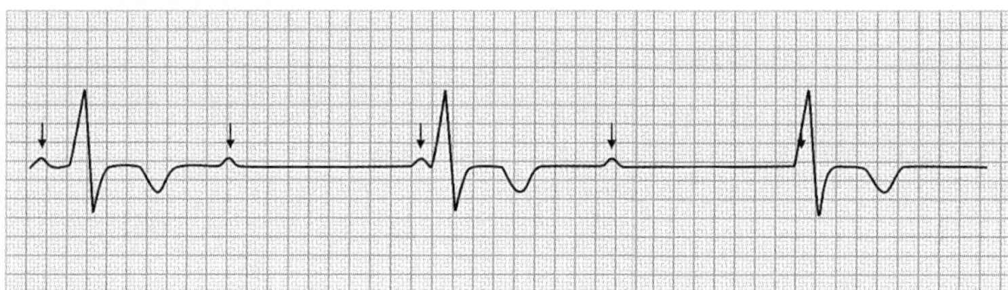

FIG. 5: Third-degree AV block (complete heart block).

Management of Bradyarrhythmias

- Patients with symptomatic bradycardia should be administered atropine 1 mg intravenous (IV) bolus immediately (**Table 5**). The therapeutic options are:
  - Atropine: first-line therapy
  - Infusion of a chronotropic agent (adrenaline or dopamine)
  - Transcutaneous pacing
  - Transvenous pacing.
- Look for and treat any reversible causes like hypoxia, hypokalemia, hyperkalemia, and other organ involvement (pneumothorax, raised intracranial pressure).
- If symptomatic bradycardia persists despite administering atropine, start a chronotropic agent infusion and prepare for a transcutaneous pacing.
- If neither option works, seek expert opinion and prepare for transvenous pacing.
- Atropine is ineffective in patients with a high-degree AV block (second-degree Mobitz type 2 or third-degree AV block; **Figs. 4** and **5**). Do not administer

TABLE 5: Therapeutic agents for symptomatic bradycardia.

Drugs/procedure	Dosage/indications
Atropine	1 mg IV stat. The dose may be repeated every 3–5 minutes up to a total dose of 3 mg
Chronotropic agent infusion	If refractory to repeated doses of atropine (total 3 mg/three doses): • Dopamine infusion 5–10 µg/kg/min • Adrenaline infusion 5–10 µg/min
Transcutaneous pacing	• Unstable/symptomatic bradycardia • Mobitz type 2 second-degree AV block • Third-degree AV block • New left, right, or alternating bundle branch block or bifascicular block • Bradycardia with symptomatic ventricular escape rhythms
Transvenous pacing (temporary pacemaker insertion)	Persistent symptomatic bradycardia despite atropine, dopamine/adrenaline infusion and transcutaneous pacing

(IV: intravenous; AV: atrioventricular)

atropine in these conditions. Proceed with transcutaneous pacing and chronotropic infusion directly (**Flowchart 2**).

TRANSCUTANEOUS PACING

These are devices that pace the heart by delivering an electrical stimulus, causing electrical depolarization and subsequent cardiac contraction. Transcutaneous pacing delivers pacing impulses to the heart through the skin by use of cutaneous electrodes (**Figs. 6A** and **B**).

The goal is to stabilize the heart till the underlying problem is resolved or a more permanent means of pacing is secured.

Technique of Transcutaneous Pacing

Positioning Pacing Electrodes/Pads

- Ideally, the heart should be sandwiched between the pacing pads to mimic the heart's normal electrical axis. They may be placed anterior–posterior or anterior–lateral depending on the manufacturer. Anterior–posterior placement of pads, with one pad on the anterior chest and the other on the posterior chest is more commonly used.
- Connect the electrocardiogram (ECG) leads.
- Set the pacemaker rate to 60–80 per minute.
- Begin pacing with 10 milliamps and slowly increase by 10 milliamps till capture is noted.

Assess clinical condition, HR < 60/min and inadequate for clinical condition

Identify and treat the underlying causes

- Maintain airway and breathing
- Oxygen if hypoxic
- Connect to cardiac monitor to identify rhythm
- IV access
- 12 lead ECG if available
- Consider reversible causes

Persistent bradyarrhythmia causing signs and symptoms

- Hypotension
- Acute altered mental status
- Signs of shock
- Ischemic chest discomfort
- Acute heart failure

Monitor and observe

If pulseless arrest occurs, go to cardiac arrest algorithm. Remember the 5Hs and 5Ts

Prepare for transcutaneous pacing

- Inj atropine 1 mg IV. Can repeat every 3–5 min to a total of 3 mg
- If ineffective, begin transcutaneous pacing. Consider without delay for type II 2nd degree/3rd degree AV block
- Consider adrenaline (2–10 µg/min) or dopamine (5–20 µg/kg/min) infusion while awaiting pacing

Consider expert consultation and transvenous pacing

FLOWCHART 2: Adult bradycardia algorithm (with pulse).

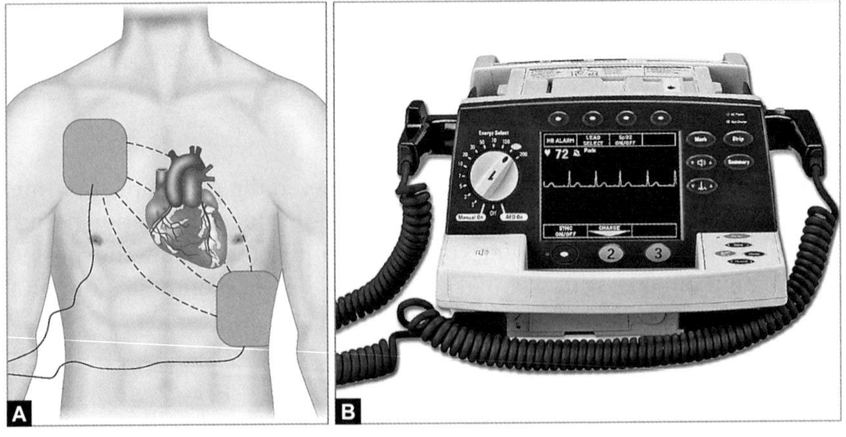

FIGS. 6A AND B: Transcutaneous pacing.

- Once pacing is captured (signified by characterized by a wide QRS complex with tall, broad T-waves on the ECG, or a palpable pulse) set the current at 5–10 milliamps above the threshold.
- External pacing can be quite uncomfortable, if the patient is awake/responsive. Consider sedation if > 50 milliamps is used for pacing.
  The success of pacing is determined by evidence of improved cardiac output: palpable pulse, rise in blood pressure, and improved level of consciousness.
- The site of application of the pads should be changed every 4 hours to prevent skin burn and discomfort.

TACHYARRHYTHMIAS

Tachyarrhythmias are defined as abnormal heart rhythms with a ventricular rate of 100 or more beats per minute (**Table 6**).

The most important clinical determination in a patient presenting with a tachyarrhythmia is whether or not the patient is experiencing signs and symptoms related to the rapid heart rate.

The following are signs of unstable tachyarrhythmia:
- Hypotension or other signs of shock
- Altered sensorium
- Active ischemic chest pain
- Acute pulmonary edema.

Initial Management of Tachyarrhythmias (Flowchart 3)

- Identify the rhythm
- Look for signs of unstable tachyarrhythmia:
  - If unstable, synchronized cardioversion is indicated
  - If stable, administer appropriate medical therapy and monitor the patient. Look for and treat reversible causes (5Hs and 5Ts)
- Refer to Chapters 39 to 42 for details of management of different tachyarrhythmias.

TABLE 6: Classification of tachyarrhythmias.		
Tachyarrhythmia	*Narrow complex*	*Wide complex[a]*
Regular	• Sinus tachycardia • SVT • Atrial flutter with fixed conduction	• SVT with aberrancy • VT
Irregular	• Atrial fibrillation • Atrial flutter with variable conduction • Multifocal atrial tachycardia	• VF • Atrial fibrillation with aberrancy • Polymorphic VT • Torsades de pointes

[a]Any regular wide complex tachycardia can be treated as ventricular tachycardia.

(SVT: supraventricular tachycardia; VT: ventricular tachycardia)

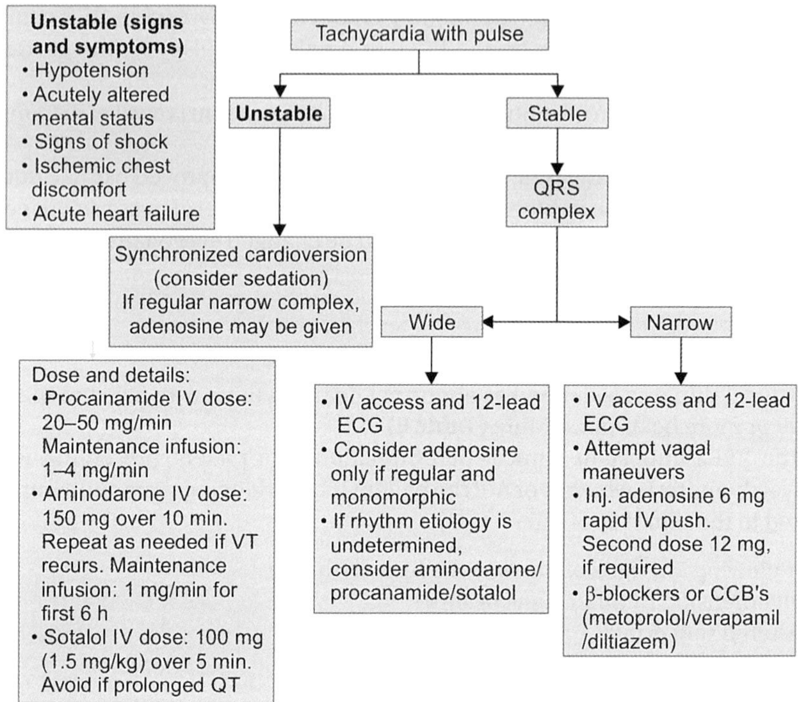

FLOWCHART 3: Adult tachycardia algorithm (with pulse).

IMMEDIATE POSTCARDIAC ARREST CARE FOR ADULTS

Systematic postcardiac arrest care after return of spontaneous circulation (ROSC) can improve the likelihood of patient survival as well as quality of survival:

- ROSC is defined as resumption of sustained cardiac activity with peripheral perfusion associated with significant respiratory effort. When ROSC is achieved, ET CO_2 abruptly increases to >40 mm Hg indicating a substantial increase in cardiac output and blood flow to the lungs.

The main objectives are:

- Control body temperature to optimize survival and neurological recovery
- Manage airway by early placement of ET tube
- Identify and treat acute coronary syndromes (ACS)
- Optimize mechanical ventilation to minimize lung injury
- Support organ function to reduce the risk of multiorgan injury.

The following are the steps to be followed for postcardiac arrest care:

1. Confirm ROSC.
2. Optimize ventilation and oxygenation:
   - Target oxygen saturation 92–98%
   - Intubate the patient (advanced airway), if not already done

- Do not hyperventilate. Give breaths at the rate of 10 per minute
- Confirm and monitor ET tube placement by waveform capnography.
3. Treat hypotension (systolic blood pressure < 90 mm Hg):
    - Give 1–2 L intravenous or intraosseous bolus of cold normal saline if inducing hypothermia (use 4°C fluid)
    - Consider vasopressor infusion
    - Target SBP > 90 mm Hg or MAP > 65 mm Hg
    - Consider and treat the reversible causes (5Hs and 5Ts)
    - Take a 12-lead ECG.
4. Assess sensorium:
    - If the patient does not follow commands, induce therapeutic hypothermia using cold saline infusion and shift the patient for advanced critical care.
    - *Targeted temperature management (TTM):* Mild therapeutic hypothermia must be induced for unconscious patients after a cardiac arrest by cold NS infusion and other cooling devices. Maintain a target temperature of 32–36°C for the first 24 hours post arrest. Monitor core body temperature (esophageal or rectal)
    - If the patient follows commands, treat ST-elevation myocardial infarction or ACS as needed and shift the patient for advanced critical care.

CARDIAC ARREST IN PREGNANCY

Cardiac arrest in a pregnant patient poses a unique challenge for resuscitation. Though rare, ED physicians must be aware of features peculiar to the pregnant state. Knowledge of anatomic and physiologic changes in pregnancy is important (refer Chapter 116).

The main priority of resuscitation remains the mother, but it must be remembered that another life is at stake. Estimate the gestational age to determine the viability of the fetus. If deemed nonviable, resuscitation can be wholly focused on the mother.

As soon as a cardiac arrest is anticipated, assemble the *'maternal cardiac arrest team'* that includes an obstetrician and a neonatologist (**Flowchart 4**).

Maternal Resuscitation

- Standard resuscitation algorithm should be followed with a few modifications to factor in the anatomical and physiological changes of pregnancy.
- Establish intravenous access above the diaphragm so that drug delivery to the heart is not impeded by the gravid uterus compressing the inferior vena cava (IVC).
- During CPR, tilt the patient 15–30° to the left and gently pull the gravid uterus to the left to relieve compression on the IVC, thus increasing venous return.
- The position and dosage of defibrillation remains the same. Remove fetal monitors prior to defibrillation.

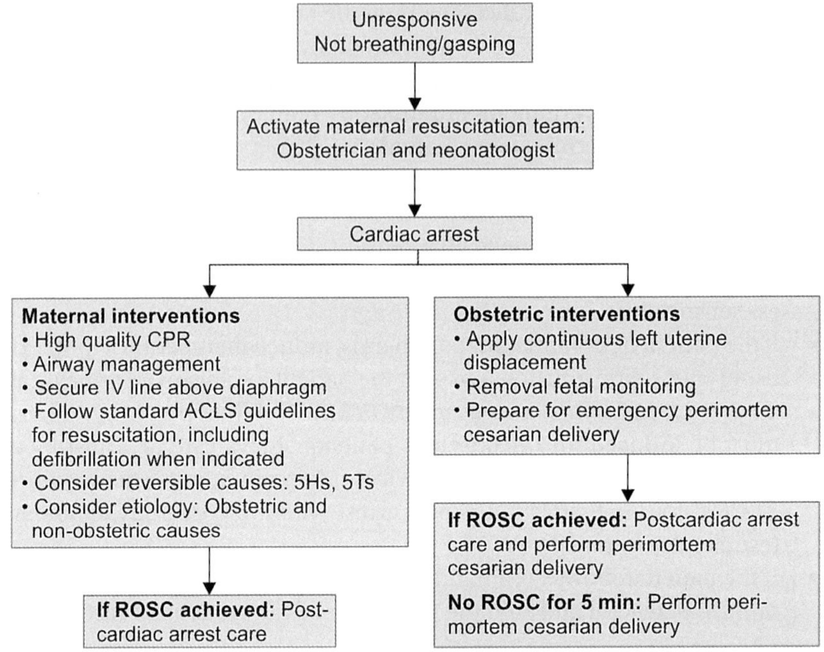

FLOWCHART 4: Maternal cardiac arrest algorithm.

- As pregnant patients are more prone to hypoxia, oxygenation and airway management should be prioritized during resuscitation.
- Due to changes in gastrointestinal motility and changes in sphincter tone, the risk of aspiration increases. Consider RSI early during resuscitation to secure the airway and prevent aspiration. Provide adequate preoxygenation.
- The pregnant airway is more prone to injury, trauma and failed intubation.

Fetal Monitoring

Fetal monitoring should not be done during cardiac arrest in pregnancy after maternal resuscitation, any fetus considered viable (GA > 20 weeks) should be monitored with fetal tocodynamometry. Look for early signs of fetal distress: tachycardia, loss of beat-to-beat variability or late decelerations.

Perimortem Cesarean Delivery

- In case of maternal mortality, perform a perimortem cesarean delivery within 5 minutes of no ROSC.
- If the mother attains ROSC and if signs of fetal distress persist, perform perimortem cesarean delivery within 5 minutes. Delivery of the fetus not only increases chances of fetal survival but also increases chances of maternal recovery.

Potential Causes of Maternal Arrest

Consider the following causes of maternal cardiac arrest and address them, in addition to the usual 5Hs and the 5Ts:

- **Obstetric causes:** Peripartum hemorrhage, pregnancy induced hypertension, peripartum cardiomyopathy, amniotic fluid embolism.
- **Nonobstetric causes:** Pulmonary embolism, infection/sepsis, trauma, myocardial infarction.

Targeted Temperature Management (TTM)

Maintain a target temperature of 32–36°C for the first 24 hours postarrest while continuously monitoring fetal heart during this phase.

PEDIATRIC CARDIAC ARREST

- In contrast to adults, cardiac arrest in children usually results from progressive respiratory failure or shock and often referred to as hypoxic/asphyxia/hypoxic-ischemic arrest. A primary cardiac cause (arrhythmias) is seen in only 10% of all pediatric arrests.
- During cardiac arrest resuscitation, the C-A-B sequence must be followed but securing airway, oxygenation and ventilation should be given high priority (**Flowchart 5**).
- Use a compression-ventilation ratio of 30:2 for single rescuer and 15:2 for 2 or more rescuers.
- After an advanced airway is established, continue chest compressions at a rate of 100–120/min and give 1 breath every 6 seconds (10 breaths/min).
- When available, use End tidal CO_2 (ET CO_2) to monitor the quality of chest compressions. ET CO_2 <10–15 mm Hg indicates inadequate cardiac output during CPR resulting in inadequate delivery to the lungs. Target ET CO_2 more than 10–15 mm Hg during CPR.
- During defibrillation, allow at least 3 cm between the paddles. The recommended paddle size based on weight and age is given below:
    - >1 year old/>10 kg: Large adult paddles (8–13 cm)
    - <1 year old/<10 kg: Small infant paddles (4.5 cm).

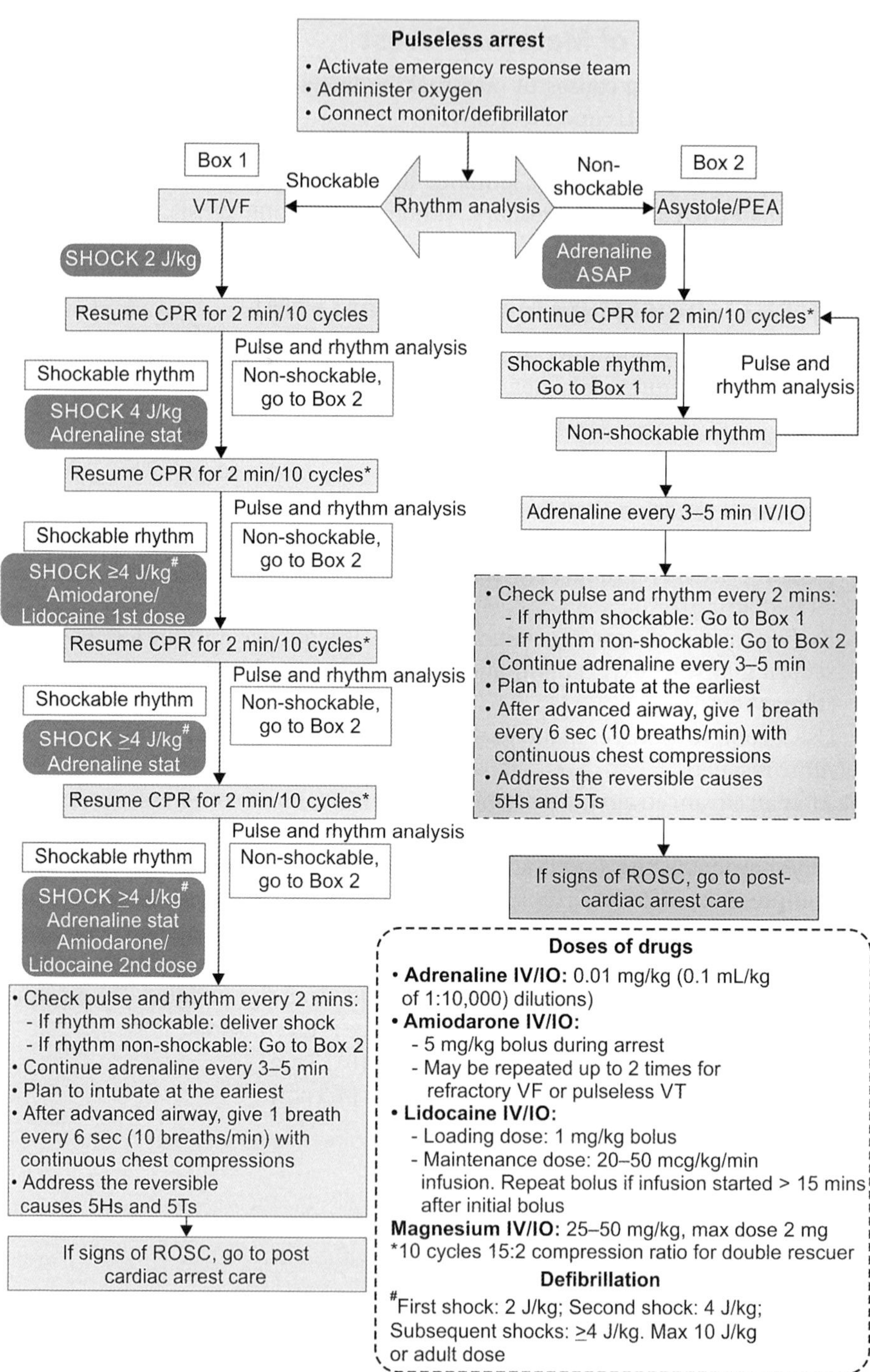

FLOWCHART 5: Pediatric cardiac arrest algorithm.

Anaphylaxis, Shock and Airway

Anaphylaxis

3

CHAPTER

INTRODUCTION

Anaphylaxis is defined as a serious allergic or hypersensitivity reaction that is rapid in onset, mediated by immunoglobulin E (IgE) and may cause death. Anaphylaxis is highly likely when any one of the three criteria given in **Table 1** is fulfilled.

The following are the organ systems involved in anaphylaxis:
- *Skin and integumentary system*: 90% of episodes
- *Respiratory system*: 70% of episodes
- *Gastrointestinal system*: 45% of episodes
- *Cardiovascular system*: 45% of episodes.

TABLE 1: Criteria for diagnosis of anaphylaxis.

Criterion 1	Acute onset of an illness (minutes to several hours) involving the skin, mucosal tissue, or both (e.g., generalized hives, pruritus or flushing, swollen lips, tongue, or uvula) and at least one of the following: • Respiratory compromise (e.g., dyspnea, wheeze, bronchospasm, stridor, reduced peak expiratory flow, hypoxemia) or • Reduced blood pressure (BP) or associated symptoms and signs of endorgan dysfunction (e.g., collapse, syncope)
Criterion 2	Fulfilled if two or more of the following occur rapidly after exposure to a likely allergen within minutes to a few hours: • Involvement of the skin-mucosal tissue (e.g., generalized hives, itch, swollen lips, tongue, or uvula) • Respiratory compromise (e.g., dyspnea, wheeze, bronchospasm, stridor, reduced peak expiratory flow, hypoxemia) • Reduced BP or associated symptoms and signs (e.g., collapse, syncope) • Persistent gastrointestinal symptoms and signs (e.g., abdominal cramps, vomiting)
Criterion 3	• Reduced BP after exposure to a known allergen (minutes to several hours) • Reduced BP in adults is defined as a systolic BP <90 mm Hg or >30% decrease from the patients baseline

Source: Sampson HA, Muñoz-Furlong A, Campbell RL, Adkinson NF Jr, Bock SA, Branum A, et al. Second National Institute of Allergy and Infectious Disease/Food Allergy and Anaphylaxis Network symposium definition and management of anaphylaxis. J Allergy Clin Immunol. 2006;117(2):391.

Caution: Concurrent administration of certain medications such as β blockers, angiotensin converting enzyme (ACE) inhibitors, and alpha adrenergic blockers may increase the likelihood of severe or fatal anaphylaxis and may also interfere with the patient's ability to respond to treatment.

MANAGEMENT OF ANAPHYLAXIS

- Remove the trigger for anaphylaxis immediately (e.g., blood transfusion, antibiotic, antisnake venom).
- *Maintain airway.* Intubate if angioedema is present. If intubation is expected to be difficult, keep tracheostomy, or cricothyroidotomy set ready.
- *Check SpO_2.* Start supplementary oxygen by mask to maintain a target SpO_2 > 94–98%.
- *Assess circulation.* If the patient is hypotensive, start a rapid infusion of 1–2 litres of normal saline (NS). Children should be given NS in boluses of 20 mL/kg, each over 5–10 minutes, and repeated, as needed. Large volumes of fluid (up to 100 mL/kg) may be required.
- Place the patient in the supine position with the lower extremities elevated, unless there is evidence of upper airway swelling necessitating the patient to remain upright (and often leaning forward). If the patient is vomiting, place the patient semirecumbent with lower extremities elevated. Place pregnant patients on their left side.
- Administer injection adrenaline 0.3–0.5 mg (0.3-0.5 mL) intramuscular (IM) (1:1,000 dilution) in the anterolateral thigh. The dose can be repeated every 5–15 minutes, if hemodynamically stable up to a maximum of 3 doses.
  The following are the dosages of adrenaline in children:
  - *<6 years*: 0.15 mg IM
  - *6–12 years*: 0.3 mg IM
  - *>12 years*: 0.5 mg IM
- If hypotension persists, administer adrenaline bolus (0.1–0.5 mg IV in 1:10,000 dilution) followed by an infusion at the rate of 0.1 µg/kg/min (e.g., for a 60 kg man start at 6 µg/min).
- *Antihistamines*:
  - *H1 blockers*: Injection avil (chlorpheniramine maleate) 1–2 mL slow intravenous (IV)/IM; injection phenergan (promethazine): 25 mg IV/IM stat; and
  - *H2 blockers*: Injection ranitidine 50 mg IV stat and q8h.

Other agents that may be used in anaphylaxis are given here:
- Injection hydrocortisone 100–200 mg IV. (Onset of action: 20 minutes. Not useful in acute stage. Blocks late response). Should be considered in acute stage only if adrenaline is not available or if the anaphylaxis is severe.

- *Bronchodilators*: Salbutamol nebulization (5 mg in 5 mL saline) if broncho-spasm present despite adrenaline.
- Glucagon 1–5 mg IV over 5 minutes, followed by infusion of 5–15 µg/min is useful in patients on regular β blockers.

  Observe patients with mild symptoms for 4–6 hours, discharge, if stable.

> Steroids (Hydrocortisone) do not relieve the initial symptoms and signs of anaphylaxis and is given to prevent the biphasic or protracted reactions that occur in some cases.
>
> Epinephrine decreases mediator release from mast cells and is the only medication that prevents or reverses obstruction to airflow in the upper and lower respiratory tracts and prevents or reverses cardiovascular collapse.
>
> *Therefore, do not substitute epinephrine with hydrocortisone during the initial management.*

If the patient is stable, discharge on the following medications:
- Tablet levocetirizine 5–10 mg hs OD for 3–5 days
- Tablet ranitidine 150 mg BD for 3–5 days
- Tablet prednisolone 0.5 mg/kg OD for 3 days.

Overview of Shock

CHAPTER 4

DEFINITION

Shock is a state of hypoperfusion that causes cellular and tissue hypoxia. This may be due to decreased oxygen delivery to the tissues or increased oxygen consumption.

CLASSIFICATION AND EXAMPLES OF TYPES OF SHOCK

- *Distributive shock*: Septic shock, neurogenic shock, anaphylactic shock, toxic shock syndrome, Addisonian crisis
- *Cardiogenic shock*: Myocardial infarction, atrial and ventricular arrhythmias, valve, or ventricle septal rupture
- *Hypovolemic shock*: Hemorrhage, diarrhea, vomiting, heat stroke, burns
- *Obstructive shock*: Pulmonary embolism, pulmonary hypertension, tension pneumothorax, constrictive pericarditis, restrictive cardiomyopathy.

STAGES OF SHOCK

- *Preshock (compensated/cryptic shock)*: In this stage, compensatory responses (tachycardia and peripheral vasoconstriction to blood loss) to decreased tissue perfusion are initiated by the body. This stage can be reversed, if the subtle signs are identified and timely and appropriate interventions are initiated immediately.
- *Shock*: This stage is characterized by signs of organ dysfunction as the compensatory mechanisms are overwhelmed. These include tachycardia, hypotension, dyspnea, restlessness, oliguria, metabolic acidosis, diaphoresis, cold, and clammy skin.
- *End stage*: Multiorgan failure and irreversible organ damage occurs, if the stage of shock is prolonged. Patients become obtunded or comatose progressing to death (**Flowchart 1**).

VASOPRESSORS AND INOTROPES

Vasopressors are drugs that cause vasoconstriction and improve the mean arterial pressure in patients with shock. Inotropes are drugs that increase cardiac contractility. There is an overlap in the inotropic and vasopressor effects of many drugs.

- *Vasopressors*: Noradrenaline, adrenaline, and phenylephrine
- *Inotropes*: Dopamine and dobutamine (**Table 1**).

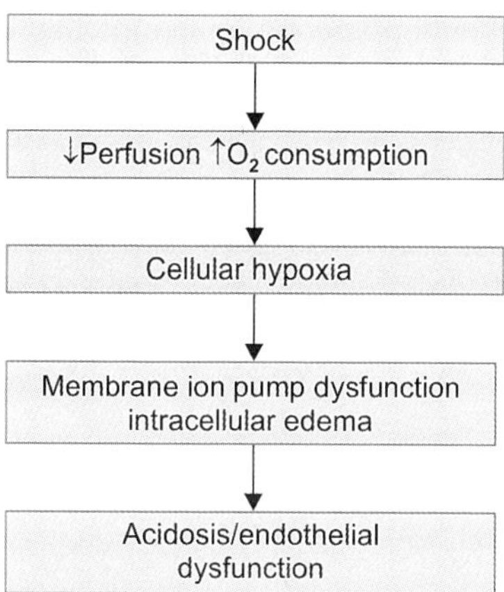

FLOWCHART 1: Mechanism of shock.

TABLE 1: Inotropes and vasopressors.

Drug (receptors)	Initial dose	Maximum dose	Indications	Complications
Noradrenaline (α1, β1)	5 µg/min	35–100 µg/min in refractory shock	First-line agent in septic, cardiogenic and hypovolemic shock	Hyperglycemia, bradyarrhythmias
Adrenaline (α1, β1, β2)	5 µg/min	35 µg/min	First-line agent in anaphylactic shock. Add on to noradrenaline in septic shock	Tachyarrhythmias, ischemia, mesenteric ischemia, hyperglycemia
Dopamine (D1, D2, α1, β1)	5 µg/kg/min	50 µg/kg/min	Second-line agent in septic, cardiogenic and hypovolemic shock	Tachycardia, arrhythmia
Dobutamine (β1, β2)	5 µg/kg/min	20 µg/kg/min	First-line agent in cardiogenic shock. Add on to noradrenaline in septic shock for augmentation of cardiac output in patients with myocardial dysfunction	Hypotension, tachyarrhythmia

Note:
- Indication for starting vasopressors/inotropes infusion in a patient with tissue hypoperfusion (**Table 2**).
  - Mean arterial pressure ≤ 60 mm Hg or
  - Drop in systolic blood pressure ≥ 30 mm Hg from baseline.

- The efficacy of some subcutaneous injections like heparin and insulin can come down due to cutaneous vasoconstriction.

Hypovolemia should be corrected with IV fluids before starting a vasopressor.

TABLE 2: Clinical algorithm to shock management.

Type of shock	Peripheries	Heart rate	JVP	SBP	DBP	Pulse pressure	Management
Hypovolemic	Cold	↑	↓	↓	↓	Normal	• Attain hemostasis in hemorrhage • Aggressive fluid resuscitation • Blood products in hemorrhage
Septic	Warm	↑	↔	↔ or ↓	↓↓	Wide	• Early empiric antibiotic therapy • Fluid resuscitation • Vasoconstrictors (noradrenaline, vasopressin) and inotropes (adrenaline, dopamine)
Cardiogenic	Cold	↑ or ↔ or ↓	↑	↓↓	↔ or ↓	Narrow	Inotropic support (Adrenaline, dobutamine, noradrenaline)
Obstructive	Cold/ normal	↑ or ↔	↑↑	↓↓	↔	Narrow	Therapeutic intervention (e.g., Pericardiocentesis, thrombolysis of PE, needle thoracostomy, etc.)
Neurogenic	Warm	↓	↔	↔ or ↓	↓↓	Wide	Fluid resuscitation Vasoconstrictors (Dopamine, Noradrenaline)
Hypoadrenal crisis	Cold	↓	↔	↓	↓	Normal	• IV glucocorticoid replacement • Fluid resuscitation Inotropic support (Dopamine, adrenaline)

(JVP: jugular venous pressure; SBP: systolic blood pressure; DBP: diastolic blood pressure)

Septic Shock   5

INTRODUCTION

Sepsis is a potentially life-threatening clinical condition characterized by systemic inflammation due to an infectious etiology. The severity ranges from early sepsis to fatal septic shock.

Systemic inflammatory response syndrome (SIRS) is an inflammatory response that may be elicited by an infectious or a noninfectious etiology. SIRS associated with a suspected infection constitutes sepsis.

DEFINITION OF SYSTEMIC INFLAMMATORY RESPONSE SYNDROME

- Temperature > 38.3 or < 36ºC
- Heart rate > 90 bpm
- Respiratory rate > 20 breaths/min
- WBC count >12,000/mm^3 or <4,000/mm^3

Though this definition has been in use for many decades and is easy to use, it lacks sensitivity and specificity and is now considered outdated.

The Third International Consensus Definitions for Sepsis and Septic Shock 2016 (Sepsis-3) defined sepsis as a life-threatening organ dysfunction caused by a dysregulated host response to infection.

Organ dysfunction is defined as an acute change in total Sequential Organ Failure Assessment (SOFA) score of 2 or more points as a result of infection. In patients with no known organ failure, the baseline SOFA score can be taken as 0. Patients with organ dysfunction can be expected to have a hospital mortality of 10%.

Septic shock is defined as a subset of patients with sepsis in whom circulatory, cellular, and metabolic abnormalities are severe enough to significantly increase mortality. Patients in septic shock have persisting hypotension requiring vasopressors to maintain mean arterial pressure (MAP) >65 mm Hg and have a serum lactate level >2 mmol/L (18 mg/dL) despite adequate volume resuscitation. This condition is associated with a mortality rate >40%. The term severe sepsis is currently considered redundant.

qSOFA (Quick SOFA) and SOFA Scores

These are predictive scoring systems that measure disease severity and are used to predict outcomes, mainly mortality. All patients with suspected sepsis should

TABLE 1: Sequential Organ Failure Assessment (SOFA) score.

	0	*1*	*2*	*3*	*4*
P/F ratio	>400	≤400	≤300	≤200	≤100
BP	No hypotension	MAP < 70 mm Hg	Dopa < 5	Dopa > 5/ Adr < 0.1	Dopa > 15/ Adr > 0.1
GCS	15	13–14	10–12	6–9	<6
Creatinine (mg%)	<1.2	1.2–1.9	2–3.4	3.5–4.9	>5
Platelet count (cells/mm³)	>150,000	100,000–150,000	50,000–100,000	20,000–50,000	<20,000
Bilirubin (mg%)	<1.2	1.2–1.9	2–5.9	6–11.9	>12

(Adr: adrenaline infusion μg/min; BP: blood pressure; Dopa: dopamine infusion μg/kg/min; MAP: mean arterial pressure)

Source: Vincent JL, Moreno R, Takala J, Willatts S, De Mendonça A, Bruining H, et al. The SOFA (Sepsis-related Organ Failure Assessment) score to describe organ dysfunction/failure. Intensive Care Med. 1996; 22(7):707-10.

have qSOFA score checked at triage. qSOFA score is a simple bedside score to identify adult patients with suspected infection who are likely to have a poor outcome. This should alert the ED physicians to further investigate for organ dysfunction. SOFA score may then be calculated and used to initiate or escalate appropriate therapy. This score may also be used to admit patients quickly in the intensive care unit (ICU) or to referral to a higher center, if adequate facilities are not available. The higher the SOFA score, the worse the outcome of patients (**Table 1; Flowchart 1**).

qSOFA Criteria (>2 Suggests Sepsis)

- Respiratory rate > 22/min
- Altered sensorium
- Systolic blood pressure < 100 mm Hg.

NATIONAL EARLY WARNING SCORE 2

National Early Warning Score 2 (NEWS2) is an aggregate score made up of six physiological parameters, with the aim of improving detection and response to clinical deterioration in acutely unwell patients (**Table 2**). Parameters measured are:

- Respiratory rate
- Oxygen saturation
- Systolic BP
- Pulse rate
- Level of consciousness (ACVPU score)
- Temperature

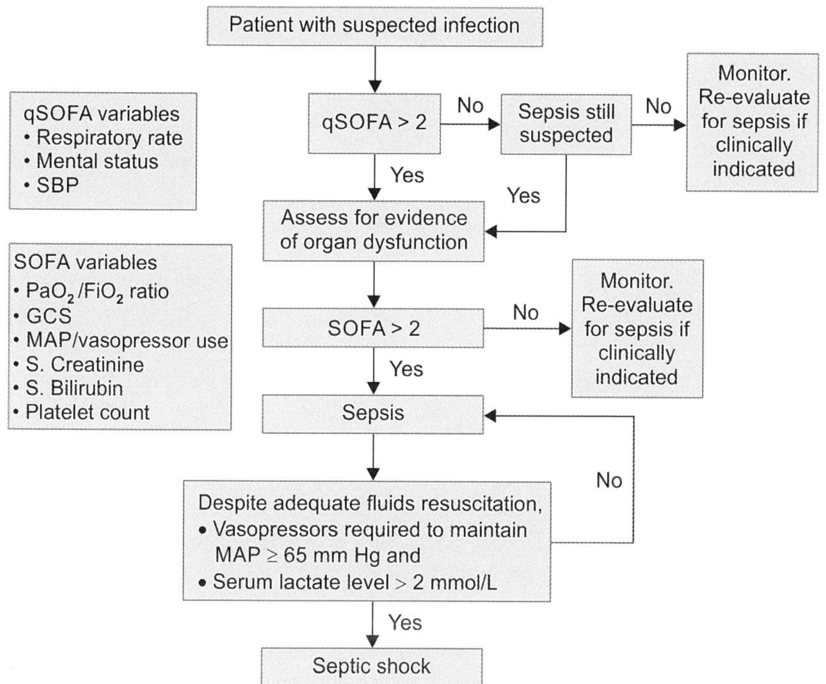

FLOWCHART 1: Evaluation of a patient with suspected sepsis.

Sepsis should be considered in any patient with a NEWS2 score of ≥5 in the presence of known infection, signs or symptoms of infection, or who are at elevated risk of infection.

MANAGEMENT OF SEVERE SEPSIS AND SEPTIC SHOCK

Patients in septic shock should be managed aggressively in the resuscitation room. The four main therapies to be immediately initiated are: (1) Fluid resuscitation, (2) antibiotic administration, (3) control of septic focus, and (4) temperature control.

Fluid Resuscitation

- Administer crystalloids (NS or RL) at a dose of 10–20 mL/kg per bolus (maximum 30 mL/kg) over the first hour. Assess the patient after every fluid bolus for increase in blood pressure and signs of fluid overload.
- In patients with ARDS or sepsis, a restrictive approach to IV fluid administration has been shown to decrease the duration of mechanical ventilation and ICU stay, compared to a more liberal approach.
- *Vasopressor*: Noradrenaline is the vasopressor of choice in septic shock. Adrenaline or vasopressin can be added as second line vasopressors to achieve the target MAP of 65 mm Hg.

TABLE 2: National Early Warning Score 2.

Physiological parameter	Score						
	3	2	1	0	1	2	3
Respiratory rate (per min)	≤8		9–11	12–20		21–24	≥25
SpO$_2$ (%) Scale 1*	≤91	92–93	94–95	≥96			
SpO$_2$ (%) Scale 2#	≤83	84–85	86–87	88–92 ≥93 on air	93–94 on oxygen	95–96 on oxygen	≥97 on oxygen
Air/Oxygen		Oxygen		Air			
SBP (mm Hg)	≤90	91–100	101–110	111–219			≥220
Pulse (per min)	≤40		41–50	51–90	91–110	111–130	≥131
Consciousness				Alert			CVPU
Temperature (°C)	≤35		35.1–36.0	36.1–38.0	38.1–39.0	≥39.1	

*Scale 1 is used in patients without risk of Type 2 failure.

#Scale 2 is used in patients with risk of Type 2 failure (COPD, neuromuscular disease) in whom target saturation is 88%.

(CVPU: confusion, voice, pain, unresponsive; SBP: systolic blood pressure)

Source: Reproduced from Royal College of Physicians. National Early Warning Score (NEWS) 2: Standardizing the assessment of acute-illness severity in the NHS. Updated report of a working party. London: RCP, 2017.

- *Inotrope*: Adrenaline or dobutamine can be started, if the cardiac contractility is low.
- *Glucocorticoid therapy*: In refractory shock not responding to fluids and vasopressors, injection hydrocortisone 100 mg q6h should be initiated.

Antibiotic Therapy

- Broad-spectrum antimicrobial therapy should be started within 6 hours, preferably 1 hour of ED admission after two blood cultures are taken from two different sites.
- Injection Piperacillin–Tazobactam, if blood pressure is normal/injection meropenem 1 g, if patient is in shock.

Control of Septic Focus

The probable focus of sepsis (e.g., diabetic foot, abscess, perforation) should be removed.

Temperature Control

Fever control with external cooling and antipyretics.

Other Measures and Monitoring

- *Management of hyperglycemia*: Target blood glucose level < 200 mg/dL
- Transfuse blood products if hemoglobin < 7 g/day
- *Lactate clearance:* This is defined by the equation [(initial lactate – lactate > 2 hours later)/initial lactate] × 100. Lactate clearance every 6 hours has been shown to a reliable marker for effective resuscitation.
- Arterial blood gas should be repeated at the end of 1 hour of resuscitation to look for:
  - *Partial pressure of oxygen or P/F ratio:* Worsening gas exchange may be to a clue to the presence of pulmonary edema from excessive fluid resuscitation and also help to detect other complications including pneumothorax from central catheter placement, acute respiratory distress syndrome, or venous thromboembolism.
  - *pH and lactates:* Resolution of metabolic acidosis and development of hyperchloremic acidosis.

AIRWAY MANAGEMENT IN THE EMERGENCY DEPARTMENT

Airway management in the emergency department (ED) is quite challenging as patients are sick and the time for preparation is shortened. Hence, all airways should be considered as difficult and difficult airway management cart should be kept ready for usage.

ASSESSMENT OF AIRWAY

ED physicians can use certain pneumonics to assess a patient's airway for difficulty. MOANS is the pneumonic used for assessing difficult mask ventilation and LEMON is a pneumonic used to predict a difficult laryngoscopy.[1]

Difficult Mask Ventilation Assessment: MOANS

- *M—Mask seal*: Facial injuries, beard, blood make a mask seal very difficult
- *O—Obesity/obstruction*: It is difficult to bag mask obese patients
- *A—Age >55 years*: The elderly may have physiological conditions that decrease compliance and hence are difficult to bag mask
- *N—No teeth*: Missing supporting structures that are necessary to seal the mask make mask ventilation difficult in edentulous patients
- *S—Stiff lungs*: Patients with chronic obstructive pulmonary disease or asthma have stiff lungs making mask ventilation difficult.

Difficult Airway Assessment: LEMON

- *L—Look externally*: Look for abnormal faces, burns, facial injuries, or a thick beard
- *E—Evaluate the 332 rule* (**Figs. 1A** to **C**): Successful laryngoscopy depends on normal relative anatomy. In patients with normal relative anatomy the following applies:
  - Normal mouth opening is three fingerbreadths. It indicates good temporomandibular joint mobility.
  - The distance between the mentum and the hyoid bone should be three fingerbreadths. It indicates good mandibular space capacity to accommodate the tongue during laryngoscopy.
  - Notch of the thyroid cartilage should be two fingerbreadths below the hyoid bone. Absence indicates a high/anterior larynx, which would be hard to visualize.

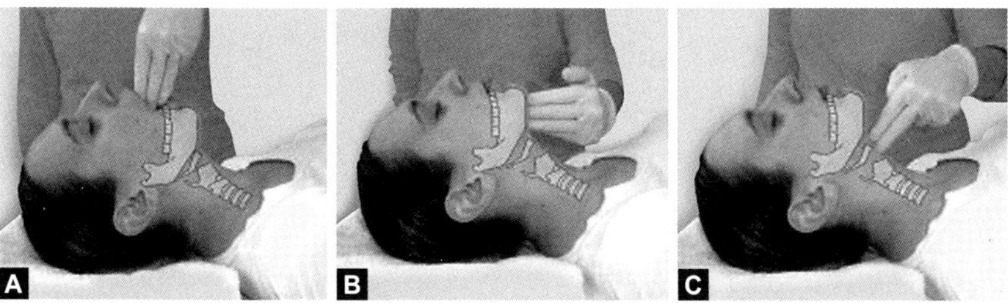

FIGS. 1A TO C: Evaluating the 332 rule.

- *M—Mallampati score*: This evaluation of an awake patient in a sitting position assesses the anatomical structures during mouth opening and classifies the airway into four grades: 1 being easy airway and 4 being very difficult airway
- *O—Obesity/obstruction*: Look for signs of anatomical obstruction like stridor, foreign bodies
- *N—Neck mobility*: Assess both flexion and extension of neck as it may be difficult to align the airway structures during intubation in a patient with limited neck mobility.

> Diabetics have cervical mobility restriction, hence predicting difficult airway.
>
> If a patient has dentures, they can be left in place for mask ventilation for better seal and removed immediately before intubation to avoid displacement and aspiration.

Identification of Compromised Airway

Look for the following clinical signs that suggest a compromised airway
- Inspiratory stridor
- Gurgling
- Snoring
- Tracheal tug and subcostal retractions
- Hoarseness, expiratory phonation
- Paradoxical chest wall movement
- Rapid shallow breathing
- Central cyanosis

Expect a difficult airway in the following clinical scenarios:
- *Maxillofacial trauma*: Due to bleeding or fractured segments
- *Burns*: Due to acute edema of glottis or tracheobronchial mucosa, neck contracture, mouth opening
- *Neoplasms*: Laryngeal or oral cancer-causing airway stenosis
- *Arthritis*: Temporomandibular joint or cervical spine (ankylosing spondylitis)
- *Infections*: Croup, supraglottitis, quincy, retropharyngeal abscess, Ludwig's angina, angioedema.

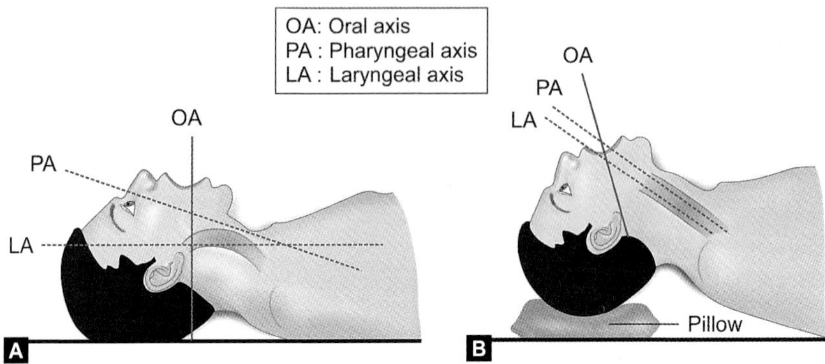

FIGS. 2A AND B: Positioning of a patient during intubation.

Preparation for Endotracheal Intubation

Make sure that the following are in place before attempting endotracheal (ET) intubation (**Fig. 2**)

- *Position*: Flexion of the neck, extension of the head
- *Pillow*: Below the occiput in adults (10 cm height)
- *Drugs*: Refer intubation protocol (Chapter 487)
- *Equipment*: Bag valve mask, suction catheter, ET tube, syringe, laryngoscope, laryngeal mask airway, Bougie, and Stylet
- Communication with the team is important.

To intubate a patient, the path from the incisor teeth to the larynx should be in a straight line. The angle of the axis of the mouth to the larynx is 90 degree. That of the pharynx to the trachea is obtuse.

When an average, nonobese patient's head is raised 10 cm off the bed by placing a folded sheet under the head, the pharyngeal and laryngeal axes align. Once the patient's head is optimally positioned, tilt the head into the extension with your right hand to bring all the axes into alignment.

- In patients with an unstable cervical spine, manual inline stabilization is required.
- In obese patients, a ramped position may have to be used by placing pillows or sheets under the patient's shoulders and torso (**Fig. 3**).

Cormack and Lehane Grading

This is a commonly used grading system to describe laryngeal view during direct laryngoscopy.

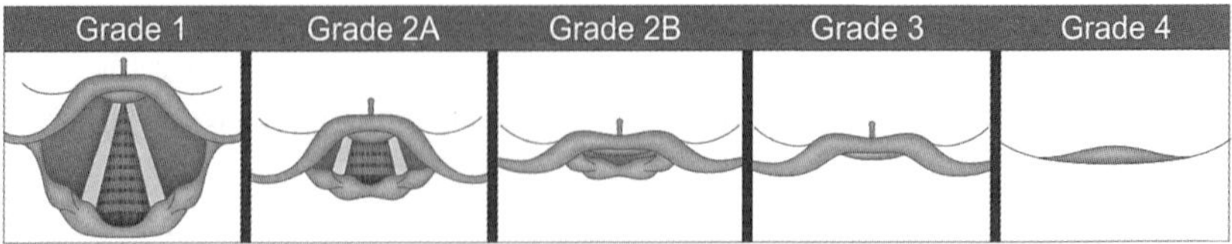

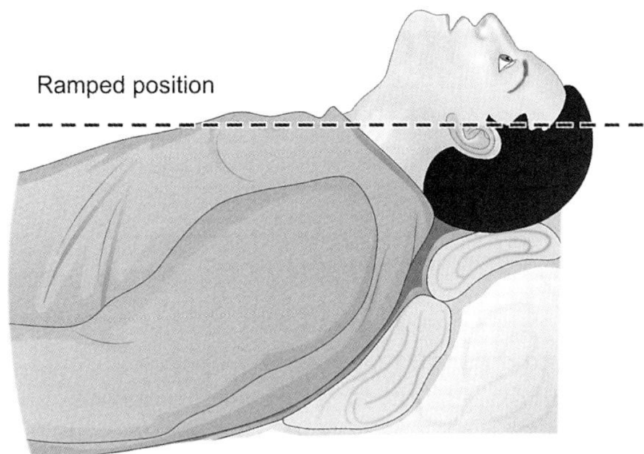

FIG. 3: Ramped position.

Grade 1: Full view of the glottis (easy)
Grade 2A: Partial view of the glottis (easy)
Grade 2B: Arytenoids/posterior part of the cords are just visible (restricted)
Grade 3: Only epiglottis is visible (difficult)
Grade 4: No glottis structure is visible (difficult)

LARYNGEAL MASK AIRWAY

Laryngeal mask airway (LMA) is a supraglottic airway device that is designed to rest inside the hypopharynx and thus allowing relative isolation of the trachea to aid positive pressure ventilation. It can be used as an alternative to intubation in the ED or during prehospital care for the following indications:

- For short duration procedures without requirement of neuromuscular blockade
- As a means of airway rescue in cases of failed endotracheal intubation.
- For blind intubation of anticipated difficult airway, in the absence of alternate/advanced equipment

  LMA is available in sized 0 (infant) to 5 (adult >80 kg). Practically, use size 3 for adult females or size 4 for adult males.

REFERENCE

1. Walls RM, Murphy MF. Manual of Emergency Airway Management, 3rd Edn. Philadelphia: Lippincott, Williams and Wilkins; 2009; pp.. 9-10.

INTRODUCTION

Oxygen can be administered conveniently by oronasal devices such as nasal catheters, cannulae, and different types of masks:

- Use face masks with oxygen flow meter or venturi masks.
- FiO_2 can be calculated by the formula 20 + [4 × O_2 flow rate (L/min)].
- PaO_2 of 60 mm Hg is equivalent to SpO_2 of 90%. However, in patients with metabolic acidosis, a higher PaO_2 should be targeted.
- Oxygen flow rates must be adjusted and delivered using appropriate delivery devices.
  - *Nasal cannula*: Oxygen flow rate up to 4 L/min.
  - *Simple face mask*: Oxygen flow rates 6–10 L/min.
  - *Venturi mask*: Oxygen flow rates 2–15 L/min.
  - *Non rebreather mask/face mask with reservoir bag*: Oxygen flow rates 10–15 L/min.

DANGERS OF OXYGEN THERAPY

- *Physical risks*: Oxygen being combustible, the risk of fire hazard and tank explosion is always present. This is more with high concentration of oxygen. Dry and nonhumidified gas can cause dryness and crusting of the oral and nasal mucosa.
- *Functional risks*: Patients who have lost sensitivity to CO_2 and depend upon the hypoxic drive for inspiration are in danger of ventilatory depression as seen in patients with chronic obstructive pulmonary disease (COPD).
- *Cytotoxic damage*: In the lungs, structural damage occurs from high FiO_2 as the oxygen can lead to the release of various reactive species, which attack the DNA.

  Respiratory support is needed for critically ill patients who have either oxygenation problem or ventilation failure.

- *Type 1 respiratory failure*: This is most widely defined as PaO_2 <8 kPa or 60 mm Hg (equivalent to SaO_2 of approximately 90%) with a normal or low $PaCO_2$ level.
- *Type 2 respiratory failure*: This is most widely defined as presence of hypercapnia with or without hypoxia. Hypercapnia is an elevated level of $PaCO_2$ (normal range: 34–46 mm Hg or 4.6–6.1 kPa).

Two types of ventilation are used in the ED; noninvasive ventilation (NIV), if the patient is conscious and cooperative or invasive ventilation in unconscious patients or if a trial of NIV fails.

NONINVASIVE VENTILATION

Noninvasive ventilation is a mode of positive pressure ventilation delivered through a noninvasive interface like nasal mask or face-mask rather than an invasive interface like endotracheal tube or a tracheostomy. It can be delivered using either a standard ventilator or continuous positive airway pressure (CPAP)/bilevel positive airway pressure (BiPAP) machine. While on NIV, patients must initiate all breaths.

When a ventilator is available, it can be used for delivering NIV, for both Type 1 and Type 2 respiratory failure. If ventilator is not available, patients with Type 1 respiratory failure can be managed by a CPAP machine.

Straps hold the interface in place and should be adjusted to avoid excessive pressure on the nose or face. Generally, the straps should be loose enough to allow one or two fingers to pass between the face and the strap. When nasal mask or prongs are used, a chin strap is usually necessary to maintain closure of the mouth.

Noninvasive ventilation can be delivered in two ways:
1. Noninvasive positive pressure ventilation (NIPPV)
   - NIPPV using a standard ventilator
   - BiPAP using BiPAP machine
   - CPAP using CPAP machine.
2. Noninvasive negative pressure ventilation (no longer used).

Indications for NIV include the following:
- Acute exacerbation of COPD with a respiratory acidosis (pH 7.25–7.35)
- Cardiogenic pulmonary edema unresponsive to medical management
- Hypercapnic respiratory failure secondary to chest wall deformity (scoliosis, thoracoplasty) or neuromuscular diseases
- Weaning from tracheal intubation
- Decompensated obstructive sleep apnea.

Contraindications of NIV:
- Comatose patient (Glasgow Coma Scale <8)
- Upper airway obstruction
- Extensive facial surgery/trauma
- *Respiratory failure:* Needs immediate intubation
- Unstable hemodynamics on >1 inotropic support
- Extensive secretions (e.g., bronchiectasis)
- Recent upper gastrointestinal (GI) surgery

- Vomiting, upper GI bleed
- Patient in multiple organ dysfunction syndrome (MODS)
- Confused/agitated patients.

NIPPV Using a Standard Ventilator

The following should be set while initiating a patient in NIPPV using a standard ventilator:

- *Mode*: NIPPV
- *Pressure support*: 12 cm H_2O
- *PEEP*: 5 cm H_2O
- *FiO_2*: Start initially with 100% O_2 and titrate to the response to maintain a saturation of 94% for Type 1 failure and 88% in Type 2 failure.
  - In Type 1 failure, increase PEEP up to 10 cm H_2O to improve oxygenation. Monitor hemodynamics as patient may develop hypotension or pneumothorax on higher PEEP.
  - In Type 2 failure, if patient demonstrates "air hunger", increase peak inspiratory flow rate to compensate for minute ventilation.

Disadvantages

- Difficult suctioning
- Risk of aspiration.

Note: NG tube is essential in a patient on NIPPV to avoid gastric inflation. Select appropriate size face mask for patient comfort and to prevent leak.

Discontinuation of NIPPV

- If there is inadequate improvement in 1 hour, intubate the patient and start invasive ventilation.
- If there is satisfactory improvement both clinically and on arterial blood gas (ABG), supports can be slowly titrated down and removed. The following should be reached.
  - $FiO_2 < 40\%$
  - PEEP = 5
  - Pressure support of ≤ 7 cm H_2O

Bilevel Positive Airway Pressure

This mode is used in Type 2 respiratory failure (ventilator failure or CO_2 retention).

Two settings have to be adjusted. These are:

1. *IPAP*: Equivalent to pressure support + PEEP in a standard ventilator
2. *EPAP (Expiratory Positive Airway Pressure)*: Equivalent to PEEP in a standard ventilator.

Initial settings in BiPAP: IPAP 15 and EPAP 5.

Increase IPAP gradually up to 20 cm H_2O, if tolerated.

Notes:

- On a BiPAP machine, increase in EPAP will decrease effective IPAP. Hence, IPAP have to be increased to maintain desired ventilation.
- On a BiPAP machine, increase in IPAP will actually decrease the delivered FiO_2 as air is used to achieve the target pressure. In a standard ventilator, oxygen blender is used and hence, FiO_2 can be set and is stable. On a BiPAP machine, increase the FiO_2 while increasing IPAP.

Continuous Positive Airway Pressure

It is used for patients with Type 1 respiratory failure (only oxygenation failure) like pulmonary edema:

- Start with FiO_2 of 100% and PEEP of 5 cm H_2O
- Increase the PEEP gradually up to 10 if tolerated to improve oxygenation.

Monitoring During Noninvasive Ventilation

- Clinical (every 30 minutes)
  - Patient comfort
  - Level of consciousness
  - Accessory muscle activity
  - Patient ventilator synchrony
  - Respiratory rate
  - Heart rate.
- Repeat an ABG after 1 hour of initiation of NIV and adjust the ventilator settings.

  (Rise in pH and fall in $PaCO_2$ are good prognostic signs in Type 2 failure).

INVASIVE VENTILATION

Invasive ventilation should be initiated when a patient is not able to maintain oxygenation or if the patient does not have spontaneous breathing or if a trial of NIV fails.

Indications for Endotracheal Intubation

- Cardiac arrest
- Apnea
- Unconscious patient with $SpO_2 < 90\%$
- Type 2 respiratory failure with failure on NIV
- Impending respiratory arrest
- GCS < 8 in trauma
- Elective intubation for conditions like tetanus.

Initial Settings in a Standard Ventilator

- *Mode*: SIMV volume controlled with pressure support
- FiO_2 100%
- *PEEP*: 5 cm H_2O
- *Tidal volume*: Start with 6–8 mL/kg
- *Rate*: 10–15/min
- *Pressure support*: 12 cm H_2O

The following needs to be monitored:
- If the expired tidal volume is less than the set tidal volume, look for leak in the system.
- Monitor peak and plateau pressures (peak pressure should be <35 cm H_2O/ plateau pressure should be <30 cm H_2O). If these pressures are high, look for patient discomfort, secretions, tube blockage, bronchospasm, tube bite, pneumothorax.
- Do an ABG after 1 hour and adjust the settings.
- Titrate FiO_2 to avoid oxygen toxicity. Keep it <50%.

Notes:
- Provide adequate sedation for all intubated patients. Midazolam infusion 4 mg/h can be started and titrated according to the response.
- Avoid neuromuscular paralyzing agents. Use it only if the patient is not adequately oxygenating (PaO_2 <60 mm Hg) on a FiO_2 of 100% and a PEEP of 10. Sedate the patient adequately before giving paralyzing agent (vecuronium) and patch the eyes to avoid exposure keratitis.
- Ensure adequate hydration before intubation as fall in blood pressure can occur after intubation which is more marked in those with volume depletion and autonomic neuropathy (Guillain–Barré syndrome). Treat hypotension with fluids. In patients with fluid overload, use inotropes instead of fluids. Vasopressors can be used to treat hypotension in volume overloaded patients.
- Oxygenation of a patient can be increased by:
  - Increasing FiO_2
  - Increasing PEEP
  - Physiotherapy and recruitment maneuvers to open the collapsed alveoli.
- Ventilation (regulating CO_2) can be done by adjusting the tidal volume and respiratory rate.
- Treat the primary cause (e.g., asthma—use of bronchodilators will improve the ventilator parameters).

Fluid and Electrolytes

Fluid Therapy

INTRODUCTION

Water comprises approximately 60% of the human body weight and the other 40% being lean body mass. Water is distributed in the two main compartments of the body: intracellular and extracellular compartments. The extracellular compartment comprises of interstitial fluid and plasma (intravascular space). These fluid compartments are in constant interchange with each other due to movement of fluids and electrolytes across the membranes (**Fig. 1**).

CHOICE OF INTRAVENOUS FLUIDS

Many crystalloids and colloids can be used for fluid resuscitation in the emergency department. The fluid administered is distributed between the intracellular and extracellular compartments (**Table 1**). The composition of the different crystalloids commonly used is shown in **Table 2**.

- *0.9% normal saline (NS)*: NS is an isotonic crystalloid and is the resuscitation fluid of choice in trauma and in dehydrated patients. It expands extracellular volume with no change in intracellular volume. Risks include hyperchloremic acidosis.
- *Ringer lactate (RL)*: RL is an isotonic crystalloid and is the resuscitation fluid of choice for acute gastroenteritis (AGE). It expands extracellular volume with minimum change in the intravascular volume. Avoid in patients with diabetic ketoacidosis due to increase in serum lactate levels.

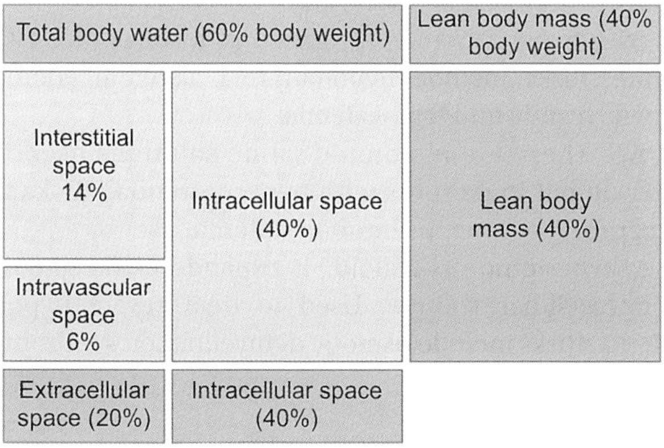

FIG. 1: Fluid compartments in the body.

TABLE 1: The net effect of infusing 500 mL of each of the solutions.					
	Normal saline (NS, 0.9%)		*Glucose containing crystalloids (DNS/5%D)*		*Colloid (albumin, dextran, and haemaccel)*
Intracellular fluid (ICF)	Negligible		333 mL (2/3rd)		Nil
Extracellular fluid (ECF)	500 mL		167 mL (1/3rd)		500 mL
	Interstitial	375 mL	Interstitial	125 mL	Interstitial — Negligible
	Intra-vascular	125 mL	Intra-vascular	42 mL	Intra-vascular — 500 mL

TABLE 2: Profile of crystalloids (1 L).					
	Na (mmol/L)	*Cl (mmol/L)*	*HCO_3 (mmol/L)*	*mOsm*	*pH*
0.9% NS	154	154		308	4.5–7
DNS	154	154		586	3.5–6.5
3% NS	512	512		1026	4.5–7
½ NS	77	77		154	4.5–7
RL	130	109		273	5.1
5% Dextrose				278	5
7.5% $NaHCO_3$	1283		1283	2566	8.3

- *Dextrose normal saline (DNS)*: A mixed crystalloid solution used for resuscitation if sugars are low and the patient needs calorie replacement. Usually used for postoperative patients.
- *5% Dextrose*: Not the initial choice for resuscitation as majority of the fluid goes into the intracellular and interstitial compartments. Only 10% is retained in the intravascular space. Used for correction of free water deficit in patients with hypernatremia. Also used as a solvent for IV infusions like noradrenaline. Risks include hyponatremia, cerebral edema, pulmonary edema, hyperglycemia and hypokalemia.
- *1/2 or 1/4 NS*: These are hypotonic saline solutions used for correction of free water deficit in patients with hypernatremia. Risks include hyponatremia, cerebral edema, pulmonary edema.
- *3% NaCl*: A hypertonic crystalloid, it expands extracellular volume and decreases intracellular volume. Used to treat severe hyponatremia and cerebral edema. Risks include osmotic demyelination syndrome.

Sodium   9

INTRODUCTION

This chapter discusses about the electrolyte, sodium. The normal level of sodium is 135–145 mEq/L.

HYPONATREMIA

Hyponatremia is a condition that occurs when the serum sodium level is less than 135 mmol/L. The causes and management of hyponatremia are given in **Table 1**.

Symptoms

The symptoms of hyponatremia are headache, nausea, vomiting, fatigue, gait disturbances, confusion, seizures, obtundation, coma, and respiratory arrest.

Management

Pseudohyponatremia: High concentration of intravascular protein or lipid may falsely result in laboratory hyponatremia. This occurs with hyperglycemia,

TABLE 1: Causes and management of hyponatremia.

Volume status of the patient (ECF)	Causes	Management
True hyponatremia		
Depletional Both H_2O and Na decreased (Na > H_2O)	• *Gastrointestinal loss*: Vomiting diarrhea • *Renal*: Renal tubular disease, diuretic therapy • Cerebral salt wasting	• *Mild*: Oral correction • *Severe*: IV fluid correction with normal saline • Calculate Na replacement and correct over 48–72 hours
Euvolemic H_2O increased and Na stable	• *SIADH*: Syndrome of inappropriate antidiuretic hormone • Hypothyroidism • Adrenal insufficiency	• Restrict fluids to 500–800 mL/day • Increase salt intake
Dilutional H_2O increased and Na increased (H_2O > Na)	• CHF • Cirrhosis • Nephrotic syndrome	• 3% NaCl IV • Restrict fluids • Cautious use of diuretics

(IV: intravenous)

hyperproteinemia (multiple myeloma), uremia, and hypertriglyceridemia. This must be considered before correcting hyponatremia. Apply the following corrections for pseudohyponatremia:
- Every 100 mg/dL of glucose decreases serum Na by 1.6 mEq/L.
- Every 25 mg/dL increase of blood urea nitrogen (BUN) above the normal value of 25 mg/dL decreases Na by 3.3 mEq/L.

Before initiating Na correction, calculate the total sodium deficit by the following formula:

Total sodium deficit = Body weight × 0.6 × [Expected Na (135) – Measured Na].

- Hyponatremia correction should not rise by <10–12 mmol/L per 24 hours because rapid correction can cause seizures or central pontine myelinolysis. So, while calculating sodium deficit, correction for a day (expected Na – measured Na) should be taken as 10–12 mEq/L.

Note: When hyponatremia is documented to have occurred within 12–24 hours, it is safe to correct at a faster rate.

Indications for 3% NaCl intravenous correction in patients with euvolemic or dilutional hyponatremia:
- Seizure
- Low sensorium
- Very low serum Na (<120 mEq/L).

3% NaCl should be given ONLY to patients with euvolemic or dilutional hyponatremia. *Never* give 3% NaCl to a patient who is dehydrated (check tongue and skin turgor) no matter what the Na level is.

- 1000 mL of normal saline contains 154 mEq of Na.
- 100 mL of 3% NaCl contains 51.2 mEq of Na.

The following investigations are helpful in the evaluation of hyponatremia:
- *Urine osmolality*: To differentiate between conditions associated with impaired free water excretion and primary polydipsia.
  - <100 mOsm/kg indicates primary polydipsia.
  - >100 mOsm/kg indicates syndrome of inappropriate antidiuretic hormone secretion (SIADH) or depletional hyponatremia.
- *Urine spot sodium*: It helps to differentiate depletional hyponatremia and SIADH.
  - 20–40 mEq/L indicates increased Na excretion (SIADH/diuretic use)
  - <20 mEq/L indicates renal conservation of Na (depletional).
- *Serum osmolality*: It differentiates between true hyponatremia and pseudohyponatremia.
  - High-serum osmolality (SOsm > 295): Hyperglycemia (pseudohyponatremia).

- ○ Normal serum osmolality (SOsm: 280–295): Pseudohyponatremia from elevated lipids or proteins.
- ○ Low-serum osmolality (SOsm <280): True hyponatremia.

HYPERNATREMIA

Hypernatremia is defined as serum sodium >145 mEq/L. Causes of hypernatremia are given in **Table 2**.

Management

- Adrogue–Madias formula for calculating water deficit

$$\text{Water deficit (L)} = 0.6 \times \text{Body weight} \times \frac{(\text{Measured serum Na} - \text{Normal serum Na})}{\text{Normal serum Na}}$$

The goal of hypernatremia correction is to lower the serum Na by a maximum of 10–12 mEq/L in 24 hours. Therefore, (measured serum Na – Normal serum Na) should be 10–12 mEq/L for calculating water deficit replacement for a day. The following fluids may be used:

- 5% Dextrose if the patient is not a diabetic.
- ½ NS or ¼ NS may be used if sugars are high.
- Clear free water via nasogastric tube at 100 mL/h, if the airway is secure.

> Rapid sodium correction can cause seizures and permanent neurological abnormalities (central pontine myelinolysis).
> So, serum Na should NOT be corrected >10–12 mmol/L over 24 hours.

TABLE 2: Causes of hypernatremia.

Excess Na	Relative water deficit	
Hypertonic saline, NaHCO₃ administration	Inadequate fluid intake	
	Excess fluid loss	
	Lung/skin loss	
	Renal loss	*Reduced ADH level*: Pituitary diabetes insipidus (DI)
		Reduced ADH action: Nephrogenic DI
	Osmotic diuresis	

Potassium   **10**

INTRODUCTION

Potassium is predominantly an intracellular ion. The serum levels do not accurately reflect the body stores of potassium. The normal potassium level is 3.5–5 mEq/L.

- Acidosis and hyperthermia cause hyperkalemia
- Alkalosis and hypothermia cause hypokalemia.

HYPOKALEMIA

Causes

- *Deficit*: Gastrointestinal loss: vomiting and diarrhea
- *Renal loss*: Diuretic use, Cushing syndrome, Bartter syndrome, and Liddle syndrome
- *Redistribution*: Insulin, bicarbonate therapy, alkalosis, periodic paralysis, and β agonists.

Clinical Features

No symptoms at >3 mEq/L. Severe hypokalemia can cause muscle weakness, fatigue, muscle cramps, and constipation.

Amount of potassium needed: The relationship between total body potassium and serum potassium is not linear. At lower levels of measured potassium, much more potassium is required to increase the serum level by 1 mEq/L than at a higher level.

- If the serum potassium is >3 mEq/L, 100–200 mEq is required to increase it by 1 mEq/L.
- If the serum potassium is <3 mEq/L, 200–400 mEq is required to increase it by 1 mEq/L assuming a normal distribution between the cells and the intracellular space.
- 1 g of intravenous KCl contains 13 mEq of K.
- 5 mL of oral KCl contains 4 mEq of K.

ECG Changes

T wave inversion followed by QT prolongation, U waves, and mild ST depression.

Management

- Potassium replacement through peripheral line causes painful thrombophlebitis. Hence, use only 500 mL (with up to 3 g KCl) or 1 L (with up to 4.5 g KCl) of normal saline (NS) as the diluent.
- Administration through a central line can be given in 100 mL of fluid (3 g KCl per 100 mL). Infusion rate should not exceed 1.5 g/h (20 mEq of KCl).
- Patients tolerating orally can be given syrup KCl (20 mL stat and repeat dose after 2 h) in addition to the intravenous correction in case of severe hypokalemia.
- Hypomagnesemia often coexists with severe hypokalemia. Add magnesium to the infusate containing KCl (2–4 g $MgSO_4$).

> Always add $MgSO_4$ 2–4 g to the K correction for severe hypokalemia (K < 3 mEq/L)

- Patients on long-term diuretic therapy can have hypokalemia and this may precipitate or aggravate digoxin toxicity. Correct hypokalemia aggressively in patients on digoxin therapy.
- After correction, if the patient is stable to be discharged, advice the patient to continue syrup KCl at a dose of at least 20 mL BD till the next OPD review.

Hypokalemic Periodic Paralysis

Attacks occur suddenly with generalized weakness. Consciousness is preserved and bulbar and respiratory muscles are rarely involved. After correction, patients may be discharged on syrup KCl and tablet acetazolamide 250 mg BD (to prevent attacks).

HYPERKALEMIA

Causes

- Increased intake
- *Reduced excretion*: Renal failure, hypoadrenal state
- *Drugs*: Angiotensin-converting-enzyme (ACE) inhibitor, angiotensin-receptor blockers (ARB), K-sparing diuretics (spironolactone, amiloride), nonsteroidal anti-inflammatory drugs, cyclosporine, tacrolimus, and tri- methoprim/sulfamethoxazole (TMP-SMX)
- *Shift out of cells*: Acidosis, tissue damage
- *Pseudohyperkalemia*: Hemolyzed sample

ECG Changes

Peaked T waves, broad QRS, ST depression, and sine wave pattern.

TABLE 1: Treatment of hyperkalemia.

Goal	Drug and dose	Onset of action	Duration of action
Cardio-protective effect	10 mL of 10% calcium gluconate over 4 min	1–3 min	30–60 min
Intracellular shift	Salbutamol nebulization 5 mg every 15 min × 3 doses	30 min	2–4 hours
	50 mL of 50% dextrose with 8 units of short-acting insulin over 10 min (if RBS is high, give only insulin)	20 min	4–6 hours
Elimination from the body	Furosemide 40–80 mg IV stat and repeat after 4 hours if blood pressure is normal	15 min	2–3 hours
	Potassium binding resin (Syrup 30 g of kayexalate with 12.5 g mannitol in 100 mL water)	>2 hours	4–6 hours
	Hemodialysis	Immediate	

Clinical Features

Patients are usually asymptomatic, but may complain of fatigue, weakness, paresthesias, paralysis, or palpitations.

False hyperkalemia is very common due to hemolyzed blood sample. If there is no obvious predisposing factor, recheck serum K before intervention.

Management

The correction of hyperkalemia is shown in **Table 1**.

Potassium level may be repeated 2 hours after a correction. After correction, if the patient is stable to be discharged.

- Make sure the offending drugs are stopped (e.g., ACI/ARB/TMP–SMX).
- Advice the patient to continue diuretics and K-binding resins (once/twice daily) till the next OPD review.

Calcium   **11**

INTRODUCTION

Calcium exists in three fractions in circulation:

1. *Protein bound*: 40–50%
2. *Ionized form*: 40–45%
3. *Nonionized chelated complexes with anions*: 10–15%.

Each gram of albumin binds 0.8 mg% (0.2 mmol/L) of calcium. Serum albumin levels can alter total calcium without changing the ionized calcium levels. Ionized form is the physiologically important form of calcium.

The normal range of ionized calcium is 4.65–5.25 mg/dL (1.16–1.31 mmol/L).

> Corrected calcium = Measured calcium + (4 – serum albumin g%) × F
> F = 0.8 if serum calcium value is in mg%
> = 0.2 if serum calcium value is in mmol/L

HYPOCALCEMIA

Causes

- Hypoalbuminemia
- *Acid-base disturbances*: Acute respiratory alkalosis
- Hypocalcemia with low parathyroid hormone (PTH) (hypoparathyroidism)
  - Postoperative thyroid, parathyroid or radical neck surgery for head and neck cancer
  - Autoimmune destruction of the parathyroid glands.
- Hypocalcemia with high PTH
  - Vitamin D deficiency or resistance
  - *Chronic kidney disease*: Due to decrease in renal production of 1,25-dihydroxy vitamin D
  - PTH resistance (impaired PTH action)
- *Drugs*: Bisphosphonates, Denosumab, Foscarnet, and Cisplatin.

Clinical Features

- *Mild*: Perioral numbness, paresthesias of the hands and feet, muscle cramps
- *Severe*: Carpopedal spasm, laryngospasm, and focal, or generalized seizures.

Trousseau's Sign

Induction of carpopedal spasm by inflation of a sphygmomanometer above systolic blood pressure for 3 minutes.

Chvostek's Sign

Contraction of the ipsilateral facial muscles elicited by tapping the facial nerve just anterior to the ear.

Management

- *Severe/symptomatic hypocalcemia*: 10% calcium gluconate 10 mL IV over 4 minutes
  - In persistent hypocalcemia, calcium gluconate 10 mL can be added in 500 mL normal saline over 4 hours and to be repeated till symptomatic improvement
  - Treat concurrent hypomagnesemia if hypocalcemia is refractory. Add 4 g $MgSO_4$ to the infusate.
- *Mildly symptomatic or chronic hypocalcemia*: Oral calcium supplementation (1,500–2,000 mg of elemental calcium as calcium carbonate or calcium citrate daily, in divided doses) can be given.

HYPERCALCEMIA

Causes

Hypercalcemia is defined as increase in total serum calcium >10.5 mg% or ionized calcium >1.4 mmol/L.

Clinical Features

Bones (painful), Groans (abdominal), Moans (depression, psychosis, apathy, confusion), and stones (renal).

The clinical presentation depends on how fast and how high the calcium level rises. Mild prolonged hypercalcemia may produce mild or no symptoms, or recurring problems (renal calculi). Sudden-onset and severe hypercalcemia may cause dramatic symptoms such as lethargy, confusion, or coma.

- Among all causes (**Table 1**), primary hyperparathyroidism and malignancy are the most common, accounting for >90% of cases.
- Once hypercalcemia is confirmed, the next step is measurement of serum PTH. An elevated or high-normal value indicates primary hyperparathyroidism.

TABLE 1: Causes of hypercalcemia.

Excess parathyroid hormone	Primary, tertiary, and ectopic
Excess vitamin D	Iatrogenic, tablet overdose, granulomatous disease
Malignancy	Bone metastasis, lymphoma, myeloma
Endocrine	Thyrotoxicosis, acromegaly, adrenal insufficiency
Medication	Thiazide diuretics, lithium

TABLE 1: Rules of compensation for a primary respiratory problem.		
	Change in HCO_3 from 24 mmol/L	
Every 10 mm Hg change in $PaCO_2$ from 40 mm Hg	Acute	Chronic
$PaCO_2$ increases (acidosis)	1	4
$PaCO_2$ decreases (alkalosis)	2	5

HOW TO INTERPRET AN ARTERIAL BLOOD GAS

- *Step 1*: Ask for the basic history and determine the primary metabolic/respiratory pathology.
- *Step 2*: Look at the PaO_2. Calculate the PaO_2/FiO_2 ratio and optimize the oxygen concentration.
- *Step 3*: Look at the pH
  - <7.3 = acidosis. >7.5 = alkalosis
  - If pH is normal but CO_2/HCO_3 is abnormal, think of a mixed problem.
- *Step 4*: Look at the base excess (BE) if the patient is likely to have a metabolic problem. Normal range is between –2 and +2. If BE is more negative, it means that the patient has a primary metabolic acidosis. If the BE is more positive, the patient has primary metabolic alkalosis.
- *Step 5*: Apply rules of compensation to look for compensation (metabolic/respiratory).
- *Step 6*: If the basic pathology is a metabolic acidosis, calculate anion gap = $(Na + K) - (HCO_3 + Cl)$. Normal range is 14 ± 4.
- *Step 7*: Check the electrolytes and sugars and correct them if abnormal.
- *Step 8*: Look at the lactate and methemoglobin levels for clues about the underlying problem. Think of the underlying cause and correct the cause (**Flowchart 1**).

Arterial Blood Gas versus Venous Blood Gas

- *pH*: The venous pH closely reflects arterial pH for most metabolic conditions including diabetic ketoacidosis, uremia. pH value does not correlate well in a cardiac arrest. As cardiac output decreases, the differences between arterial and venous measurements increase. However, in clinical practice, knowledge of either the arterial or venous pH or pCO_2 during cardiac arrest does not alter management.
  Pooled mean difference is +0.035 pH units.
- *Lactate*: When lactates are elevated (>2), there is a close correlation between arterial and venous lactate levels. A normal venous lactate measurement predicts a normal arterial level. The bottom line is that venous lactate levels are similar to those found in arterial samples.
  Mean difference 0.08. (–0.27 to 0.42 95% CI).

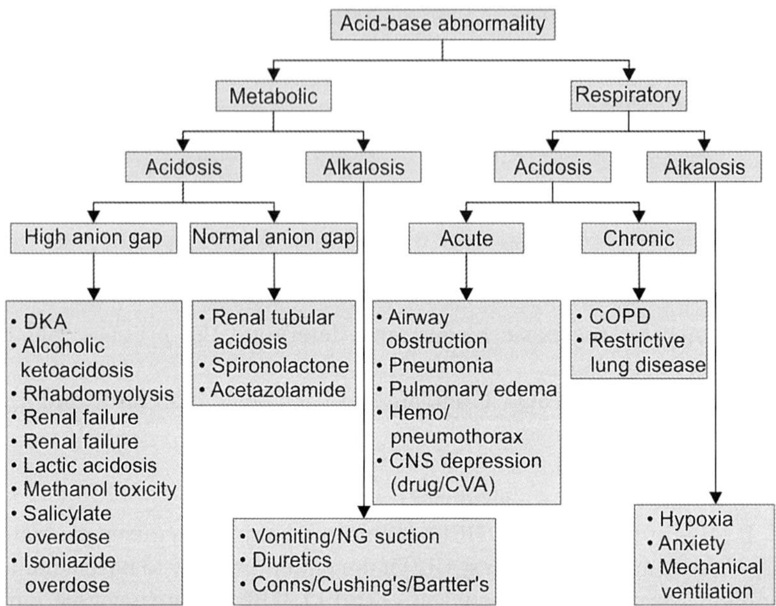

FLOWCHART 1: Causes of acid-base disturbances.

- HCO_3: Similar in both ABG and VBG.
  Mean difference −1.41 mmol/L (−5.8 to +5.3 mmol/L 95%CI).
- pCO_2: Venous pCO_2 levels are significantly higher than arterial pCO_2 levels and hence presence or absence of clinically significant hypercarbia cannot be decided by a VBG.
- pO_2: Venous pO_2 levels do not reflect the arterial pO_2 levels and therefore is a poor surrogate to determine oxygen delivery to tissues.

> Neither an ABG nor a VBG is required in most of the patients who present to the ED. A good history and clinical examination gives much more information than any laboratory test.
> Do not be over dependent on ABG to make a diagnosis.

- When to do a VBG?
  In our ED, a VBG is sufficient for most of the cases. Indications are:
  - Suspected DKA to determine the pH, lactate levels.
  - Acute severe pancreatitis in shock
  - Renal failure (acute/chronic) to determine the pH and need for dialysis.
  - To determine electrolyte abnormalities (K, Mg) in patients with arrhythmias or impending cardiac arrest.
- When to do an arterial blood gas?
  Venous blood gas is easier to perform and gives most of the essential information for most cases. The following are the *only* indications when an ABG is required.

- ○ In a patient chronic obstructive pulmonary disease with exacerbation and suspected type 2 failure, to decide on the need for noninvasive ventilation/mechanical ventilation.
- ○ SpO_2 is usually sufficient for clinical decision making unless pulse oximetry is unreliable for other reasons (shock, methemoglobinemia, etc.) A VBG/ABG is not needed for any decision making in a patient on Venturi mask (up to 8 L/min or 60% oxygen). An ABG may be warranted in some patients who require high flow oxygen (>8 L/min)
- ○ In patients with type 1 respiratory failure on NIV/mechanical ventilation to decide on adjusting the flow rate of oxygen.

To summarize, the only two indications to do an ABG and not a VBG in the ED are:

- A patient suspected to have type 2 failure to know the pCO_2 levels that may determine the need to intubate or not
- A patient on high flow oxygen to determine the PaO_2/FiO_2 ratio and decide the need for NIV/intubation.

Infectious Diseases

Antibiotic Protocol for Common Conditions

INTRODUCTION

Febrile illnesses and infections are common presentations to the emergency department (ED). **Table 1** shows the antibiotic protocol for commonly seen infections in the ED.

TABLE 1: Antibiotic protocol for commonly seen infections in the emergency department.

Condition	Etiology (most likely pathogens)	First choice	Alternatives
Acute gastroenteritis	Viral entero-toxigenic *Escherichia coli* Enteropathogenic *Escherichia coli*	Not indicated	
Cholera	*Vibrio cholerae*	Doxycycline 300 mg PO × 1 dose	• Tablet azithromycin 1 g × 1 dose • Tablet ciprofloxacin 500 mg bd × 3 days
Bacillary dysentery	*Shigella* species	None needed for previously healthy patient with mild symptoms	Ciprofloxacin 500 mg PO bd × 3 days in patients with severe symptoms or immunocompromised patients
Giardiasis	*Giardia lamblia*	Tinidazole 2 g PO × 1 dose	
Helminthiasis	*Ascaris, Enterobius,* and *Ankylostoma*	Albendazole 400 mg PO × 1 dose Repeat dose after 2 weeks for *Enterobius*	
Typhoid fever	*Salmonella typhi* *Salmonella paratyphi* A	Azithromycin 1 g PO × 14 days or Injection Ceftriaxone 2 g IV od × 14 days	• Tablet cotrimoxazole 1 ds tablet PO bd × 14 days • Tablet chloramphenicol 500 mg PO q6h × 14 days

Continued

Continued

Condition	Etiology (most likely pathogens)	First choice	Alternatives
Cholangitis	Enterobacteriaceae	Piperacillin-Tazobactam 4.5 g IV q6–8h × 7 days Ertapenem 1 g IV od × 7 days (if qSOFA ≥2)	Cefoperazone-Sulbactam 3 g IV q12h
Acute cholecystitis	Enterobacteriaceae	Piperacillin-Tazobactam 4.5 g IV q6–8H × 7 days Ertapenem 1 g IV od × 7 days (if qSOFA ≥2)	Cefoperazone-Sulbactam 3 g IV q12h
Spontaneous bacterial peritonitis	Enterobacteriaceae (most often *E. coli*)	Piperacillin-Tazobactam 4.5 g IV q6-8h × 7 days Ertapenem 1 g IV od × 7 days (if qSOFA ≥ 2)	Cefoperazone-Sulbactam 3 g IV q12h
Secondary peritonitis (bowel perforation)	Enterobacteriaceae Anaerobes (*Bacteroides* species)	Ertapenem 1 g IV od × 5–7 days	Cefoperazone-Sulbactam 3 g IV q12h
Intra-abdominal abscess	Enterobacteriaceae Anaerobes (*Bacteroides* species)	Ertapenem 1 g IV od × 5–7 days	• Cefoperazone-Sulbactam 3 g IV q12h • Tigecycline 100 mg IV × 1 dose, then 50 mg IV q12h
Cellulitis	*Streptococcus pyogenes, Staphylococcus aureus*	Cloxacillin 1 g IV q6h Cefuroxime 1.5 g IV q8h (for moderately ill patients)	Cloxacillin 500–1000 mg PO q6H × 7–10 days or Cephalexin 500 mg PO q6h × 7–10 days
Furunculosis	*S. aureus*	Cloxacillin 500 mg PO q6h × 7–10 days	Cephalexin 500 mg PO q6h × 7–10 days
Diabetic foot— mild (localized cellulitis, no or mild systemic symptoms)	*S. aureus*	Cefuroxime 1.5 g IV q8h × 7–10 days	Cloxacillin 500–1,000 mg PO q6h × 7–10 days OR Cephalexin 500 mg PO q6h × 7–10 days

Continued

Continued

Condition	Etiology (most likely pathogens)	First choice	Alternatives
Diabetic foot—moderate-to-severe (limb threatening)	Polymicrobial—*S. aureus*, Group A *Streptococcus*, aerobic gram-negative bacilli, anaerobes	Piperacillin-Tazobactam 4.5 gIV q6-8h + Vancomycin 15 mg/kg IV q12h	Piperacillin-Tazobactam 4.5 g IV q6-8h Ertapenem 1 g IV od
Necrotizing fasciitis (life-threatening infection)	Group A *Streptococcus*	Meropenem 1 g IV q8h + Vancomycin 15 mg/kg IV q12h	Piperacillin-Tazobactam 4.5 g IV q6-8h + Clindamycin 900 mg IV q8h
Chickenpox	Varicella zoster virus	Valacyclovir 1,000 mg PO tid × 7 days	Acyclovir 800 mg PO 5 times/day × 7 days
Acute osteomyelitis	*S. aureus* polymicrobial	Cloxacillin 2 g IV q4H	Cefazolin 2 g IV q8h
Septic arthritis	*S. aureus*	Cloxacillin 2 g IV q6H × 14–28 days	Cefuroxime 1.5 g IV q8h
Acute pharyngitis	Respiratory viruses Gb A *Streptococcus*	Amoxycillin 500 mg PO tid x 10 days	Azithromycin 500 mg PO od × 5 days
	Group A β-hemolytic streptococci	Benzathine penicillin 12 L units intra-muscularly (IM) × 1 dose For penicillin allergsic patients: Erythromycin 500 mg PO q6h × 10 days	Amoxicillin 500 mg PO q8h × 10 days
Acute epiglottitis	*Haemophilus influenzae*	Ceftriaxone 1–2 g IV od × 7–10 days	
Ludwig's angina Vincent's angina	Polymicrobial (oral anaerobes)	Amoxicillin-clavulanate 1.2 g IV q12h × 14 days	Clindamycin 600 mg IV q8h × 2 weeks
Acute bronchitis	Viral	Not required	
Acute bacterial rhinosinusitis	*S. pneumoniae* *H. influenzae* *Moraxella catarrhalis*	Amoxicillin clavulanate 1,000 mg PO bd × 7 days	
Leptospirosis	*Leptospira interrogans*	Crystalline penicillin 15 L units IV q6H for 7 days Anicteric form (mild disease): Doxycycline 100 mg PO bd × 7 days	Ceftriaxone 1 g IV od × 7 days

Continued

Continued

Condition	Etiology (most likely pathogens)	First choice	Alternatives
Scrub typhus	*Orientia tsutsugamushi*	Doxycycline 100 mg PO bd × 7 days	Azithromycin 500 mg PO od × 7 days
Acute bacterial meningitis (community acquired)	*S. pneumonia Neisseria meningitidis*	Ceftriaxone 2 g IV q12H + Vancomycin 15–20 mg/kg IV q8-12h + Dexamethasone10 mg IV q6h × 4 days; first dose 15 minutes before or along with the first dose of antibiotic.	If *Listeria* is suspected, add Ampicillin 2 g IV q4h
Bites (cat, dog, human, and rat)	*Pasteurella multocida Eikenella S. viridans Spirillum minus Streptobacillus*	Amoxicillin-clavulanate 625 mg PO tid for 3–5 days	

INTRODUCTION

Dengue fever is an arthropod-borne (*Aedes aegypti*) viral infection caused by dengue virus (DENV) endemic in many parts of India during the monsoon season (July–November). Incubation period is 3–7 days. There are four serologically distinct DENV types of the genus Flavivirus, called DENV-1, DENV-2, DENV-3, and DENV-4 with transient cross-protection among the four types. Therefore, a person can possibly get infected with DENV a maximum of 4 times.

The management of dengue is based on clinical assessment of severity. In the absence of warning signs, management is mostly symptomatic and supportive. The WHO case definition of dengue fever is shown in **Table 1**.

TABLE 1: Case definitions and grading.

Case definitions and grading	Clinical features	HCT and platelet count	Tourniquet test
Dengue fever	Fever of 2–7 days with two or more of the following— headache, retro-orbital pain, myalgia, arthralgia, and no evidence of plasma leakage	May have mildly increased hematocrit (HCT) and mild throm-bocytopenia, with or without leukopenia	Negative
Dengue hemorrhagic fever (grade I)	Above plus positive tourniquet test and evidence of plasma leakage	• HCT >20% of baseline • Platelets <100,000	Positive
Dengue hemorrhagic fever (grade II)	Above plus some evidence of spontaneous bleeding (skin or other organs) and abdominal pain	• HCT >20% of baseline • Platelets <100,000	Positive
Compensated dengue shock syndrome (grade III)	Above plus circulatory failure (weak rapid pulse, narrow pulse pressure, hypotension, cold clammy skin, restlessness)	• HCT >20% of baseline • Platelets < 100,000	Positive
Uncompensated dengue shock syn drome (grade IV)	DHF with profound shock with undetectable blood pressure or pulse	• HCT >20% of baseline • Platelets <100,000	Positive

Source: WHO. National Guidelines for Clinical Management of Dengue Fever. New Delhi: WHO; 2015.

Tourniquet test: Apply a blood pressure (BP) cuff, inflated for 5 minutes mid- way between systolic blood pressure and diastolic blood pressure. Positive test is petechiae >10/sq. inch on forearm.

WARNING SIGNS IN DENGUE FEVER

Look for the following warning signs of dengue fever. These signs and symptoms indicate severity and disease progression and warrant aggressive resuscitation and monitoring.
- Abdominal pain or tenderness
- Persistent vomiting
- Clinical or radiological fluid accumulation (ascites or pleural effusion)
- Mucosal bleeding
- Lethargy, restlessness
- Hepatomegaly
- *Laboratory*: Increase in hematocrit (HCT) associated with rapid decrease in platelet count.

INVESTIGATIONS

Complete blood count, urea, creatinine, electrolytes, and liver function test. Diagnosis is clinical. Tests such as reverse transcription–polymerase chain reaction and NS1 antigen-based ELISA are helpful in early infection (days 1–5). Dengue IgM and dengue IgG ELISA tests should be sent only after 5–7 days of the onset of symptoms.

MANAGEMENT

Management of dengue fever depends on the grade of severity.
- *Dengue fever*:
  - Advice bed rest, tepid sponging, oral paracetamol, adequate oral hydration with ORS
  - Avoid nonsteroidal anti-inflammatory drugs (NSAIDs)
  - Explain warning signs
  - Monitor HCT and platelets on an OPD basis.
- *Dengue hemorrhagic fever (DHF) (Grade I and II)*:
  - Admit the patient, look for warning signs and signs of shock
  - Monitor HCT and platelet count
  - Start hydration with intravenous (IV) crystalloids and titrate therapy to clinical improvement as evidenced by a fall in HCT, decrease in pulse rate, stable BP, and good urine output
  - However, if HCT falls rapidly with signs of internal hemorrhage, transfuse packed red cells.

- *Dengue shock syndrome (DSS) with compensated shock (Grade III):*
  - Start aggressive resuscitation with IV crystalloid infusion and titrate therapy to clinical improvement
  - If the clinical condition deteriorates (rise in HCT, decrease in platelets with signs of shock), continue aggressive fluid resuscitation and initiate inotropic support
  - Transfuse packed red cells if there is evidence of hemorrhage.
- *DSS with profound shock (Grade IV):*
  - Assess and stabilize airway, breathing, circulation (ABC)
  - Start aggressive resuscitation with IV crystalloid bolus (10 mL/kg) and titrate therapy to clinical improvement
  - Reassess and repeat fluid bolus, if necessary
  - If the shock is refractory to fluid resuscitation, initiate inotropic support
  - Transfuse packed red cells, if there is evidence of hemorrhage.

INDICATIONS FOR BLOOD PRODUCTS IN DENGUE

Severe bleeding in dengue shock may necessitate transfusion of packed red cells or whole blood. Platelet transfusion has not been shown to be effective at preventing or controlling hemorrhage but may be warranted in patients with severe thrombocytopenia and shock. The following are the only indications for transfusing platelets in dengue fever.

- For major or life-threatening hemorrhage, transfuse platelets regardless of platelet count as there may be platelet dysfunction in DHF.
- Shock with coagulopathy.
- Prophylactic platelet transfusion may be considered in patients without bleeding manifestations only if the platelet count is less than $10,000/mm^3$.

Scrub Typhus   16
CHAPTER

INTRODUCTION

Scrub typhus is a rickettsial infection, caused by *Orientia tsutsugamushi*, which is spread by bite of the larva (chigger) of trombiculid mites, which thrives in scrub vegetation. Ask for history of exposure to vegetation like working in the fields, trekking, etc., which is essential for a person acquiring the infection.

EPIDEMIOLOGY

Scrub typhus is no longer restricted to the classical '*Tsutsugamushi* triangle' with cases being reported in South America, Africa, and Europe. In India, it is endemic in many states, especially Tamil Nadu, Andhra Pradesh, Kerala, Maharashtra, Rajasthan, Himachal Pradesh, the Himalayan belt, and the North–Eastern states.

CLINICAL FEATURES

The mean duration of fever before presentation is usually 8 days. Clinical features include fever, myalgia, nausea, breathlessness, abdominal pain, headache, and altered sensorium. Severe cases may be associated with multiple organ failure (renal failure, hepatic failure, shock, acute respiratory distress syndrome, meningitis, and meningoencephalitis).

The basic pathogenesis is vasculitis and perivasculitis of the small blood vessels, resulting in multiple organ involvement.

Classical Finding

Eschar: A thorough search should be done as many eschars are found in the genital region, inguinal region, axilla, and inframammary folds. An eschar may be seen on any part of the body (**Fig. 1**). The finding of an eschar on the body provides the most vital clue for diagnosing Scrub typhus.

INVESTIGATIONS

Complete blood count (CBC), electrolytes, creatinine, urea, and liver function test (LFT).

The typical abnormalities are leukocytosis, thrombocytopenia, hyper-bilirubinemia, low albumin, elevated liver enzymes, and alkaline phosphatase.

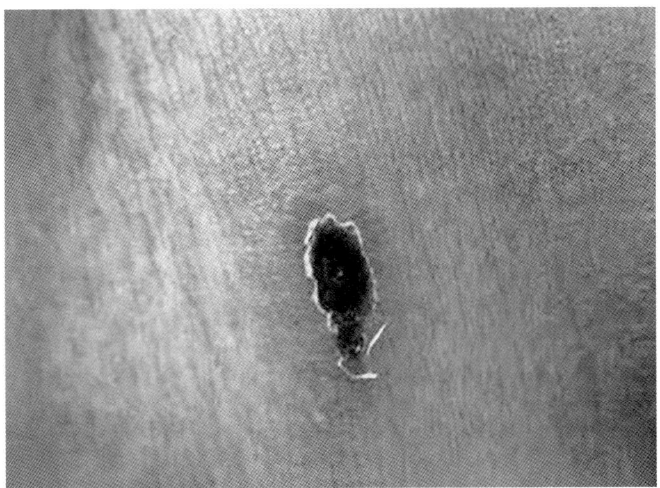

FIG. 1: Eschar of scrub typhus. *(For colour version see Plate)*

Cerebrospinal fluid analysis may show an aseptic meningitis picture with elevated counts (Mean: 80 cells/cumm; range: 5–740) with a lymphocyte predominance and elevated protein (Mean: 105 mg%; range: 13–640) and low sugars.

DIAGNOSIS

Diagnosis can be confirmed by Scrub IgM ELISA positivity with or without a pathognomonic eschar. However, ELISA test must be done only after 5 7 days after onset of symptoms.

MANAGEMENT

- *Severe cases*: Doxycycline 200 mg intravenous (IV) stat in 100 mL normal saline with 1 ampoule ascorbic acid over 30 minutes followed by 100 mg IV q12h × 7 days.
- *Mild cases*: Tablet doxycycline 100 mg PO bd × 7 days.
- *Alternate drug*: Tablet/injection—azithromycin 500 mg od × 7 days. Doxycycline is contraindicated in pregnancy. Azithromycin can be given.
- Supportive care for multi organ failure as indicated.

Malaria 17

INTRODUCTION

Malaria is a protozoan infection cause by the bite of infected female *Anopheles* mosquitoes. Four species of Plasmodium (*P. vivax, P. falciparum, P. ovale* and *P. malariae*) cause malaria with most severe infections caused by *P. falciparum*. Ask for history of travel to an endemic area.

Patients with one or more of the following clinical criteria are considered to have "severe malaria" and should be treated with intravenous (IV) antimalarials.

- *Impaired consciousness*: GCS < 11
- Convulsions
- *Metabolic acidosis*: Base deficit > 8 mEq/L or HCO_3 level < 15 mmol/L or lactate ≥5 mmol/L
- Hypoglycemia
- *Severe anemia*: Hb < 5 g%
- *Renal failure*: Serum creatinine >3 mg% or serum urea >20 mmol/L
- *Jaundice*: Serum bilirubin >3 mg%
- Acute respiratory distress syndrome
- Shock
- Disseminated intravascular coagulation
- *Plasmodium falciparum parasitemia*: Parasitic index (PI) >5%.

HOW TO INTERPRET THE RESULT OF MALARIAL PARASITE (MP) TEST?

- Look for the presence of ring forms or schizonts on the peripheral smear.
- Presence of only gametocytes (without ring forms or schizonts) on the smear does not suggest active infection. It only means that the patient can pass on the infection through mosquito bites. Radical cure with primaquine is then warranted for *Plasmodium vivax* gametocytes or artesunate or artemether for *P. falciparum* gametocytes.
- Look for PI in the case of falciparum malaria. A PI above 5% is indicative of severe malaria.

Antigen-based rapid diagnostic tests (RDTs) are widely available and are used in resource-poor settings. RDTs detect one or more of the following antigens: histidine-rich protein 2 (HRP2), plasmodium lactate dehydrogenase (pLDH), and aldolase. RDTs that detect HRP2 are somewhat more sensitive for *P. falciparum* than those that detect pLDH.

MANAGEMENT

- Antimalarial therapy as per **Table 1**.
- Consider exchange transfusion for patients with parasitemia above 10%.
- *Look for, and treat complications*: Acute respiratory distress syndrome, renal failure, shock, disseminated intravascular coagulation, and anemia.
- *Uncomplicated malaria in pregnancy*:
  - Chloroquine sensitive *P. falciparum*: All trimesters – Chloroquine
  - Chloroquine resistant *P. falciparum*: First trimester: Quinine + Clindamycin Second and third trimesters: Artemesinin combination therapy
- *Complicated malaria in pregnancy*: All trimesters – Artesunate + Clindamycin. Alternate options: Artemether or quinine

TABLE 1: Antibiotic therapy for *P. vivax* and *P. falciparum*.

Malaria	*P. vivax*	Chloroquine phosphate • *Day 1*: 1,000 mg PO (600 mg base) (4 tablets) • *Day 2*: 1,000 mg PO (600 mg base) (4 tablets) • *Day 3*: 500 mg PO (300 mg base) (2 tablets) • *For radical cure*: Primaquine phosphate 30 mg PO od × 14 days
	P. falciparum	Artemether 20 mg + Lumefantrine 120 mg (co-formulated tablets) 4 tablets bd × 3 days
Severe malaria	*P. falciparum*	• Artesunate 2.4 mg/kg IV given as a bolus at 0, 12, and 24 hours, and then once daily + Doxycycline 100 mg PO q12h or clindamycin 450 mg q8h • Give IV Artesunate for a minimum of 24 hours and then switch to oral therapy

DRUGS RECOMMENDED FOR TRAVELERS FOR PROPHYLAXIS OF MALARIA

- *Chloroquine*: Prophylaxis only in areas with chloroquine-sensitive malaria. 300 mg base (500 mg salt) orally, once/week. Begin 1–2 weeks before travel. Continue for 4 weeks after leaving the area.
- *Mefloquine*: 228 mg base (250 mg salt) orally, once/week. Begin 1–2 weeks before travel. Continue for 4 weeks after leaving the area.
- *Doxycycline*: 100 mg orally, daily. Begin 1–2 days before travel. Continue for 4 weeks after leaving the area.
- *Atovaquone (200 mg)–proguanil (100 mg)*: One tablet daily. Begin 1–2 days before travel. Continue for 1 week after leaving the area.

Community-acquired Pneumonia

18
CHAPTER

INTRODUCTION

Community-acquired pneumonia (CAP) is a lower respiratory tract infection. It should be differentiated from hospital-acquired pneumonia (hospitalized in the past 90 days) as the choice of antibiotics is very different.

ETIOLOGY

Streptococcus pneumoniae, Haemophilus influenzae, Staphylococcus aureus, gram-negative bacilli, *Legionella* species, *Mycoplasma pneumoniae, Chlamydia pneumoniae,* and viruses.

CLINICAL FEATURES

Patients usually present with fever, cough with expectoration, breathing difficulty, fatigue, or pleuritic chest pain.

Use the CURB-65 score to assess the severity of the pneumonia.

Assessment of severity: CURB-65 score: 6-point score (range 0–5). Gives one point each for:

- Confusion (abbreviated mental test score <8 or new disorientation in person, place, or time)
- Urea > 42 mg/dL
- Respiratory rate > 30 breaths/min
- Low blood pressure (systolic blood pressure < 90 mm Hg or diastolic blood pressure <60 mm Hg)
- Age > 65 years.

The choice of antibiotics and the setting of care depends on the CURB-65 score (**Table 1**).

SETTING OF CARE

- *CURB-65 score 0 or 1 (Low risk of death)*: Outpatient
- *CURB-65 score 2 (moderate risk of death)*: Inpatient (ward)
- *CURB-65 score >3 (high risk of death)*: Inpatient (ICU).

TABLE 1: Antibiotic management of community-acquired pneumonia.

CURB score	Preferred	Alternatives
CURB-65 score 0 or 1	Amoxicillin 500 mg PO q8h × 5–7 days	Levofloxacin 750 mg PO od × 5–7days Azithromycin 500 mg PO od × 3 days Doxycycline 100 mg PO bd × 5 days
CURB-65 score 2	Ceftriaxone 1g IV od + Azithromycin 500 mg IV od + Oseltamivir 75 mg PO bd × 5–7 days	Crystalline Penicillin G 20 Lakh units IV q4h + Azithromycin 500 mg IV od + Oseltamivir 75 mg PO bd × 5–7 days
CURB-65 score 3 or more	Piperacillin tazobactam 4.5 g IV q8h + Azithromycin 500 mg IV OD + Oseltamivir 75 mg PO bd × 5–7 days	

LUNG ABSCESS

Lung abscess (necrotizing pneumonia) refers to necrosis of the lung parenchyma resulting in a localized collection of pus.

- *Etiology*: Oral anaerobes (*peptostreptococcus, prevotella,* bacteroides, *Fusobacterium*)
- *Antibiotic of choice*: Amoxicillin clavulanate 1.2 g IV q8h
- *Alternative choice*: Clindamycin 600 mg IV q8h.

EMPYEMA THORACIS

Empyema thoracis refers to collection of pus in the pleural space often as a complication of pneumonia, tuberculosis or a subphrenic abscess. May present with fever, cough and pleuritic chest pain. Intercostal tenderness may be noted with decreased breath sounds and dullness on percussion.

Etiology: *Streptococcus milleri, Streptococcus pneumoniae,* oral anaerobes

Empiric antibiotic: Amoxicillin clavulanate 1.2 g IV q8h or crystalline penicillin 20 lakh units IV q4h.

If MRSA suspected, add vancomycin 10–20 mg/kg IV q12h.

Chest tube drainage is required to facilitate drainage of thick pus.

BIBLIOGRAPHY

1. Lim WS, van der Eerden MM, Laing R, Boersma WG, Karalus N, Town GI, et al. Defining community acquired pneumonia severity on presentation to hospital: an international derivation and validation study. Thorax. 2003;58(5):377-82.

INTRODUCTION

- Seasonal influenza is an acute respiratory viral infection that is spread by respiratory secretions. It is caused by influenza A or B viruses, members of *Orthomyxoviridae* family. Influenza viruses are further subtyped on the basis of the surface hemagglutinin (H) and neuraminidase (N) antigens.
- The H1N1 strain of influenza A is responsible for the 2008 pandemic flu. It causes a mild self-limiting respiratory illness in the majority. However, high-risk population may develop a severe respiratory illness with systemic symptoms.

Incubation period: 1–4 days.

Period of infectivity: 3–5 days

CLINICAL FEATURES

Fever, coryza, sore throat, cough, breathlessness, myalgia, and pharyngeal congestion may be seen. Patients with severe disease may have tachypnea, diffuse crepitations, hypotension, hypoxemia, and signs of respiratory failure.

INVESTIGATIONS

Investigations include complete blood count, urea, creatinine, electrolytes, liver function test, chest X-ray, and arterial blood gas (ABG).

Leukopenia, mild transaminitis, and azotemia may be noted.

Chest X-ray may show features of consolidation or diffuse fluffy alveolar infiltrates. ABG may show hypoxemia and respiratory alkalosis in early disease and mixed respiratory failure in very severe disease.

Confirmatory test: Influenza panel polymerase chain reaction on a nasal or throat swab.

Caution: Do not wait for results to initiate treatment, if indicated.

HIGH-RISK CATEGORY FOR COMPLICATIONS OF INFLUENZA/H1N1

- Pregnancy
- Underlying respiratory illness
- Extremes of age (<2 years and >65 years)

- ○ *Unfractionated heparin*: 5,000 units subcutaneously BD
  - ○ Fondaparinux 2.5 mg subcutaneously OD (consider dose adjustment in renal failure)
- Antivirals, anti-inflammatory agents and antibiotics
  - ○ *Primary antivirals against SARS-CoV-2*: Many drugs like hydroxychloroquine, ivermectin, ritonavir, remdesevir and favipiravir, have been tried for their antiviral properties against SARS-CoV-2 and have now fallen out of favor with most guidelines and recommendations.
  - ○ *Anti-inflammatory agents for host-directed therapy*: Several targeted immunomodulatory drugs have shown promise against SARS-CoV-2 induced cytokine storm. These include tocilizumab (IL-6 inhibitor), Canakinumab (IL-1 inhibitor) and Baricitinib (Janus Kinase inhibitor).
  - ○ *Empiric antibiotics*: Administer broad spectrum empiric antibiotics (piperacillin-tazobactam/meropenem) only for patients with severe and critical illness to cover secondary bacterial infections.

PREVENTION

- Good hand hygiene, wearing face masks, physical distancing, and contact prevention. Quarantining and other public health measures advised.
- Appropriate PPE use for high-risk procedures to prevent transmission to healthcare workers (HCW).
- Mass national vaccination campaigns from all over the world have shown a clear benefit of vaccines preventing death and severe disease, and help attain herd immunity.
- Vaccines currently available include mRNA vaccines (Pfizer, Moderna), nonreplicating vector vaccines (AstraZeneca/Covishield, Sputnik), and inactivated viral vaccines (Covaxin).

ANIMAL RESERVOIRS

- Dogs account for 90% or more of reported cases of rabies transmitted to humans.
- Other animals that can transmit rabies are cats, bats, raccoons, skunks, and foxes.
- Small rodents, such as gerbils, chipmunks, guinea pigs, squirrels, rats, mice, and rabbits have not been conclusively proven to have transmitted rabies.

Incubation period: Average is 1–3 months after exposure, but can range from several days to several years.

CLINICAL FEATURES

- *Encephalitic (furious) rabies*: (80%) fever, hydrophobia, pharyngeal spasms, agitation with hyperexcitability, opisthotonos and autonomic hyperactivity leading to paralysis, coma, and death.
- *Paralytic (dumb) rabies*: (20%) ascending paralysis, which can mimic Guillain-Barré syndrome. Paralysis is usually more prominent in the bitten limb. It may then spread either symmetrically or asymmetrically eventually resulting in death.

MANAGEMENT

Management of a dog bite includes the following:
- Wound care
- Postexposure prophylaxis (PEP) for rabies [rabies immunoglobulin (RIG) and rabies vaccine]
- Tetanus prophylaxis.
  The classification of wounds and recommended therapy is shown in **Table 1**.

Wound Care

Wounds should be washed thoroughly. Flush and irrigate the wounds with sterile water or saline using a 26-gauge needle to disinfect immediately.
- Wounds that are better managed by delayed primary closure after 72 hours:
  - Deep wounds
  - Wounds on the hand and feet
  - More than 12 hours old (24 h old on face)
  - Puncture wounds.

TABLE 1: Classification of wounds and recommended therapy.			
Category	Description	PEP vaccine	RIG
I	Touching, feeding of animals or licks on intact skin	No exposure, therefore, no prophylaxis (if history reliable)	Not required
II	Minor scratches or abrasions without bleeding or nibbling of uncovered skin	Patients NOT immunized previously: Full 5 dose schedule	Not required
		Patients who have been immunized before*: 2 doses on day 0 and 3	Not required
III	Single or multiple transdermal bites or scratches, licks on broken skin, contamination of mucous membrane with saliva (i.e., licks) and suspect contacts with bats	Patients NOT immunized previously: Full 5 dose schedule	Administer RIG
		Patients who have been immunized before*: 2 doses on day 0 and 3	Not required

*Previously immunized patients include those who received pre-exposure prophylaxis and those who completed a post-exposure vaccine regimen >3 months back.

- Wounds that can be considered for immediate primary closure:
  - Clinically uninfected wounds
  - Less than 12 hours old (24 h on the face)
  - Wounds on parts of the body other than on the hands or feet.

However, most studies do not show any difference in the rates of infection between immediate suturing and late primary closure.

Wound care should be followed up by antibiotic prophylaxis (amoxicillin–clavulanate 625 mg tid × 5 days).

Post-exposure Prophylaxis

- Pregnancy, infancy, and concurrent infections are not contraindications for post-exposure prophylaxis (PEP).
- PEP vaccine must be provided regardless of duration since bite. Even if it has been months after been bitten, the same PEP vaccination as for recent contact must be administered.
- If the involved animal (dog or cat) remains healthy 10 days after the exposure has occurred, PEP may be discontinued.
- Even immunized animals can transmit rabies because of the possibility of vaccine failure. Therefore, immunization status of the animal is not a factor in deciding administration of PEP.
- PEP includes rabies vaccine and/or RIG.

Rabies Immunoglobulin

- Maximum possible dose of RIG should be infiltrated into the depth and around the wounds. If the wound is small, infiltrate as much as possible into the wound and inject the remainder intramuscularly at a site (anterior thigh) distant from that of the rabies vaccine.

- *Dose of RIG*: 20 IU/kg for human RIG or 40 IU/kg for equine RIG (ERIG).
- If the wounds are large or multiple, dilute the RIG two to threefold in sterile normal saline to be able to infiltrate all the wounds. Make sure you do not exceed the total recommended dose.
- If RIG is not available at presentation, it can be administered up to 7 days from the date of the first dose of vaccination. After the seventh day, antibody response to the vaccine would have occurred and the RIG is likely to be ineffective. RIG is not indicated in previously vaccinated individuals.
- Even though the currently manufactured ERIG is highly purified and adverse events are significantly less, it is safer to perform a skin sensitivity test prior to its administration. Human RIG does not require any prior skin sensitivity testing.
- Human monoclonal antibodies, with fewer side effects can also be administered for the same indication at a recommended dose of 3.3 IU/kg.

Rabies Vaccine

- Postexposure prophylaxis for unvaccinated persons: Two intramuscular schedules may be used for category 2 and 3 exposures:
  - *The 5-dose intramuscular regime*: One dose of the vaccine should be administered on days 0, 3, 7, 14, and 28 in deltoid region or, in small children, into the anterolateral area of the thigh muscle.
  - *The 2 1 1 regimen* may also be used. Two doses are given on day 0 in the deltoid muscle, right and left arm. In addition, one dose is given on day 7 and one on day 21 in the deltoid muscle.
  - Vaccines should not be injected into the gluteal region.
- Postexposure prophylaxis for previously vaccinated persons:
  - Previously immunized patients includes those who have received pre-exposure prophylaxis and those who have completed a post-exposure vaccine regimen >3 months ago. For PEP, administer two intramuscular doses of rabies vaccine; on day 0 or at the earliest and the second dose 3 days later.
  - RIG is not indicated for previously immunized people.

Tetanus Prophylaxis

- If the patient completed three doses of the primary series of tetanus-diphtheria (Td) vaccine but the last dose/booster was <5 years ago: No need for a Td vaccine or tetanus immunoglobulin (TIG).
- If the patient completed three doses of the primary series of Td vaccine but the last dose was >5 years ago: Administer Td vaccine alone. No need for TIG.
- If the patient took less than three doses of the primary series of Td vaccine or if the vaccine status is unknown: Administer Td and TIG. Advice the patient to take two more doses of Td at least 2 weeks apart.

Food Poisoning and Acute Gastroenteritis

INTRODUCTION

Food poisoning is caused by the consumption of food or water contaminated with bacteria and/or their toxins, parasites, viruses, or chemicals. The pathogenesis of diarrhea in food poisoning is broadly classified into either non-inflammatory or inflammatory types.

Noninflammatory diarrhea: It caused by the enterotoxin-producing organisms [*Vibrio cholerae*, enterotoxigenic *Escherichia coli* (ETEC), *Clostridium perfringens*, *Bacillus cereus*, and *Staphylococcus* organisms] or by organisms that disrupt the absorptive and/or secretory processes of the enterocytes by attaching to the mucosa (rotavirus, Norwalk virus, adenovirus, *Giardia lamblia*, and *Cryptosporidium*). There is no mucosal inflammation or destruction.

Inflammatory diarrhea: This type of diarrhea can be caused by two types of organisms: cytotoxin-producing noninvasive organisms [enteroinvasive *E. coli* (EIEC), *Yersinia enterocolitica*, *C. difficile*] or by invasive organisms (*Salmonella*, *Shigella*, *Campylobacter*, and *Entamoeba histolytica*).

MANAGEMENT

Oral hydration is the treatment of choice for mild-to-moderate dehydration. Oral rehydration solution (ORS), 200 mL after each loose stool should be encouraged. This may also be achieved by using sports beverages, fruit juices (orange, banana, coconut), soups or a balanced clear liquid diet at home.

For severe dehydration or shock, insert a 18-G cannula in the antecubital fossa and start IV infusion of Ringer lactate. Pediatric patients should be given a bolus of 20 mL/kg of NS/RL and repeated as indicated.

- If vomiting is present, injection ondansetron 8 mg IV may be given along with IV pantoprazole/omeprazole
- Monitor urine output. If decreased, suspect acute kidney injury. Monitor electrolytes and correct any imbalance, especially sodium and potassium.

- Antibiotics are *not* indicated in *most* cases of acute gastroenteritis (AGE)
- Most cases of diarrhea settle down with just oral fluid rehydration
- If cholera is suspected (large volume, watery loose stools): Give doxycycline 300 mg stat followed by 100 mg PO bd × 3 days, if hanging drop preparation is positive for *vibrio cholerae*
- If bacillary dysentery is suspected (bloody diarrhea, fever, tenesmus, abdominal pain)—Give tablet azithromycin 1g as a single dose or ciprofloxacin 500 mg bd for 3 days.
- If amoebic dysentery is suspected, send stool sample for ova and parasites and start metronidazole therapy.

- Discharge the patient on ORS once frequency of loose stools or vomiting decreases.
- Avoid anti-motility agents such as loperamide when infective or invasive diarrhea is suspected.

ETIOLOGY OF FOOD POISONING/AGE BASED ON INCUBATION PERIOD

Very Short Incubation Period (1–6 Hours)

- *Bacillus cereus* and staphylococcal species are the usual pathogens responsible for food poisoning with a very short incubation period.
- Results from eating improperly refrigerated rice, meat, ham, poultry, eggs, and salads.
- Severe nausea, vomiting, abdominal pain, and cramps are the usual symptoms. Diarrhea is rare.
- Antibiotics are not indicated and treatment is mainly supportive care.

Short Incubation Period (10–48 Hours)

- Rotavirus, calicivirus, astrovirus, adenovirus, parvovirus, *C. perfringens*, and *C. botulinum* are the usual pathogens.
- Watery diarrhea, nausea, and abdominal cramps are the usual symptoms.
- Treatment is mainly supportive.

Long Incubation Period (1–5 Days)

- *Vibrio cholerae, Y. enterocolytica, Y. pseudotuberculosis, Salmonella, Shigella,* ETEC, enterohemorrhagic *E. coli* (EHEC), nontyphoidal *Salmonella* species, and *Campylobacter jejuni* are the usual pathogens causing AGE with a longer incubation period.
- Antibiotics are needed for cholera, salmonellosis, bacillary dysentery, and severe ETEC infections.

Urinary Tract Infections

INTRODUCTION

The term urinary tract infection (UTI) covers a heterogeneous group of conditions with different etiologies, which have as their common factor the presence of bacteria in the urinary tract, associated with variable clinical symptoms.

The first and the most important step after making a diagnosis of UTI is to differentiate between cystitis and pyelonephritis (**Flowchart 1**).

- *Lower UTI (cystitis)*: Infections that are localized to the lower urinary tract (urethra, bladder). Symptoms are dysuria, frequency, urgency, and urinary incontinence.
- *Upper UTI (acute pyelonephritis)*: The most important symptom is fever. Other symptoms include nausea and vomiting, loin and back (flank) pain. Costovertebral angle tenderness may be elicited. The patient is systemically ill with signs of sepsis and shock.

Cystitis presents only with lower urinary tract symptom. Fever is not a feature of cystitis. Presence of fever with chills with urinary symptoms indicates acute pyelonephritis. Oral antibiotics are adequate for cystitis; IV antibiotics are preferred for pyelonephritis.

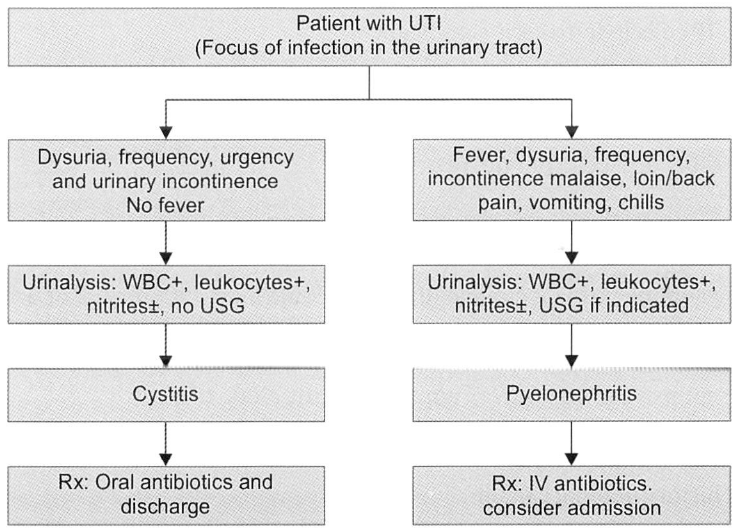

FLOWCHART 1: Diagnosis and management of urinary tract infection (UTI).

ASYMPTOMATIC BACTERIURIA

Asymptomatic bacteriuria is defined as isolation of a specified quantitative count of bacteria in an appropriately collected urine specimen from an individual without symptoms or signs of UTI.

- In asymptomatic women or men, bacteriuria is defined as two consecutive clean-catch voided urine specimens with isolation of the same organism in quantitative counts of $\geq 10^5$ cfu/mL.
- In asymptomatic catheterized men or women, bacteriuria is defined as a single catheterized specimen with isolation of a single organism in quantitative counts of $\geq 10^5$ cfu/mL.

Whom to treat: Screening for and treatment of asymptomatic bacteriuria is appropriate for pregnant women and for patients undergoing urologic procedures in which mucosal bleeding is anticipated.

Whom not to treat: There is no role for screening for or treating asymptomatic bacteriuria in populations other than pregnant women or patients undergoing urologic procedures expected to cause mucosal bleeding.

Investigations to be sent: For lower urinary tract infections, confirm with urine analysis and microscopy. Complete blood count, electrolytes, creatinine, liver function test, blood culture and sensitivity (c/s), urinalysis, and urine c/s may be sent for suspected pyelonephritis.

HOW TO INTERPRET URINALYSIS?

- *Look for the urine white blood cell count*: More than 5 cells in males and more than 10 cells in females is significant.
- *Leukocyte esterase* may be used to detect more than 10 leukocytes per high-power field (sensitivity of 75–96%; specificity of 94–98%).
- *The nitrite test* is fairly sensitive and specific for detecting $\geq 10^5$ cfu of Enterobacteriaceae per mL of urine.

ULTRASONOGRAPHY OF THE KIDNEYS

Acute pyelonephritis is a clinical diagnosis confirmed with results of urinalysis. An ultrasonography (USG) of abdomen is not needed for most cases of community-acquired pyelonephritis or for cystitis. The indications for an urgent USG are:

- Unresponsive to 48 hours of appropriate antibiotic therapy
- Patients with known urogenital tract abnormalities
- Catheter-acquired UTI
- Past history of renal calculi
- Elevated creatinine (acute worsening of renal functions).

Presence of renal angle tenderness without the above-mentioned conditions is *not* an indication for requesting an USG abdomen.

A complicated UTI is defined as being associated with one of the following: Diabetes mellitus, pregnancy, symptoms >7 days, renal failure, urinary tract obstruction, renal transplantation, immunosuppression, nosocomial infection, and indwelling urethral catheter or stent.

MANAGEMENT OF UNCOMPLICATED UTI

- *Cystitis*:
  - Oral antibiotics [nitrofurantoin, fluoroquinolones, and trimethoprim/sulfamethoxazole (TMP/SMX)]
  - Amoxicillin–clavulanate, cefpodoxime, and cefaclor are alternatives but are less effective
  - Ampicillin or amoxicillin should not be used (high-resistance rates).
- *Pyelonephritis*:
  - Outpatient management with oral fluoroquinolones is acceptable for patients with mild-to-moderate illness. IV ceftriaxone is an alternative
  - Patients requiring hospitalization should receive beta lactams + beta-lactamase inhibitor or carbapenems.

MANAGEMENT OF COMPLICATED UTI

- *Cystitis*:
  - Oral fluoroquinolones (ciprofloxacin 500 mg bd/levofloxacin 750 mg od)
  - Nitrofurantoin, TMP/SMX, oral beta-lactams are poor choices (high resistance rates)
  - Parenteral therapy with once daily regimen of levofloxacin (500 mg), ceftriaxone (1 g), ertapenem (1 g), or an aminoglycoside (3–5 mg/kg of gentamicin) may be tried.
- *Pyelonephritis*:
  - Patients with complicated pyelonephritis should be managed as inpatients with carbapenems (**Table 1**).

TABLE 1: Antibiotics for urinary tract infection (UTI).

Acute uncomplicated cystitis in women (dysuria and frequency in healthy, adult, non-pregnant women with normal urinary tract)	*Escherichia coli*	Nitrofurantoin 100 mg PO qid × 5–7days	Alternate choice: Ciprofloxacin 500 mg PO bd × 3 days
Pyelonephritis— uncomplicated [no underlying genitourinary (GU) disease]	*E. coli*	Mild-to-moderate illness: Piperacillin tazobactam 4.5 g IV q6-8h or Cefoperazone/sulbactam 3 g IV q12h	Severe illness (qSOFA ≥ 2): Ertapenam 1 g IV od
Complicated UTI (underlying GU disease)	*E. coli, Proteus Pseudomonas Acinetobacter*	Meropenem 1 g IV q8h; de-escalate as per c/s	

Acute Central Nervous System Infections

INTRODUCTION

Acute central nervous system (CNS) infections includes meningitis, encephalitis and brain abscess. Meningitis refers to inflammation of the leptomeningitis surrounding the brain, while encephalitis refers to inflammation of the brain parenchyma itself.

ETIOLOGY

- *Pyogenic meningitis*: *Streptococcus pneumoniae, Neisseria meningitidis*; Group B *Streptococcus, Haemophilus influenzae*, and *Listeria monocytogenes*.
- *Viral meningitis* or *encephalitis*: Herpes simplex virus (HSV), enteroviruses (coxsackie, echovirus, other nonpoliovirus enteroviruses), varicella zoster virus (VZV), mumps, HIV, lymphocytic choriomeningitis (LCM) virus.

MENINGITIS VERSUS ENCEPHALITIS

The presence or absence of normal brain function is the important distinguishing feature between encephalitis and meningitis.

- *Meningitis*: Patients usually have fever, headache, lethargy, vomiting, and neck stiffness.
  Cerebral function remains normal initially in patients with meningitis.
- *Encephalitis*: Patients present with fever, altered mental status, motor or sensory deficits, personality changes, speech or movement disorders or seizures.
  Abnormalities in brain function are common and an early feature of encephalitis.
- *Meningoencephalitis*: The distinction between the two entities is frequently blurred since some patients may have both a parenchymal and meningeal process with clinical features of both.

Patients with pyogenic meningitis are usually toxic and clinically deteriorate rapidly within 3–5 days of onset of fever.

Patients with aseptic meningitis usually present later and have milder symptoms.

Patients with viral encephalitis present early but are usually nontoxic and have altered mental status or seizures.

CLINICAL EXAMINATION

Classic examination finding of meningitis is neck stiffness. Remember that the elderly may have a significant amount of neck stiffness due to cervical spondylopathy. Other classical signs of meningitis include Kernig's sign and Brudzinski's sign.

Presence of papilledema on fundoscopy can be an indicator of raised ICP and is a contra indication for a diagnostic lumbar puncture in resource limited settings.

INVESTIGATIONS

- Complete blood count, electrolytes, creatinine, liver function test, blood culture and sensitivity (c/s), and CT brain (plain).
- Chest X-ray if respiratory symptoms are present.
- Prothrombin time (PT), activated partial thromboplastin time (aPTT) if patient is in systemic inflammatory response syndrome or shock.
- *Cerebrospinal fluid (CSF) analysis*: CSF total count (TC), differential count (DC), protein, sugar, routine c/s, and multiplex polymerase chain reaction (PCR) (if aseptic meningitis suspected). Check concomitant RBS during the lumbar puncture (LP).

MANAGEMENT

Acute management of a bacterial CNS infection includes immediate administration of an empiric antibiotic with anti-epileptics if required and supportive care. Most viral infections resolve without specific anti-virals but could lead to long term sequelae. Empiric anti-viral drugs are warranted for herpes encephalitis/meningitis. Empiric antibiotic therapy in the ED depends on the suspected etiology.

- *Pyogenic meningitis*: Ceftriaxone 2 g IV q12h + vancomycin 15–20 mg/kg IV stat

  Dexamethasone 10 mg IV first dose 15 minutes before first dose of antibiotic
- *Viral meningitis or encephalitis*: Injection acyclovir 10 mg/kg IV stat and q8h
- *Scrub typhus meningoencephalitis*: Injection doxycycline 200 mg IV stat.

The approach to an acute CNS infection and the empiric antibiotic choice is shown in **Flowchart 1**.

Before doing a LP, make sure that there is no papilledema or contraindication for LP on CT scan.

In general, the presence of unequal pressures between the supratentorial and infratentorial compartments is a contraindication for a LP.

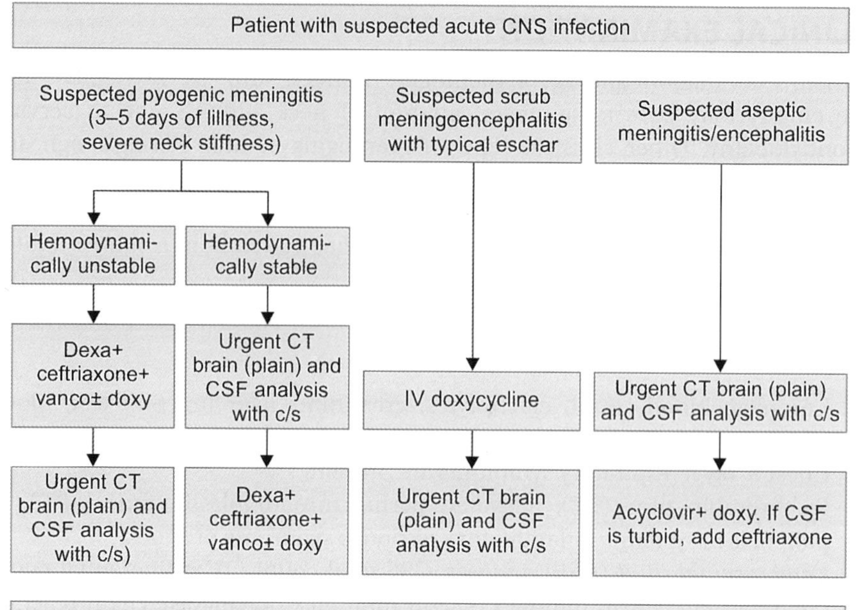

FLOWCHART 1: Approach and empiric antibiotic choice in a patient with suspected acute central nervous system infection.

CONTRAINDICATION FOR A LUMBAR PUNCTURE AS DEFINED BY CT BRAIN

- Midline shift
- Cerebral hemorrhage/subarachnoid hemorrhage/epidural or subdural hemorrhage
- Brain abscess
- Posterior fossa mass
- Loss of suprachiasmatic and basilar cisterns
- Loss of the superior cerebellar or quadrigeminal plate cistern.

Tetanus   **25**

CHAPTER

INTRODUCTION

- Tetanus is a nervous system disorder characterized by muscle spasms that are caused by the toxin-producing anaerobe *Clostridium tetani*, which is found in the soil.
- The incubation period of tetanus can be as short as 2 days or as long as 38 days, with most cases occurring at a mean of 7–10 days following exposure.
- The severity of tetanus can be assessed by the Patel and Joag score (**Table 1**)

THERAPY

- Injection tetanus immunoglobulin (Tetglob) 500 U intravenous (IV) stat
- Injection tetanus immunoglobulin (Tetglob) 250 U intrathecal
- Injection crystalline penicillin 20 L U IV q4h × 10 days or injection metronidazole 500 mg IV q6h × 7 days.

TABLE 1: Assessment of severity: Tetanus score (Patel and Joag score).

Parameter	Score
Age >60 years	1
Postabortal	1
Incubation period <7 days	1
Period of onset <24 hours	1
Dysphagia	1
Rigidity	1
Reflex spasms	1
Spontaneous spasms	1
Autonomic hyper-reactivity (variable heart rate, fluctuating blood pressure, diaphoresis)	2
Total score	
<4	Mild
4–6	Moderate
>6	Severe (requires elective intubation)

GENERAL MEASURES

- Secure airway and breathing. Intubate if necessary and possible or perform a tracheostomy, if indicated (based on the scoring system).
- Isolate the patient to a quiet environment without triggers of spasm.
- *Liberal sedation and muscle relaxation*: Diazepam 10–20 mg IV/po q1–2 hours (up to 500 mg/day).
- Supportive care.

ACTIVE IMMUNIZATION

Tetanus is one of the few bacterial diseases that do not confer immunity following recovery from acute illness. All patients with tetanus should receive active immunization with a total of three doses of tetanus ± diphtheria toxoid spaced at least 2 weeks apart, commencing immediately upon diagnosis. Tetanus toxoid should be administered at a different site than tetanus immunoglobulin.

TETANUS PROPHYLAXIS

Tetanus prophylaxis should be administered as soon as possible following a wound but should be given even to patients who present after a few months for medical attention (**Table 2**).

TABLE 2: Tetanus prophylaxis.

Previous doses of TT	Clean and minor wound		All other wounds	
	TT	Human TIG	TT	Human TIG
<3 doses or unknown	Yes[*]	No	Yes[*]	Yes[#]
≥3 doses	Only if last dose given ≥10 years ago	No	Only if last dose given ≥5 years ago	No

[*]The vaccine series should be continued and three doses at 2-week intervals should be completed.
[#]The dose of human TIG is 250–500 U intravenous stat with part infiltrated around the wound.
(TT: tetanus toxoid; TIG: tetanus immunoglobulin)

Antibiotic Doses and Spectrum

26

It is important to know the etiology of any infection and the antimicrobial spectrum of commonly used antibiotics in order to be able to choose the most appropriate empiric antibiotic in the emergency department (**Table 1**).

TABLE 1: Dosages of commonly used antibiotics and their antimicrobial spectrum.

Antibiotic	Dose	Antimicrobial spectrum
Crystalline penicillin	20 L U IV bolus	• *Gm-pos*: Strep group A, B, C, G, *Streptococcus pneumoniae, Enterococcus*, and *Listeria* • *Gm-neg*: *Neisseria meningitidis* and *Haemophilus ducreyi* • *Anaerobes*: *Actinomyces, Prevotella, Clostridium*, and *Peptostreptococcus*
Amoxicillin/ ampicillin	500 PO q8h	• *Gm-pos*: Strep group A, B, C, G, *S. pneumoniae, Enterococcus*, and *Listeria* • *Gm-neg*: *N. meningitidis* and *Proteus* • *Anaerobes*: *Clostridium, Fusobacterium*, and *Peptostreptococcus*
Cloxacillin	500–1,000 mg PO q6h	• *Gm-pos*: Strep group A, B, C, G, *S. pneumoniae, Staphylococcus aureus* (MSSA), and *Staph epidermidis* • *Anaerobes*: *Peptostreptococcus*
• Piperacillin–tazobactam • Cefoperazone–sulbactam		• *Gm-pos*: Strep group A, B, C, G, *S. pneumoniae, S. aureus* (MSSA), *S. epidermidis*, and *Enterococcus* • *Gm-neg*: *N. meningitidis, Moraxella, H. influenzae, E. coli, Klebsiella, Enterobacter, Serratia, Salmonella, Shigella, Proteus, Citrobacter, Aeromonas*, and *Pseudomonas* • *Anaerobes*: *Bacteroides, Prevotella, Clostridium, Fusobacterium*, and *Peptostreptococcus*
Amoxicillin-clavulanate	625 mg PO TID or Augmentin duo 1.2 g BD	• *Gm-pos*: Strep group A, B, C, G, *S. pneumoniae, Staph. aureus*, (MSSA), and *Enterococcus* • *Gm-neg*: *Neisseria gonorrhoeae, N. meningitidis, Moraxella, H. influenzae, E. coli, Klebsiella, Salmonella, Shigella, Proteus, Aeromonas*, and *H. ducreyi* • *Anaerobes*: *Actinomyces, Bacteroides, Prevotella, Clostridium, Fusobacterium*, and *Peptostreptococcus*

Continued

Continued

Antibiotic	Dose	Antimicrobial spectrum
Cefazolin (first generation) IV	1–1.5 g IV q8h	• *Gm-pos*: Strep group A, B,C, G, *S. pneumoniae, S. viridans*, and *Staph. aureus* (MSSA) • *Gm-neg*: *Neisseria gonorrheae, H. influenzae, E. coli, Klebsiella*, and *Proteus*
Cefalexin (first generation) oral	250–1,000 mg PO q6h	• *Gm-pos*: Strep group A, B, C, G, *S. pneumoniae, S. viridans*, and *S. aureus* (MSSA) • *Gm-neg*: *H. influenzae, E. coli, Klebsiella*, and *Proteus* • *Anaerobes: Peptostreptococcus*
Cefuroxime (second generation) IV/oral	125–500 mg PO/IV q12h	• *Gm-pos*: Strep group A, B, C, G, *S. pneumoniae, S. viridans, S. aureus* (MSSA) • *Gm-neg*: *Neisseria gonorrheae, Moraxella, H. influenzae, E. coli, Klebsiella, Proteus*, and *Aeromonas*
Ceftriaxone (third generation) IV	1–2 g IV stat	• *Gm-pos*: Strep group A, B, C, G, *S. pneumoniae, S. viridans*, and *S. aureus* (MSSA) • *Gm-neg*: *Neisseria gonorrheae, N. meningitides, Moraxella, H. influenzae, E. coli, Klebsiella, Salmonella, Shigella, Proteus, Aeromonas, Y. enterocolitica*, and *H. ducreyi* • *Anaerobes: Actinomyces, Clostridium*, and *Peptostreptococcus*
Ceftazidime (third generation) IV	1–2 g IV q8h	• *Gm-pos*: Strep. group A, B, C, G, *S. pneumoniae* • *Gm-neg*: *Moraxella, H. influenzae, E. coli, Klebsiella, Salmonella, Shigella, Proteus, Aeromonas, Pseudomonas, Burkholderia cepacia*, and *H. ducreyi* • *Anaerobes: Clostridium* and *Peptostreptococcus*
Cefixime (third generation) oral	200–400 mg PO q12h	• *Gm-pos*: Strep. group A, B, C, G, *S. pneumoniae*, and *S. viridans* • *Gm-neg*: *Moraxella, H. influenzae, E. coli, Klebsiella, Salmonella, Shigella, Proteus, Aeromonas, Y. enterocolitica*, and *H. ducreyi* • *Anaerobes: Peptostreptococcus*
Vancomycin	1–2 g IV bolus in 100 mL normal saline (NS) and q12h	• *Gm-pos*: Strep group A, B, C, G, *S. pneumoniae, Enterococcus, S. aureus* (MSSA), *S. aureus* (MRSA), *S. epidermidis*, and *Listeria* • *Anaerobes: Clostridium, Peptostreptococcus*
Linezolid	600 mg q12h PO/IV	• *Gm-pos*: Strep group A, B, C, G, *S. pneumonia, Enterococcus, S. aureus* (MSSA), *S. aureus* (MRSA), *S. epidermidis*, and *Listeria* • *Anaerobes: Peptostreptococcus*

Continued

Continued

Antibiotic	Dose	Antimicrobial spectrum
Ciprofloxacin	500–750 mg PO bd 200–400 mg IV q8h	• *Gm-pos*: S. aureus (MSSA), S. epidermidis, Listeria • *Gm-neg*: N. meningitidis, Moraxella, H. influenzae, E. coli, Klebsiella, Enterobacter, Salmonella, Shigella, Proteus, Aeromonas, Pseudomonas, Y. enterocolitica, Legionella, Chlamydia, and Mycoplasma pneumoniae
Levofloxacin	750 PO od	• *Gm-pos*: Strep group A, B, C, G, S. pneumoniae, Enterococcus, S. viridans, S. aureus (MSSA), S. epidermidis, Listeria • *Gm-neg*: N. meningitidis, Moraxella, H. influenzae, E. coli, Klebsiella, Enterobacter, Salmonella, Shigella, Proteus, Aeromonas, Pseudomonas, Y. enterocolitica, Legionella, Chlamydia, and Mycoplasma pneumoniae • *Anaerobes*: Clostridium and Peptostreptococcus
Azithromycin	500 mg PO od or 500 mg IV in 500 mL 5% D over 1 hour	• *Gm-pos*: Listeria • *Gm-neg*: Moraxella, H. influenzae, Legionella, Haemophilus ducreyi, Chlamydia, Mycoplasma pneumoniae, Mycobacterium avium, and Rickettsia • *Anaerobes*: Actinomyces, Clostridium, Prevotella, and Peptostreptococcus
Doxycycline	100 mg BD PO/IV	• *Gm-pos*: Strep pneumoniae, Listeria • *Gm-neg*: Neisseria meningitidis, Moraxella, H. influenzae, Aeromonas, E. coli, Brucella, Chlamydia, Mycoplasma pneumoniae, and Rickettsia • *Anaerobes*: Actinomyces, Clostridium, Prevotella, and Peptostreptococcus
Meropenem	1 g IV in 100 mL NS	• *Gm-pos*: Strep group A, B, C, G, S. pneumoniae, Enterococcus, S. viridans, S. aureus (MSSA), S. epidermidis, and Listeria • *Gm-neg*: N. meningitidis, Moraxella, H. influenzae, E. coli, Klebsiella, Enterobacter, Salmonella, Shigella, Proteus, Aeromonas, Morganella, Citrobacter, and Pseudomonas • *Anaerobes*: Bacteroides, Clostridium (nondifficile), Prevotella, Fusobacterium, and Peptostreptococcus

Continued

Continued

Antibiotic	Dose	Antimicrobial spectrum
Ertapenem	1 g IV in 100 mL NS bolus	• *Gm-pos*: Strep group A, B, C, G, *S. pneumoniae*, *Enterococcus*, *S. viridans*, *S. aureus* (MSSA), *S. epidermidis*, and *Listeria* • *Gm-neg*: *N. meningitidis*, *Moraxella*, *H. influenzae*, *E. coli*, *Klebsiella*, *Enterobacter*, *Salmonella*, *Shigella*, *Proteus*, *Aeromonas*, *Morganella*, and *Citrobacter* • *Anaerobes*: *Bacteroides*, *Clostridium* (nondifficile), *Prevotella*, *Fusobacterium*, and *Peptostreptococcus*
Gentamicin	1.5–2 mg/kg IV in 100 mL NS bolus and od	• *Gm-pos*: *S. aureus* (MSSA) • *Gm-neg*: *Moraxella*, *H. influenzae*, *E. coli*, *Klebsiella*, Enterobacter, Shigella, Serratus, Proteus, Aeromonas, Pseudomonas, *Y. enterocolitica*, and *Francisella tularensis*
Amikacin	15 mg/kg IV in 100 mL NS bolus and od	• *Gm-pos*: *S. aureus* (MSSA) • *Gm-neg*: *Moraxella*, *H. influenzae*, *E. coli*, *Klebsiella*, Enterobacter, Shigella, Serratus, Proteus, Aeromonas, Pseudomonas, *Y. enterocolitica*, *Francisella tularensis*, and *Mycobacterium avium*
Clindamicin	15–20 mg/kg IV in 100 mL 5% od	• *Gm-pos*: Strep group A, B, C, G, *S. pneumoniae*, *S. aureus* (MSSA) • *Anaerobes*: *Actinomyces*, *Clostridium*, *Prevotella*, *Fusobacterium*, and *Peptostreptococcus*
Metronidazole	500 mg PO q8h/400 mg IV q8h	• *Anaerobes*: *Bacteroides*, *Clostridium difficile*, *Prevotella*, and *Fusobacterium*
Nitrofurantoin	100 PO q6h	• *Gm-pos*: Strep group A, B, C, G, *S. pneumoniae*, *Enterococcus*, *S. aureus* (MSSA), and *S. aureus* (MRSA) • *Gm-neg*: *Neisseria gonorrhoeae*, *E. coli*, and *Salmonella*

(Gm-pos: gram-positive; Gm-neg: gram-negative; Strep: *Streptococcus*; MSSA: methicillin-susceptible *S. aureus*; MRSA: methicillin-resistant *S. aureus*)

All the above doses are for patients with normal renal function. Dose adjustments may be needed for some of the antibiotics in the presence of renal failure.

Toxicology

General Measures

27
CHAPTER

INTRODUCTION

History is often the most valuable tool because many patients (e.g., children, suicidal or psychotic adults, patients with altered consciousness) cannot provide the required reliable information; friends, relatives, and rescue personnel should be questioned. Even, seemingly reliable patients or relatives may incorrectly report the amount or time of ingestion. When possible, the patient's living quarters should be inspected for clues (e.g., partially empty pill containers, evidence of recreational drug use). Pharmacy and medical records may provide useful information. Decontamination is an emergency procedure done to decrease and minimize absorption of toxins into the systemic circulation. These include gastrointestinal (GI), skin and mucosal decontamination.

GASTRIC LAVAGE

Gastric lavage is a GI decontamination procedure in which toxic contents in the stomach are removed by repetitive instillation and aspiration of small amounts of fluid. Most patients present beyond the window period of 1–2 hours and hence lavage may not be helpful in decreasing the gastric absorption. It must be done only after ensuring that the airway is secured.

Indications

- Potentially life-threatening poisoning (or if history is not available) and unconscious presentation
- Potentially life-threatening poisoning and presentation within 1 hour
- Potentially life-threatening poisoning due to drug with anticholinergic effects and presentation within 4 hours
- Ingestion of sustained release preparation of significantly toxic drug
- Large amount of salicylate poisoning presenting within 12 hours
- Iron or lithium poisoning.

Do not perform a gastric lavage in drowsy or unconscious patients unless the airway is secured because of the high risk of aspiration.

Technique

- Insert a large (16F) nasogastric tube and check its placement by air insufflations and auscultating the epigastrium

- Place the patient in the left lateral decubitus position
- Instill 100–200 mL of warm tap water slowly through the NG tube
- Drain the fluid with the stomach contents into a dependent bucket placed at the head end
- Repeat the process of instilling and draining of the fluid till the draining fluid is clear
- Usually, 500–3,000 mL of tap water is required to perform a good lavage.

ACTIVATED CHARCOAL

Activated charcoal is a highly adsorbent powder that is produced by pyrolysis of organic material and steam cleaning (activation) to increase its surface area. It adsorbs toxins in the gut lumen, thereby decreasing GI absorption.

It is indicated for poisonings that fulfill the following criteria:
- Drug ingested is adsorbed by charcoal and has significant potential for toxicity
- Time since ingestion is less than 1–2 hours
- Drug has significant enterohepatic circulation
- Drug delays gastric emptying and time with ingestion less than 4 hours
- Drug is in a controlled release preparation with ingestion less than 12–18 hours.

Dose: Mix 50 g of activated charcoal 100 mL of water and leave it in the stomach.

Multidose Activated Charcoal

The use of repeated activated charcoal is likely to produce a meaningful clinical outcome for the following drugs: Carbamazepine, clonidine, colchicine, dapsone, digitoxin, phenobarbitone, phenytoin, quinidine, salicylate, tricyclic antidepressants (TCA), theophylline, verapamil, and warfarin.

Dose: 25–50 g (0.5 g/kg) mixed in 100 mL water every 4 hours.

Contraindications for Activated Charcoal

- Depressed mental status without airway protection (risk of aspiration)
- Late presentation
- Suspected esophageal or gastric perforation.

Drug Overdose

INTRODUCTION

Drug overdose is usually intentional, but may be accidental in children. Many self-poisonings involve multiple drugs or coingestion with alcohol. History may be unreliable. Insist that the relatives go back and search for evidence such as empty pill covers or bottles that may have been discarded by the patient near the place of incident.

GENERAL MANAGEMENT OF DRUG OVERDOSE

- Assess airway, breathing and circulation (ABC)
- Obtain intravenous access and start fluid resuscitation
- Send the blood investigations including drug levels, if available
- Perform gastric lavage or activated charcoal if indicated (usually for patients presenting within 1 hour of consumption)
- Provide supportive care.
- Administer specific antidotes, if available (**Table 1**)

ACETAMINOPHEN OVERDOSE

Acetaminophen (N-acetyl-p-aminophenol or paracetamol) is one of the most widely used drugs for deliberate self-poisoning. Doses up to 4,000 mg per day are considered therapeutic. The toxic dose is usually more than 150 mg/kg of paracetamol (7.5–10 g in adults)

TABLE 1: Common specific antidotes.

Toxin	Antidote
Acetaminophen	N-Acetylcysteine
Benzodiazepines	Flumazenil
Carbamates	Atropine
Digitalis glycosides (digoxin, digitoxin, and oleander)	Digoxin-specific Fab fragments
Ethylene glycol	Ethanol
Methanol	Ethanol and fomepizole
Opioids	Naloxone
Organophosphates	Atropine and pralidoxime
Tricyclic antidepressants	$NaHCO_3$

Clinical Presentation

The initial manifestations are often mild and nonspecific and include nausea, vomiting or anorexia. Initial laboratory investigations may be normal. Acute liver failure usually develops 24–36 hours after ingestion at which time laboratory evidence of hepatotoxicity and occasionally nephrotoxicity become apparent.

Measure serum paracetamol levels 4 hours postingestion and then 4 hours later to determine the 'possible risk' of hepatotoxicity using the modified Rumack-Matthew treatment nomogram.

Management

- Gastric lavage ± activated charcoal if patient presents within 1 hour of ingestion
- If the patient likely ingested >7.5–10 g or has features of hepatotoxicity, administer intravenous N-acetyl cysteine as an antidote
- *Dose*:
  - 150 mg/kg in 200 mL of 5% dextrose over 15 minutes, then
  - 50 mg/kg in 500 mL of 5% dextrose over 4 hours, then
  - 100 mg/kg in 1 L 5% dextrose over 16 hours
- Administer vitamin K1 10 mg IV stat

TRICYCLIC ANTIDEPRESSANT OVERDOSE

Tricyclic antidepressants (TCA) commonly used for DSP are amitriptyline, imipramine, desipramine, lofepramine

Clinical Presentation

Patients often present with anticholinergic symptoms like dry mouth, dilated pupils, blurred vision, tachycardia, urinary retention, agitation, seizures or coma. Cardiac conduction abnormalities are common due to inhibition of the fast sodium channels in the His-Purkinje system and myocardium.

ECG changes: Sinus tachycardia, QRS prolongation>100 ms, prolongation of PR and QT intervals, VT, VF

Venous blood gas analysis: Look for metabolic acidosis which indicates severe toxicity

Management

- Monitor the patient closely for cardiac conduction delays, arrhythmias and hypotension.
- If QRS prolonged/metabolic acidosis/hypotension/arrhythmias, $NaHCO_3$ is the primary initial therapy for cardiotoxicity. Administer $NaHCO_3$ 50–100 mL IV bolus followed by 10 mL/h infusion.

- Hypotension may be refractory, primarily secondary to peripheral alpha-1 adrenergic receptor antagonism: If present, rush in a fluid bolus and administer Glucagon: 5 mg IV bolus, repeat after 10 minutes. Then start glucagon infusion at 1–5 mg/h or vasopressors like nor-adrenaline
- Ventricular dysrhythmias unresponsive to alkalinization: $MgSO_4$ 2 g IV over 20 minutes
- *Respiratory failure*: Intubate and secure the airway
- *Seizures/agitation*: Midazolam/diazepam
- Lipid emulsion therapy may be considered in patients who do not respond to the above standard therapies

The clinical features and management of some other common drug overdoses are shown in **Table 2**.

TABLE 2: Clinical features and specific management of common drug overdose.

	Symptoms and signs	Specific treatment
Benzodiazepines	Drowsiness, slurred speech, nystagmus, hypotension, ataxia, respiratory depression, coma	Flumazenil • 0.2–0.3 mg bolus, repeat dose every 5 min till patient is rousable up to a max of 3 mg, followed by • 0.1–0.4 mg/h infusion
Barbiturates	Respiratory depression, hypotension, shock, and urinary retention	• Maintain airway and breathing. Intubate if severe respiratory depression • Fluid resuscitation and forced alkaline diuresis • Hemodialysis if renal failure/anuria
Beta-blockers	Sinus bradycardia, hypotension, bronchospasm, seizures, cardiac failure, cardiac arrest drowsiness, hallucinations, coma	• Bradycardia: Atropine 1 mg IV, repeat every 3–5 min. Max dose: 3 mg. If persists and in shock: cardiac pacing • *Seizures*: Midazolam 5 mg IV or diazepam • *Bronchospasm*: Salbutamol nebulization/terbutaline infusion 0.05 µg/kg/min • *In severe cases, administer high dose insulin therapy*: 1 U/kg insulin bolus followed by 1–4 U/kg/h insulin infusion in 10% dextrose (improves myocardial contractility and systemic perfusion). Monitor sugars and potassium • *Hypotension*: Glucagon 5 mg IV bolus, repeat after 10 min. Then start infusion at 1–5 mg/h • Calcium gluconate loading, then add 10 mL to the IV fluids every 4 hours.

Continued

Continued

	Symptoms and signs	Specific treatment
Calcium channel blockers (CCB) • Nifedipine and amlodipine • Verapamil and diltiazem	• *General*: Nausea, vomiting, dizziness, confusion, seizures • *Metabolic*: acidosis, hypocalcemia, and hyperkalemia • *Cardiac*: hypotension, bradycardia, AV block, complete heart block, pulmonary edema	• Calcium gluconate loading, then add 10 mL to the IV fluids every 4 hours • *Glucagon*: 5 mg IV bolus, repeat after 10 minutes. Then start infusion at 1–5 mg/h • *Hypotension*: elevate foot end of bed and give fluid challenge. Inotropes (noradrenaline) if severe hypotension persists • *Bradycardia*: Atropine 1 mg IV, repeat every 3–5 min. Max dose: 3 mg. Consider pacing if required • *In severe cases, administer 'High dose insulin therapy'*: 1 U/kg insulin bolus followed by 1–4 U/kg/h insulin infusion in 10% Dextrose (improves myocardial contractility and systemic perfusion). Monitor sugars and potassium • Correct acidosis (pH <7) with $NaHCO_3$
Copper sulfate (powerful oxidizing agent)	Acute: Nausea, vomiting, hemorrhagic gastroenteritis. After 24 hours: Hemolysis, hepatic failure, coagulopathy, cardiovascular collapse, rhabdomyolysis, renal failure, coma	• *Corrosive esophageal burns*: Early UGI scopy. Treat like corrosive poisoning • D-Penicillamine 1,000–1,500 mg/day in three divided doses for 1–2 weeks • *If methemoglobinemia (MetHb)*: Give methylene blue 1–2 mg/kg IV bolus. Repeat dose after 1 hour if MetHb level still elevated. Administer oxygen
Digoxin	• Anorexia, nausea, vomiting, any cardiac arrhythmia, visual changes, diplopia, photophobia, xanthopsia (objects appear yellow) • Hypokalemia, hypomagnesemia, renal failure precipitates toxicity • *ECG changes*: Down sloping ST depression, shortened QT interval, Flat, inverted or biphasic T waves	• Digoxin specific antibody (Fab) fragments, if available • *Bradyarrhythmia's*: Atropine 1 mg IV, repeat every 3–5 min. Max dose: 3 mg. Consider transcutaneous pacing • *Hypotension*: IV fluid bolus • Correct hypokalemia, hypomagnesemia or hypercalcemia if present • *Life-threatening ventricular arrhythmias*: Manage as per ACLS protocol

Continued

Continued

	Symptoms and signs	*Specific treatment*
Iron	GI irritation, abdominal pain, hepatic failure, coagulopathy, seizures, shock	• Desferrioxamine IV 15 mg/kg/h for a max dose of 80 mg/kg (5 h infusion) • Treat coagulopathy with blood products • Hemodialysis for severe toxicity • Consider early decontamination of the gut by Whole bowel irrigation if X-ray abdomen shows radio-opaque iron tablets beyond the pylorus
Lithium	Thirst, polyuria, diarrhea, vomiting, tremors, seizures, arrhythmias, hypotension	• *Li level <1.4 mmol/L*: Supportive care • *Li level >1.4 mmol/L*: Hemodialysis is indicated • Ensure adequate hydration • *Do not* give diuretics
Phenytoin therapeutic range: 20–40	• *Rapid loading*: hypotension, bradyarrhythmias, and asystole • *Increased levels*: nystagmus, ataxia, slurred speech, lethargy, confusion, coma	• Stop the drug • Supportive care • Treat seizures with barbiturates/benzodiazepines • *In severe cases*: Dialysis may be helpful

(IV: Intravenous)

ORGANOPHOSPHORUS COMPOUNDS

There are more than a hundred organophosphorus (OP) compounds in common use. These are classified according to their toxicity and clinical use.

- High toxicity (e.g., tetraethyl pyrophosphates and parathion): These are mainly used as agricultural insecticides.
- Intermediate toxicity (e.g., coumaphos, chlorpyrifos, and trichlorfon): These are used as animal insecticides.
- Low toxicity (e.g., diazinon, malathion, and dichlorvos): These are used for household application and as field sprays.

Clinical Features of Organophosphorus Poisoning

- SLUDGE/BBB—salivation, lacrimation, urination, defecation, gastric emesis/ bronchorrhea, bronchospasm, bradycardia
- DUMBELS—defecation, urination, miosis, bronchorrhea/bronchospasm/ bradycardia, emesis, lacrimation, salivation (**Table 1**).

Neurological Manifestations

- Type I paralysis or acute paralysis.
- *Type II paralysis or intermediate syndrome*: This syndrome develops 24–96 hours after the poisoning. Following recovery from the acute cholinergic crisis, and before the expected onset of delayed neuropathy, some patients develop a state of muscle paralysis. The cardinal feature of the syndrome is

TABLE 1: Symptoms and features of organophosphorus poisoning.

Muscarinic receptors	Nicotinic receptors	Central receptors
• **Cardiovascular:** Bradycardia, hypotension • **Respiratory:** Rhinorrhea, bronchorrhea bronchospasm, cough • **Gastrointestinal:** Nausea/vomiting, increased salivation, abdominal cramps, diarrhea, fecal incontinence • **Genitourinary:** Urinary continence • **Eyes:** Blurred vision, increased lacrimation, miosis • **Glands:** Excessive salivation	• **Cardiovascular:** Tachycardia Hypertension • **Musculoskeletal:** Weakness Fasciculations Cramps Paralysis	• **General effects:** Anxiety, restlessness ataxia, convulsions insomnia, dysarthria, tremors • **Coma** • **Absent reflexes** • **Respiratory depression** • **Circulatory collapse**

muscle weakness affecting the proximal limb muscles and neck flexors. One of the earliest manifestations in these patients is the inability to lift their head from the pillow (due to a marked weakness in neck flexion).

- Type III paralysis or organophosphate-induced delayed polyneuropathy (OPIDP): characterized by distal weakness occurring 2–4 weeks after OP exposure with recovery in weeks to months.

Cardiovascular Manifestations

Seen in two-thirds of patients, common ECG manifestations include QTc prolongation, ST-T segment changes and T wave abnormalities. Death due to cardiac causes is either due to an arrhythmia or due to severe refractory hypotension.

Diagnosis

- Diagnosis is confirmed by a low-plasma pseudocholinesterase levels.
- Red blood cells cholinesterase is more accurate, but plasma cholinesterase is easier to assay and is more readily available.
- Cholinesterase levels do not always correlate with severity of clinical illness.
- Falsely depressed levels of plasma cholinesterase are observed in liver dysfunction, low-protein conditions, neoplasia, hypersensitivity reactions, use of certain drugs (succinylcholine, codeine, and morphine), pregnancy, and genetic deficiencies.

Management

The treatment should be initiated immediately on clinical suspicion, without waiting for blood investigations.

- Skin decontamination
- Airway protection, if indicated
- Gastric lavage if patient presents within 1 hour of ingestion
- Anticholinergics
    - *Atropine*: IV bolus of 2 mg, then double the dose every 5 minutes till atropinization targets are achieved. Central nervous system (CNS) side effects include psychosis and restlessness.
    - *Glycopyrrolate*: It is equally effective, with less CNS side effects than atropine. The standard dose used is 100 µg as bolus every 2–5 minutes.
    - After all the above targets are achieved, start atropine infusion at a rate of 20–30% (mL/h) of the total dose required for atropinization.

Atropinization targets:
- Heart rate >80/min
- Pupils not constricted
- No secretions. Dry lungs (Note: Focal crepitations may suggest aspiration)
- Systolic blood pressure (SBP) >80 mm Hg.

- *Cholinesterase reactivator (oximes)*: The use of oximes is controversial and they are not widely used.

ORGANOCHLORIDE COMPOUNDS

Chlorinated hydrocarbon (organochlorine) compounds are used in pesticides, solvents, and fumigants. Organic chlorines lower the seizure threshold or remove inhibitory influences to produce CNS stimulation. Dichloro-diphenyl-trichloroethane (DDT) is a commonly used organochloride.

Clinical Presentation

Features of CNS stimulation, seizures, agitation, lethargy, nausea, vomiting, hyperaesthesia of the mouth and face, tongue, extremities, headache, dizziness or myoclonus.

Management

- General measures and gastric lavage, if patient presents within 1–2 hours
- Secure airway
- Seizure control with benzodiazepines, phenytoin, barbiturates or propofol
- Atropine is *not* indicated in organochloride toxicity.

CARBAMATES

OP and carbamates are the two groups of cholinesterase-inhibiting insecticides commonly used that can cause cholinergic toxicity. Medical carbamate compounds include physostigmine, pyridostigmine and neostigmine. However, these agents are transient cholinesterase inhibitors, which spontaneously hydrolyze from the cholinesterase enzymatic site within 48 hours. As such, the duration of cholinergic symptoms in carbamate poisoning is <48 h. However, severe complications may persist.

Clinical Presentation

- SLUDGE/BBB—salivation, lacrimation, urination, defecation, gastric emesis, bronchorrhea, bronchospasm, bradycardia
- DUMBELS—defecation, urination, miosis, bronchorrhea/bronchospasm/bradycardia, emesis, lacrimation, salivation.

Management

- General measures and gastric lavage if patient presents within 1–2 hours
- Treatment is with atropine but smaller doses and shorter courses are adequate
- Carbamates do not produce intermediate and late syndromes.

PYRETHROIDS

Pyrethroids are synthetic derivatives of the natural pyrethrins extracted from the flower Chrysanthemum. These are contact poisons and exert their toxicity on ion channels by prolonging neuronal excitation. Two basic poisoning syndromes are seen.

- Type I pyrethroids produce reflex hyperexcitability and fine tremor.
- Type II pyrethroids produce salivation, hyperexcitability, choreoathetosis, and seizures. Both produce potent sympathetic activation.

Management

- General measures and gastric lavage if patient presents within 1–2 hours
- Seizure control with benzodiazepines, Phenytoin, barbiturates or propofol
- Atropine is not indicated in pyrethroid toxicity.

PARAQUAT POISONING

Paraquat (dipyridylium) is a highly lethal herbicide when ingested, while causing only limited, localized injury on dermal exposure. It is a highly polar and corrosive substance, which upon absorption, rapidly diffuses and concentrates in tissues like lung, kidney, liver, and muscle. Swallowing about 30 mL of 20–24% paraquat concentrate is usually lethal.

Clinical Presentation

- Patients present with a painful mouth and difficulty in swallowing, nausea, vomiting and abdominal pain.
- Respiratory symptoms suggest systemic toxicity.
- Patients who ingest large doses (50–100 mL) present with fulminant multi-organ dysfunction syndrome (MODS) with pulmonary edema, cardiac, hepatic, renal failure and central nervous system involvement with seizures with a high case fatality rate.

Management

- There is no antidote and management is mainly supportive care addressing airway, breathing and circulation.
- Gastric lavage is not recommended as paraquat is corrosive in nature. Naso-gastric tube should be inserted early.
- Treat multi-organ dysfunction as indicated with supportive care like ventilation, blood products, etc.
- Hemodialysis can reduce the plasma load of paraquat but may not reduce the toxic effects on the target organs, with no evident mortality benefit.

  The commonly available insecticide compounds and their trade names are shown in **Table 2**.

TABLE 2: Commonly available compounds and trade names in India.

	Chemical names	Trade names
Organo phosphates	Parathion, malathion, fenthion, ethion, fensulfothion, diazinon, trichlorfon, disulfoton, terbu fos, dichlorvos, monocrotophos, coumaphos, chlorpyriphos, bromophos, triazophos, quinalphos, fenamiphos, cyanophos, azinphos, fonophos, mevinphos, dichrotophos, fenchlorphos, temaphos, dimethoate, crufomate, phenthoate, phorate, TEPP, acephate, demeton, thionazin, and schradan	Brahma, Chlorex, Chase, Cythion, Ekalux, and Rogor, Kaycermal and Tarzen
Organo chlorides	• DDT and related analogs • *Cyclodienes*: Aldrin, dieldrin, endrin, heptochlor and endosulfan • Hexachlorocyclohexane (lindane) • Mirex and chlordecone	Hildan and Thiodan
Carbamates	Aldoxycarb, aminocarb, asalum, barban, bendiocarb, bufencarb, butacarb, benomyl, Carbofuran, carbaryl, carbetamide, carbendazim, chlorbufam, dochlormate, dimetilan, hoppcide, methomyl, oxamyl, propoxur, propham, thiofanox, terbucarb and thiophenateethyl	Furadan
Pyrethroids	Allethrin, bifenthrin, cyfluthrin, cyhalothrin, cypermethrin, DPhenothrin, deltamethrin, flumethrin, fenpropathrin, fenvalerate, flucythrinate, permethrin, resmethrin, tetramethrin and transfluthrin (all out)	Ambush, All out, Good Night, and Karate
OP + Pyrethroid	Chlorpyriphos + Cypermethrin Prophenphos + Cypermethrin Ethion + Cypermethrin	Anaconda, Rocket, Korasha
Other newer compounds	Imidacloprid, cartap hydrochloride, avermectin, amitraz, fipronil, and azadirachtin (neem oil)	Atom

Rodenticides **30**

INTRODUCTION

Rodenticides are commonly used across India for deliberate self-harm. Anticoagulant rodenticides are relatively innocuous while phosphorous-based compounds are highly lethal to human beings.

TYPES OF RODENTICIDES

- *Anticoagulants*:
  - First-generation compounds: Warfarin, coumachlor, and coumatetralyl
  - Second-generation compounds: Chlorophacinone, diphacinone, bromadiolone, difethialone, and brodifacoum.
- *Inorganic rodenticides*: Zinc phosphide, aluminum phosphide, yellow phosphorus, and thallium.
- *Others*: Strychnine, cholecalciferol.

ANTICOAGULANTS (WARFARIN AND RELATED COMPOUNDS, COUMARINS, AND INDANDIONES)

These compounds depress the hepatic synthesis of vitamin K-dependent blood-clotting factors [II (prothrombin) and VII, IX, and X], which results in mucosal or internal bleeding.

The second-generation compounds, also called super-coumarins, have a longer half-life and hence may require monitoring of the PT with international normalized ratio (INR) for many days. Some agents such as brodifacoum may not show an elevation of PT with INR until 48 hours after ingestion.

Treatment

- Prolonged INR with no bleeding: Inj. vitamin K1 10 mg IV OD or 10–50 mg orally, two to four times per day till INR normalizes. However, patients ingesting large doses of second-generation coumarins may require higher doses (100–400 mg oral) of vitamin K1 and a longer duration of treatment (weeks to months).
- Prolonged INR with significant bleeding manifestations: Vitamin K1 and fresh frozen plasma as required. Refer to Chapter 70 on Anticoagulation for details of management.

PHOSPHORUS COMPOUNDS

Aluminum and Zinc Phosphides

- Aluminum and zinc phosphides are highly effective insecticides and rodenticides.
- Commonly found in powder, pellet, or tablet form.
- Acute poisoning with these compounds may be direct due to ingestion of the salts or indirect from accidental inhalation of phosphine generated during their approved use.
- Both forms of poisoning are mediated by phosphine, which has been thought to be toxic because it inhibits cytochrome c oxidase.
- Mortality often occurs rapidly within the first day of severe metallic phosphide poisoning regardless of therapy. Death typically results from cardiac arrhythmias or refractory shock and cardiac failure.

Clinical Features

There is usually only a short interval between ingestion of phosphides and the appearance of systemic toxicity in case of aluminum phosphide toxicity while there is a latent period in zinc phosphide toxicity.

- *Cardiac*: Impaired myocardial contractility leading to circulatory collapse and shock
- *Pulmonary*: Pulmonary edema, either cardiac or noncardiac
- *Hepatic*: Hepatic necrosis and fulminant hepatic failure
- *Hematological*: DIC
- *Metabolic*: Severe metabolic acidosis

Management

- Supportive measures are all that can be offered and many patients die despite intensive care.
- Correct electrolyte abnormalities, especially hypomagnesemia as this may contribute to mortality.
- N-Acetyl Cysteine (NAC) has been proposed as an antidote and may be given if the patient presents early (<12 h).
  Dose: 150 mg/kg in 200 mL of 5% dextrose over 15 minutes then 50 mg/kg in 500 mL of 5% dextrose over 4 hours then 100 mg/kg in 1 L of 5% dextrose over 16 hours.

YELLOW PHOSPHORUS

Elemental phosphorus exists in two forms: red and white (yellow)

- The red form, used in match stick production is not absorbed and has minimal toxicity.
- Compounds of yellow phosphorus are commonly used as everyday rodenticides, fertilizers and in fire crackers and are easily available in Tamil Nadu.

Phosphorus is readily absorbed via the gastrointestinal (GI) tract. Renal and hepatic phosphorus concentrations are elevated within hours. Yellow phosphorous is commonly commercially manufactured as RATOL: Rat killer.

Clinical Features

- Yellow phosphorus causes cardiac, hepatic, renal, and multi-organ failure similar to zinc phosphide and aluminum phosphide poisoning
- However, patients with yellow phosphorus intoxication passes through three stages:
    i. *First stage*: 24 hours. Patient is either asymptomatic or has signs and symptoms of local GI irritation
    ii. *Second stage*: 24–72 hours. An asymptomatic period
    iii. *Third stage*: >72 hours. Features of cardiac, hepatic, renal, and multi-organ failure eventually resulting in death.

Management

- Supportive measures are all that can be offered and many patients die despite intensive care.
- NAC may be given as an antidote if the patient presents early (<12 h).
  Dose: 150 mg/kg in 200 mL of 5% dextrose over 15 minutes then 50 mg/kg in 500 mL of 5% dextrose over 4 hours then 100 mg/kg in 1 L of 5% dextrose over 16 hours
- Administer vitamin K1 10 mg IV stat
- Liver transplantation if possible, may be the only lifesaving option.

OLEANDER

Yellow Oleander (Cerebra thevetia); Tamil name: Arali. The leaves, flowers, fruits, and seeds of this plant are all poisonous. The main poisonous principles are cardiac glycosides (oleandrin, neriin, thevetin, etc).

Clinical Presentation

Ingestion of the plant components results in poisoning similar to digitalis toxicity. Common symptoms include nausea, vomiting, abdominal pain, diarrhea, and restlessness.

Hyperkalemia is the most dangerous complication that may precipitate cardiotoxicity unless identified and corrected immediately

Cardiac toxicity may manifest as bradycardia with atrioventricular (AV) block, atrial tachycardias, ventricular tachycardia or ventricular fibrillation. Cardiogenic shock with myocardial depression can also occur.

Management

- Gastric lavage followed by the administration of activated charcoal and, possibly, a cathartic, if patient presents within 1–2 hours.
- Bradycardia/heart blocks may require atropine or electrical pacing. Ventricular arrhythmias could be treated with phenytoin [intravenous (IV) infusion of 3.5–5.0 mg/kg, at a rate not greater than 50 mg/min], or lignocaine (1 mg/kg slow IV bolus followed by continuous infusion of 2–4 mg/min).
- *Treat hyperkalemia*: Hyperkalemia is due to extracellular shift of K rather than increase in total body K, best treated with insulin dextrose and salbutamol nebulizations. DO NOT give calcium gluconate as calcium increases the risk of cardiac arrhythmias.
- *If patient has hypokalemia*: Hypokalemia worsens toxicity of digitalis glycosides and could be life threatening. Give KCl supplementation, oral/IV.
- *Antidote*: Digoxin-specific Fab antibody fragments have been used successfully in adult patients intoxicated with nerium oleander. However, they are very expensive and not available in India.

ODUVANTHALAI

Oduvanthalai (*Cleistanthus collinus*): *Tamil* name: Oduvan. Patients may consume fresh leaves, freshly ground leaf paste, or boiled leaf extract. Mortality is highest if

- Look for features of neurotoxicity.
  - Difficulty in lifting the neck suggests neck muscle weakness.
  - Ptosis
  - *Single breath count*: It is normally >20–30 numbers per minutes. A decreased single breath count indicates neurotoxicity.
- Look for features of hemotoxicity: Bleeding manifestations like petechiae, hematuria, gum bleed, melena, and hematemesis.
- *Whole blood clotting time*: Take 10 mL of whole blood in a glass tube and leave it by the bed side. Clotting time >10 minutes suggests coagulopathy.
- *Investigations*: Complete blood count (CBC), electrolytes, creatinine, urea, urinalysis, Prothrombin time (PT), activated partial thromboplastin time (aPTT), Creatine kinase (CK), and ECG.

MANAGEMENT

- Analgesics for pain relief (avoid NSAIDs in patients with hemotoxicity).
- *Antibiotics for infection*: Anaerobic infections should be covered. Amoxicillin-clavulanate is a good choice.
- *Tetanus prophylaxis*: Tetanus toxoid or diphtheria-tetanus (dT) vaccine 1 amp intramuscular (IM) into the deltoid.

ANTISNAKE VENOM

Antisnake venom is prepared by hyperimmunizing horses against the venoms of the 'Big four' poisonous snakes of India. Plasma obtained from the hyperimmunized horses is enzyme refined, purified, and concentrated.

Remember that most bites are *dry bites* and do not require the polyvalent ASV. It needs to be given *only* when there are features of envenomation.

- Premedication to decrease the risk of anaphylactic reactions
  - Premedication is not needed for most of the patients.
  - In those with history of atopy/reaction to equine antiserum, administer.
    - Injection chlorpheniramine maleate (avil) 1 ampoule slow intra-venous (IV).
    - Injection Adrenaline 0.25 mg IM (1:1,000 dilution) in the anterolateral thigh.
- Dose of ASV
  - *Hemotoxic bite*: 8–10 vials in 5% Dextrose over 30 minutes
    - Reassess bleeding manifestation and whole blood clotting test after 6 hours and give four to eight vials, if needed depending on the severity of symptoms.
  - *Neurotoxic bite*: 8–10 vials in 5% dextrose over 30 minutes
    - Reassess after 2 hours and if neurotoxicity persists, give 4–8 vials depending on the severity of symptoms.

- Treatment of early anaphylactic reaction
  - Stop the ASV infusion immediately
  - Injection Adrenaline 0.5 mg IM (1:1000 dilution) in the anterolateral thigh
  - Injection Chlorpheniramine maleate (Avil) 1 ampoule slow IV/IM
  - Restart the ASV slowly after 30–60 minutes after the reaction has settled.
- If respiratory failure develops, mechanical ventilation may be required.
- If significant bleeding continues despite giving ASV, send fibrinogen levels and arrange for fresh frozen plasma/cryoprecipitate.
- Shock due to myocardial depression needs to be treated with fluid resuscitation and inotropes.
- Renal failure due to rhabdomyolysis or shock may require hemodialysis.
- Ptosis due to neurotoxic snake bite may persist for 1–2 weeks. Without other neurological manifestations, there is no indication to continue ASV for just ptosis.

> Each vial of lyophilized ASV costs more than Rs. 650. Administer ASV only when indicated and use it judiciously.

Most of the venom used for the production of ASV in India is supplied by the Irula tribal society snake catchers, who catch the big four snakes from the districts of Kancheepuram and Thiruvalluvar in Tamil Nadu.

> The venom of a Russell's viper in North India is different from the venom of a Russell's viper from South India. Hence, the efficacy of ASV in other parts of India is questionable. Though there is no evidence, smaller doses may be sufficient in Tamil Nadu.

- The currently available polyvalent ASV is not effective against King Cobra envenomation, which is seen in the Himalayan belt, Eastern and Western ghats. Monovalent antivenom against King Cobra is available in some places.

33

SCORPION STING

Among the 86 species of scorpions in India, *Mesobuthus tamulus* and *Palamnaeus swammerdami* are venomous. The venom stimulates the sustained release of acetylcholine and catecholamines resulting in initial cholinergic and late adrenergic symptoms. Generally, the less venomous species cause more local reaction.

Clinical Features

- *Benign stings*: Most stings are benign and cause severe local pain with no progression of symptoms.
- Potentially dangerous stings:
  - *0 hours*: Mild local pain, paresthesia, vomiting and salivation
  - *4 hours*: (Autonomic storm) sweating, priapism, cool limbs, tachycardia, hypertension, myocardial dysfunction, arrhythmias, and pulmonary edema
  - *48 hours*: Stage of shock and death, if untreated.

Investigations: Complete blood count (CBC), electrolytes, creatinine, and ECG.

Management

- First aid consists of applying an ice bag over the area of the sting.
- Benign stings need good pain relief with intravenous/intramuscular (IV/IM) opiates or digital ring block with 2% xylocaine (*without* adrenaline).
- Administer diphtheria-tetanus (dT) toxoid intramuscularly if not adequately vaccinated. (Refer chapter 25)
- Antibiotics if signs of infection are present (cloxacillin/augmentin)
- Potentially dangerous stings with autonomic storm
  - *Prazosin*: 0.25 mg for children and 0.5 mg for adults every 3 hours till extremities become warm and dry. Usually, 2–6 doses of prazosin are needed. Administer the first dose of prazosin even if blood pressure is low. Start noradrenaline infusion concomitantly.
  - Benzodiazepines/phenobarbitones for seizures
  - Treat shock and cardiac failure with fluids and inotropes
  - Treat life-threatening arrhythmias.

CENTIPEDE BITE

Centipede bite mostly causes only local reaction, pain, anxiety, vomiting, headache, and palpitations. Symptoms are usually mild.

Management

- Adequate pain relief with NSAIDs/opiates
- Local application of ice may reduce some of the discomfort
- Antitetanus prophylaxis if not adequately vaccinated. (Refer chapter 25)
- Antibiotics if signs of infection present (cloxacillin/augmentin)
- Antihistamines may be given for local pruritic reactions.

BEE AND WASP (*HYMENOPTERA* SPECIES) STINGS

Bees, wasps, hornets and fire ants belong to the order *Hymenoptera* and frequently sting humans when disturbed. It may not always be possible to exactly identify the culprit species, but the sting is always acutely painful. Most people only develop minor local reactions (redness and swelling that usually resolves within a few hours). However, some (0.3–3%) may develop anaphylaxis and could be fatal.

Bees and wasps have a similar mechanism of delivering venom. After a single sting by a bee, the barbed venom apparatus detaches, eviscerating, and killing the bee instantly. However, the unbarbed venom apparatus of a wasp remains intact and hence a wasp can sting a person multiple times.

Management

- Uncomplicated local reactions may be treated with just cold compresses
- Large local reactions (exaggerated redness/swelling) can be treated with cold compresses, antihistamines (levocetirizine 5 mg PO OD × 1–2 days) and a nonsteroidal anti-inflammatory drug (NSAIDs). Persistent large local reactions may require 1 or 2 days of oral prednisolone at a dose of 40–60 mg PO od.
- Administer beta agonist (salbutamol) nebulizations for patients who develop wheezing
- If symptoms of anaphylaxis are observed, treat with adrenaline, antihistamines, H_2 blockers and fluid resuscitation. (Refer chapter 3)
- After a sting, the barbed sting apparatus with the venom sac remains lodged in the skin. Venom is released within seconds to minutes of the bite. Hence removal of the embedded stingers from the skin by scraping the skin with a 23-G needle or scalpel (**Fig. 1**) is useful if done immediately after the sting. However, if the patient presents after 5–10 minutes, removal of the sting apparatus is not urgent as most of the venom would have already been released into the body. All the stings should still be removed to prevent foreign body reactions.

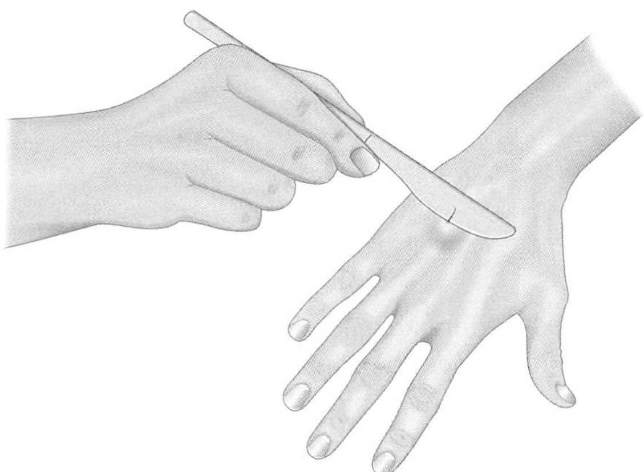

FIG. 1: Technique of *Hymenoptera* sting removal.

- Clean and disinfect the site of sting with soap and water followed by spirit
- Apply ice packs to slow down the spread of venom
- If the patient is stable to be discharged, advice calamine lotion to be applied twice daily.

OTHER INSECT BITES

Beetles, Caterpillars, and Millipedes

Some species of these arthropods cause severe burning pain, numbness, erythema, nausea, vomiting, and headache. Wash the area thoroughly with soap and water and remove any spines or hairs by using adhesive tape or glue or facial peel. Apply local ice packs and give analgesics for severe pain.

Spider Bites

Majority of spiders are non-venomous. Rate bites of *Loxosceles* and *Poecilotheria* species have been reported from India. Symptoms of a bite may include mild erythematous lesions with pruritis and swelling. The lesion may become necrotic with eschar formation in a week. Management includes local ice pack application, anti histamines and analgesics if required. Antibiotics (cloxacillin) are warranted for severe local reactions.

OPIOIDS

Opioids are prescribed legitimately for analgesia, especially for palliation. Overdose of a legitimate prescription and illicit drug abuse result in a large number of cases. Commonly abused opioids include morphine, heroin, tramadol, methadone, and oxycodone.

Symptoms and Signs of Overdose

- Central nervous system (CNS) depression, respiratory depression, and miosis are the characteristic features of opioid intoxication.
- Nausea, vomiting, orthostatic hypotension, localized urticaria, and bronchospasm may also be seen.
- Diagnosis is purely clinical based on the classic triad of respiratory depression, coma, and miosis.

Management

- Securing airway and breathing is crucial
- *Antidote*: Naloxone works by competitive inhibition of the OP_3 receptor and fully reverses the CNS and respiratory depression. Antidote can be given intravenously/intramuscularly/subcutaneously (IV/IM/SC) or intratracheally.

Intravenous Dose of Naloxone

- *Adults*: 0.4–2 mg IV bolus depending on the severity of symptoms. Repeat doses of 0.4–2 mg IV may be given every 2–3 minutes till full reversal is achieved. The maximum total dose is 10 mg.
- *Children <5 years/<20 kg*: 0.1 mg/kg.
- *Children >5 years/>20 kg*: 0.4–2 mg IV bolus.
- Depending on the severity of presentation, additional bolus doses may be required every 30 minutes to 2 hours to maintain reversal.

CANNABIS (MARIJUANA)

- Natural marijuana contains over 60 cannabinoids and include delta-9-tetrahydrocannabinol, the most psychoactive cannabinoid, cannabidiol, and cannabinol.

- Recreational use often consists of smoking the dried flower in the form of rolled cigarettes (joints) and water bongs.
- Common slang terms include *pot, grass, dope, MJ, Mary Jane, doobie, hooch, weed, hash, reefers, and ganja.*
- Synthetic cannabinoids are now widely available and are sold as *K2, spice, crazy monkey, chill out, spice diamond, spice gold, and chill X.*
- *Signs of intoxication*: Tachycardia, tachypnea, elevated blood pressure (BP), conjunctival injection, dry mouth, nystagmus, ataxia, and slurred speech.
- *Complications associated with inhalation use*: Acute exacerbations of asthma, pneumomediastinum, pneumothorax, angina, and myocardial infarction.

Management of Acute Intoxication

- Mild symptoms of anxiety may be controlled with benzodiazepines (lorazepam/midazolam)
- Cannabis hyperemesis syndrome (abdominal pain, nausea, and vomiting) may be treated with IV fluids, antiemetics (ondansetron), and benzodiazepines
- If the patient complains of sudden onset chest pain, consider ACS/pneumothorax/acute exacerbation of asthma and treat accordingly.

AMPHETAMINE

Amphetamine is widely abused for its CNS arousal effects. Complications include vasospasm and intracranial hemorrhage secondary to hypertension.

Management of Acute Intoxication

- Sedate agitated patients with a benzodiazepine (diazepam 5–10 mg IV or lorazepam 1–2 mg IV/IM). Haloperidol 5–10 mg IM may be useful in psychotic patients.
- Control seizures with benzodiazepines.
- If the patient has seizures/focal deficits, get a computed tomography (CT) scan is done to rule out intracerebral bleed/subarachnoid hemorrhage.
- Significant hypertension (diastolic blood pressure >120 mm Hg) may respond to sedation. If not, treat as a hypertensive emergency.

COCAINE

Street names include *coke, cola, dust, nose candy*, etc.

Presentation: Seizures (common), hypertension, tachycardia, CNS depression, ventricular arrhythmias, cardiorespiratory failure, and paranoid delusions (chronic use).

Complications: Angina/myocardial infarction (vasoconstrictor effects on the coronary circulation), cerebrovascular accident, and psychotic reactions.

Management of Acute Intoxication

- Sedate agitated patients with a benzodiazepine to control seizures.
- Treat hypertension as a hypertensive emergency and rapidly lower the BP with antihypertensives.
- If the patient has seizures/focal deficits, do a CT scan to look for an intracranial bleed.
- If the patient complains of sudden onset chest pain, consider an acute coronary syndrome.

ECSTASY/3,4-METHYLENEDIOXYMETHAMPHETAMINE

3,4-Methylenedioxymethamphetamine (MDMA), commonly known as ecstasy or molly, may cause life-threatening cardiac dysrhythmias, acute liver failure, cerebral infarction, and hemorrhage. Severe hyperthermia (core temperature >40°C), severe metabolic acidosis, muscle rigidity, DIC, and rhabdomyolysis may also occur.

- Treatment is mainly supportive in a quiet environment. Stabilize ABC.
- If the patient presents within 1 hour of ingestion, perform a gastric lavage and administer activated charcoal.
- Benzodiazepines can be given to control agitation, seizures, or panic reaction.
- Initiate cooling measures for hyperthermia.
- Monitor ECG and look for cardiac arrhythmias.

LYSERGIC ACID DIETHYLAMIDE (LSD)

LSD, commonly known as 'acid' is a hallucinogenic drug that causes altered thoughts, feelings and awareness of one's surroundings. Clinical features include pupillary dilatation, sweating, acute anxiety state, tachycardia, depolarization, and visual illusions. Large doses can cause convulsions, focal neurological deficit (due to vasospasm), and coma.

- Treatment is mainly supportive in a quiet environment. Stabilize ABC.
- Benzodiazepines can be given to control agitation.
- LSD is rapidly absorbed through the gastrointestinal tract. Hence, gastric lavage and activated charcoal are not beneficial and best avoided.

CORROSIVE POISONING

A corrosive is a substance that erodes and destroys any surface it comes in contact with. Acids and alkalis are the two primary types of agents which are most often responsible for caustic exposures.

- *Alkali ingestion*: Causes liquefaction necrosis.
- *Acid ingestion*: Causes coagulation necrosis.

Commonly Used Corrosives

- *Acids*: Car battery fluid (sulfuric acid), descalers/toilet bowl cleaners (hydrochloric acid), metal cleaners (nitric acid), rust removers (hydrogen fluoride), acetic acid, phenol (carbolic acid), and oxalic acid.
- *Alkalis*: Bleach (hypochlorite) and sodium hydroxide (liquid lye and paint remover/drain cleaner).
- Heavy metal salts (sublimate), formalin, and iodine tincture.

Investigations to be Sent

Complete blood count, electrolytes, creatinine, liver function test, ECG, rapid blood-borne virus screen (BBVS), chest X-ray, and X-ray neck soft tissue AP/lateral.

Management

- If the patient presents within 24 hours of ingestion
  - Do not give gastric lavage. Patients may aspirate and worsen stricture
  - Establish intravenous (IV) access and start IV fluid resuscitation
  - Remove contaminated clothes and continuously irrigate any ocular injuries
  - Injection Pantoprazole 40 mg IV and injection metoclopramide 10 mg IV stat
  - Administer adequate analgesia
  - Refer to ENT for evaluation of oropharynx and clearance for upper gastrointestinal (UGI) scopy.
  - *Diagnostic endoscopy*: Refer to gastroenterology for endoscopy-guided NG tube insertion and further management. Endoscopy must be done within 6–24 hours of ingestion. If performed earlier than 6 hours, the lesions may not manifest and if performed later than 24 hours, the risk of esophageal perforation is very high.
  - If there is evidence of esophageal perforation, start extended spectrum antibiotics: clindamycin 15–20 mg/kg IV stat or ertapenem 1 g IV stat.

- If the patient presents after 24 hours of ingestion
  - The role of endoscopic evaluation and intervention decreases, if the patient presents to the ED after 24 hours of ingestion of corrosive.
  - If the patient already has a NG tube placed outside, refer to gastroenterology for further management plan.
  - If NG tube has not been inserted even after 24 hours of ingestion, the primary treatment for severe corrosive injury is surgical. Feeding gastrostomy or feeding jejunostomy tube needs to be inserted by general surgery. The primary unit would be general surgery.

If endoscopy reveals only mild lesions, then the patient can be discharged and clinical follow-up should be done at 1 month. If severe lesions are found on endoscopy, then surgical gastrostomy is indicated, which should be followed by repeat endoscopy and dilatation after 3 weeks.

METHANOL (METHYL ALCOHOL) POISONING

Methanol toxicity occurs most commonly due to consumption of illegally produced alcohol products. It causes an initial syndrome similar to alcohol. However, the formation of toxic metabolites leads to a profound metabolic acidosis and there is also direct retinal toxicity from these metabolites (**Fig. 1**).

A dose of as little as 10 mL of pure methanol may cause significant toxicity or death.

Clinical Features

- The initial effects of methanol resemble those of alcohol with central nervous system (CNS) depression, ataxia, nausea, and vomiting. Subsequent CNS effects may be secondary to the acidosis or to the activity of the metabolites and include coma and convulsions.

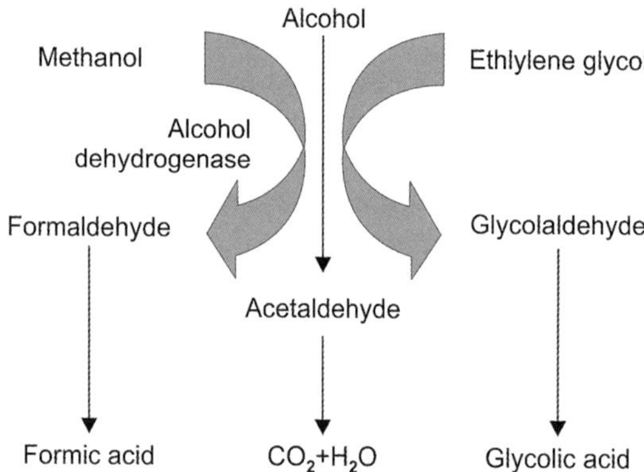

FIG. 1: Metabolism of ethanol and methanol.

- With the development of acidosis, tachycardia, tachypnea, and hypertension may occur. However, more severe toxicity is manifested by hypotension and cardiogenic shock.
- Blurred vision, photophobia, and decreased visual acuity may occur. About 25% of patients will have some degree of permanent visual loss.
- The major feature seen is a severe metabolic acidosis with a raised anion gap.

Management

- *Supportive care*: IV fluid hydration.
- Acidosis should be corrected with bicarbonate.
- Fomepizole (4-methyl pyrazole), if available should be given. Dose: 15 mg/kg IV infusion over 30 minutes, then 10 mg/kg IV q12h for four doses. Treat until ethylene glycol or methanol levels are <20 mg/dL.
- Ethanol has a higher affinity for alcohol dehydrogenase and competitively inhibits the metabolism of methanol to more toxic metabolites. Hence, ethanol should be given intravenously or orally if the IV preparation is not available. A blood alcohol level of 100 mg/dL (21.7 mmol/L) is required to maximally inhibit alcohol dehydrogenase.
  Loading dose:
  - Four standard drinks (4 × 30 mL of spirits) orally.
  - 360–420 mL of 10% ethanol by IV infusion.
- Folate is a cofactor in the further metabolism of formic acid to nontoxic metabolites. Folic acid 50 mg IV q4h (or folinic acid 50 mg q4h) should be given to patients with severe toxicity.
- *Hemodialysis*: Methanol and its metabolites are cleared by hemodialysis.
  Indications:
  - Renal failure
  - Severe metabolic acidosis (pH <7.1)
  - Methanol concentration >50–100 mg/dL.

KEROSENE POISONING

Pulmonary toxicity can occur within 1–8 hours of ingestion due to aspiration into the respiratory tract (chemical pneumonitis). Symptoms may include breathlessness, cough, nausea, vomiting, or abdominal pain. X-ray abnormalities may be evident only after 72 hours.

Management

- Avoid emesis and gastric lavage.
- Supplemental oxygen if patient is tachypneic or saturation is low.
- Patients with acute lung injury may require prophylactic antibiotics (piperacillin-tazobactam or meropenem)
- Refer to medicine for further management.

INHALATION INJURIES (CARBON MONOXIDE POISONING)

Common inhalation injuries are smoke inhalation and accompanying burns. Smoke is a complex and variable mixture of solid, liquid, and gas constituents.

Components of inhalation injury are:
- Carbon monoxide poisoning (responsible for 85% of deaths)
- Direct thermal injury
- Soot particles that cause local injury to the cilia of the respiratory tract and obstruct small airways
- *Gas products of combustion*: Oxides of sulfur, nitrogen, ammonia, chlorine, phosgene, isocyanates, aldehydes, and ketones are highly irritative and cause laryngospasm.

Clinical Features

Suspect smoke inhalation if any of the following features are present: exposure to smoke or fire in an enclosed place without adequate ventilation, confusion, altered sensorium, singed nasal hairs, oropharyngeal burns, hoarseness of voice, wheeze, dysphagia, stridor.

Severe carbon monoxide poisoning can cause neurological manifestations like seizures, syncope, or coma, myocardial ischemia, ventricular arrhythmias, pulmonary edema, and profound lactic acidosis.

Delayed neuropsychiatric syndrome can be seen in up to 40% of patients with severe CO poisoning and can occur 3 days–8 months after recovery, and are characterized by variable degrees of cognitive deficits, personality changes, movement disorders, parkinsonism features, and focal neurologic deficits.

Investigations

CBC, electrolytes, creatinine, LFT, CXR, ECG, ABG, carboxy-Hb (COHb) level.

COHb levels correlate poorly with clinical features and are not predictive of delayed neurologic sequelae.

Management

- Prompt removal from the source of carbon monoxide.
- Administer high-flow oxygen by face mask. Give the highest possible concentration of humidified oxygen. The use of hyperbaric oxygen remains controversial.
- Protect the airway. Intubate early if necessary. However, mucosal swelling in the upper airway and oropharynx can progress rapidly and necessitate a surgical airway.
- IV fluid resuscitation depending on the extent of burns
- Salbutamol nebulization if bronchospasm occurs.

CYANIDE POISONING

Cyanide is a mitochondrial toxin, which is extremely lethal.

Cyanide avidly binds to the ferric ion (Fe^{3+}) of cytochrome oxidase a3, inhibiting this final enzyme in the mitochondrial cytochrome complex. The cell must then switch to anerobic metabolism of glucose to generate ATP and this produces severe lactic acidosis.

Sources of Cyanide

- *Industrial exposure*: Plastics, photography, fumigation, metal polish, electroplating, hair removal from hides
- *Plants and fruits*: Bamboo sprout, Rosaceae family (plum, peach, pear, apple, bitter almond, cherry)
- *Drugs*: Sodium nitroprusside, laetrile
- *Others*: Artificial nail glue remover, phencyclidine synthesis.

Clinical Features

Clinical features of cyanide poisoning are dependent upon the route, duration, and amount of exposure. The CNS and CVS are mostly affected.

Headache, anxiety, confusion, vertigo, initial tachycardia and hypertension, then bradycardia and hypotension, vomiting, abdominal pain, hepatic necrosis, renal failure, coma.

Clinical features are similar to carbon monoxide poisoning, which is a strong differential for cyanide poisoning.

Management

General measures and ABC as for any poisoning. Three antidotal strategies may be used:
- *Direct cyanide binding* using hydroxycobalamin, a precursor of vitamin B12 that contains a cobalt moiety that avidly binds to intracellular cyanide with greater affinity than cytochrome oxidase.
- *Induction of methemoglobinemia* using amyl nitrite or sodium nitrite. The formation of methemoglobin (MetHb) provides an attractive alternative binding site for cyanide, in direct competition with the site on the cytochrome complex. When cyanide binds MetHb, a relatively less toxic cyanmethemoglobin is formed.
- *Sulfur donors* using sodium thiosulfate maximizes the availability of sulfur donors for rhodanese, a ubiquitous enzyme that detoxifies cyanide by transforming it to thiocyanate.

Cyanide poisoning is common among jewelers as an occupational exposure or intentional self-harm. They are usually provided the antidotes as a "cyanide kit" when they buy cyanide compounds for commercial reasons. Administer the antidote immediately, if available.

Dosages

- ○ *Amyl nitrite*: Inhaled by the patient (held under the patient's nose or via the endotracheal tube) for 30 seconds of each minute, for 3 minutes
- ○ *Sodium nitrite*: 10 mg/kg IV bolus
- ○ *Sodium thiosulfate*: 50 mL of a 25% solution (12.5 g) IV bolus
- ○ *Hydroxycobalamin*: 70 mg/kg IV bolus. A second dose of 35 mg/kg can be given depending upon the severity of poisoning or the clinical response to treatment.

METHEMOGLOBINEMIA

Methemoglobin is generated by oxidation of the heme iron moieties into ferric state (Fe^{+3}), causing a a characteristic bluish-brown muddy colour resembling cyanosis. Methemoglobin has a very high affinity for oxygen and hence virtually no oxygen is delivered to the tissues.

There are two types of methemoglobinemia: Congenital and acquired.

1. *Congenital type*: It is characterized by decreased enzymatic reduction of methemoglobin back to functional hemoglobin. Affected patients have lifelong cyanosis but are generally asymptomatic; e.g., cytochrome b5 reductase deficiency, hemoglobin M disease, cytochrome b5 deficiency.
2. *Acquired type*: Can be fatal and typically results from ingestion of specific drugs or agents that cause an increase in the production of methemoglobin (**Table 1**).

Clinical Features

Symptoms in patients with acquired methemoglobinemia result from an acute impairment in oxygen delivery to tissues:

- *Asymptomatic*: (at levels <20%)
- *Early symptoms*: (at levels >20%) pale skin, lightheadedness, headache, tachycardia, fatigue, dyspnea, and lethargy
- *At higher levels of MetHb*: (>30%) cyanosis, respiratory depression, altered sensorium, coma, shock, seizures, and death.

TABLE 1: Common precipitating agents of acquired methemoglobinemia.	
Drugs	Dapsone, Clofazimine, Chloroquine, Metoclopramide, Primaquine, Rasburicase, and Sulfonamides
Local anesthetics	Benzocaine, Lidocaine, and Prilocaine
Nitrites	Amyl nitrite, Farryl nitrite, Sodium nitrite, Nitroglycerin, Nitric oxide
Others	• Acetanilide, p-Aminosalicylic acid, Aniline, aniline dyes, Benzene derivatives, Chlorates, Naphthalene, • Nitrobenzene, Paraquat, Phenacetin, Phenazopyridine, and Resorcinol

When to Suspect Methemoglobinemia?

- Sudden onset of cyanosis with symptoms of hypoxia after administration or ingestion of an agent that can cause methemoglobinemia
- Hypoxia (low SpO_2 on pulse oximeter) that does not improve with an increased fraction of inspired oxygen
- Abnormal dark red, chocolate, or brownish coloration of the blood observed during phlebotomy.

Management

- *Asymptomatic patient with a MetHb level <20%*: No therapy other than discontinuation of the offending agent(s)
- *Symptomatic patients or if the MetHb level is > 20%*:
  - *Methylene blue*: Methylene blue 1–2 mg/kg IV bolus. Repeat dose after 1 hour if MetHb level is still elevated (>20%). The response is usually rapid and one dose is sufficient in most patients. Repeated doses may cause acute hemolysis and may worsen the methemoglobinemia.
  - *Ascorbic acid*: 10 g IV every 6 hours *or* 300–1,000 mg/day orally in divided doses may be given if methylene blue is contraindicated (G6PD deficiency). Ascorbic acid is slow to act and requires multiple doses over 24 hours for the same effect as methylene blue.

Cardiac Emergencies

CHAPTER 36

Acute Coronary Syndrome

INTRODUCTION

The term acute coronary syndrome (ACS) refers to a spectrum of clinical presentations ranging from myocardial ischemia to myocardial infarction (MI). There are three types of ACS (**Flowchart 1**):

1. ST elevation (Q-wave) MI (STEMI)
2. Non-ST elevation (non-Q wave) MI (NSTEMI)
3. Unstable angina (UA).

Angina Pectoris

- Substernal discomfort precipitated by exertion
- Radiation to the shoulder, jaw, or inner aspect of the arm
- Relieved by rest or nitroglycerin in <10 minutes.

Unstable Angina

- Rest angina, >20 minutes in duration
- New onset angina that markedly limits physical activity
- Angina that is more frequent, longer in duration, or occurs with less exertion than previous angina.

Angina Equivalents

Not all patients with ACS present with a typical chest pain. Many patients, especially diabetic patients may present with symptoms other than chest pain

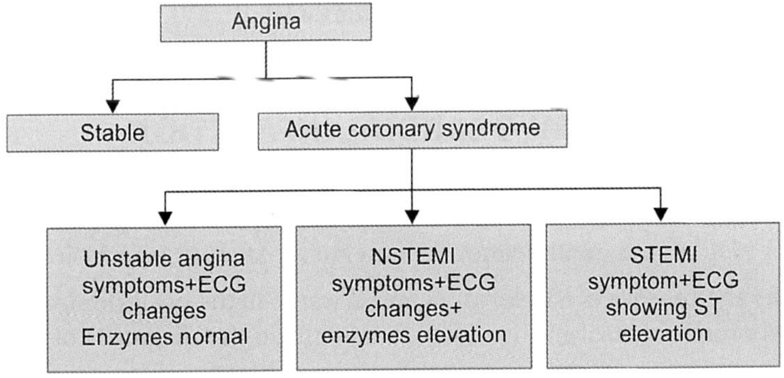

FLOWCHART 1: Spectrum of acute coronary syndromes.

that should arouse a suspicion of ACS. These symptoms, called angina equivalents include breathlessness, epigastric pain with vomiting, palpitations, presyncope and syncope.

EXAMINATION

- Look for features of hypoperfusion on examination, e.g., cold extremities, sweating, hypotension, altered sensorium, thready pulse, focal deficits
- Look for features of cardiac failure.

ECG Criteria for Diagnosis

- *STEMI*: New ST elevation at the J point in two anatomically contiguous leads with the following diagnostic cutoffs.
  - $\geq$1 mm elevation in all leads other than V_2 and V_3
  - In leads V_2 and V_3, the following ST elevation limits are needed for diagnosis
    - *In women*: $\geq$1.5 mm elevation
    - *In men >40 years*: $\geq$2 mm elevation
    - *In men <40 years*: $\geq$2.5 mm elevation
- NSTEMI/UA
  - New horizontal or down-sloping ST depression $\geq$0.5 mm in two anatomically contiguous leads or
  - T inversion 1 mm in two anatomically contiguous leads with prominent R wave or R/S ratio >1.
- Old MI (in the absence of LVH/LBBB)
  - Look for
    - Q wave in leads V_2 to V_3 $\geq$0.02 s or
    - QS complex in any 2 contiguous leads
    - Q wave $\geq$0.03 s and $\geq$1 mm deep in any two contiguous leads or
    - R wave $\geq$0.04 s in V_1 to V_2 and R/S $\geq$1 with a concordant positive T wave in the absence of a conduction defect.

Contiguous leads are defined as pairs or groups of leads that reflect the different walls of the heart. These are the inferior (II, III, aVF), lateral (I, aVL), and anterior leads (V_1–V_6).

POSTERIOR WALL MYOCARDIAL INFARCTION

Posterior infarction usually occurs along with an inferior or lateral infarction and is associated with an increased risk of LV dysfunction and death. Isolated posterior infarction is an indication for emergent coronary reperfusion.

ECG criteria: Presence of ST elevation and Q waves in the posterior leads (V_7–V_9). ST elevation of only 0.5 mm is required to confirm the diagnosis of a posterior wall MI.

INTRODUCTION

Pulmonary edema is a common and potentially fatal cause of acute respiratory distress. Patients with acute pulmonary edema need continuous cardiac monitoring.

"Flash" pulmonary edema is a term that is used to describe an acute onset of severe decompensated heart failure caused by acute increase in left ventricular (LV) diastolic pressure with rapid fluid accumulation in the pulmonary interstitial and alveolar spaces.

CAUSES

- *Cardiogenic:* Left ventricular failure, mitral stenosis
- *Noncardiogenic*: Infections (pneumonia), inhaled toxins, aspiration, acute radiation pneumonitis, hypoalbuminemia,
- *Unknown/incompletely understood*: High-altitude pulmonary edema, neurogenic pulmonary edema, narcotic overdose, postcardioversion

INVESTIGATIONS TO BE SENT

Complete blood count (CBC), electrolytes, creatinine, urea, troponin T, electrocardiogram (ECG), chest X-ray (CXR), and arterial blood gas (ABG).

MANAGEMENT

- Sit the patient up in bed.
- Start oxygen (O_2) therapy with 60–100% O_2 by face mask. Target SpO_2 94–98%
- Treat any hemodynamically unstable arrhythmia: Urgent synchronized cardioversion may be required.
- *Diuretics*: Furosemide 40–120 mg intravenous (IV) or torsemide 20–60 mg IV. Check systolic blood pressure (SBP) before giving furosemide. Administer only if SBP >100 mm Hg
- If the patient has arrhythmia/acute coronary syndrome (ACS), start heparin/ antiplatelets. If SBP >90 mm Hg, give glyceryl trinitrate (GTN) 5 mg sublingual or spray.
  Start GTN infusion at 5–10 µg/min and increase infusion rate every 15–20 minutes [target mean arterial pressure (MAP) around 70].

- If SBP is <90 mm Hg, treat as cardiogenic shock with noradrena line (0.1–0.5 µg/kg/min)/dopamine (5–20 µg/kg/min) infusion
- Consider dialysis if known oliguric renal failure or no response to furosemide in 4 hours or with rising creatinine.
- Start continuous positive airway pressure (CPAP) if severe type 1 failure [Start with FiO_2 of 100; PEEP of 5]. Invasive ventilation may be needed, if the patient deteriorates clinically.

HIGH ALTITUDE PULMONARY EDEMA (HAPE)

Exposure to high altitude (usually >2,000 meters) with physical exertion is a common cause of noncardiogenic pulmonary edema in unacclimatized yet otherwise healthy individuals. This condition is commonly seen in tourists visiting hill stations and in mountaineering expeditions and could be fatal. Symptoms include shortness of breath, nonproductive cough, headache, and decreased effort tolerance. The mechanism is unknown but hypoxia seems to play major role.

Acute mountain sickness (AMS) may manifest as nausea, vomiting, headache. High altitude cerebral edema (HACE) with features of ataxia, confusion resulting in coma may coexist with HAPE.

Management

- Descent to a lower altitude must be the highest priority
- For mild AMS, Tab. Acetazolamide 125–250 mg PO bd may help in speeding acclimatization
- Administer oxygen if available (2–4 L to maintain SpO_2 >90%)
- If oxygen is unavailable, nifedipine 10 mg PO q4-6h may be given for HAPE
- For HACE/HAPE, dexamethasone 4 mg PO/IV stat, then 4 mg q6h provides symptomatic relief
- Prophylactic inhalation of β2-agonists like Salmeterol reduces the incidence of HAPE

INTRODUCTION

Atrial fibrillation (AF) is one of the most common arrhythmias encountered in the ED and is characterized by an irregularly irregular pulse.

CLINICAL PRESENTATION

Atrial fibrillation may present with palpitations, chest pain, breathlessness, syncope, hypotension, and embolic episodes (stroke or peripheral embolus).

Management of the patient depends on the duration of the AF (if known).

There are four main types of AF:

1. *Paroxysmal*: Self terminating AF or with intervention within 7 days of onset, with recurrent episodes of variable frequency
2. *Persistent*: AF lasting more than 7 days and not self-terminating
3. *Long-term persistent*: AF lasting more than 12 months
4. *Permanent*: AF lasting more than 12 months with unsuccessful rhythm control interventions or decision made by patient and clinician not to pursue rhythm control.

ELECTROCARDIOGRAM CHARACTERISTICS

Atrial rate of about 300 beats per minute (bpm).

- Irregularly irregular rhythm
- Absent P waves
- Presence of fibrillation waves.

CAUSES

- *Underlying cardiac disease*: Rheumatic heart disease (RHD), ischemic heart disease (IHD), hypertension (HT), congestive cardiac failure (CCF), cardiomyopathy, and pericarditis.
- Thyrotoxicosis
- *Electrolyte imbalance*: Hypokalemia, and hypomagnesemia
- *Drugs*: Alcohol, and sympathomimetics.

INVESTIGATIONS TO BE SENT

- Complete blood count (CBC), electrolytes, creatinine, magnesium (Mg), thyroid-stimulating hormone (TSH), and chest X-ray (CXR)

- Cardiac enzymes and drug levels (digoxin), if needed
- Other investigations depend on suspected precipitant.

MANAGEMENT

- Stabilize airway, breathing, and circulation
- *Correct any electrolyte abnormality and metabolic acidosis*: Correct hypokalemia or hypomagnesemia if present. Sodium bicarbonate ($NaHCO_3$) for severe metabolic acidosis
- ***Rate and rhythm control*:**
  - *Patient with signs of unstable rhythm (hypotension/signs of shock/acutely altered sensorium/ischemic chest pain/acute heart failure)*: Synchronized cardioversion starting at 50 J, if no response, increase to 100 J, then 200 J, with adequate sedation (midazolam 2 mg IV or ketamine 1–2 mg/kg IV).
    - Do not attempt to cardiovert patients with known chronic AF, severe mitral stenosis (MS) and severe left ventricular (LV) dysfunction as chances of success are very low and risk of embolization is high.
    - If *DC shock fails initially*:
      - Attempt further DC shock with 200 J
      - Give Amiodarone 150 mg over 10 minutes followed by 1 mg/min infusion for 6 hours.
      - Check and correct electrolyte abnormalities.
  - *Hemodynamically stable patients or if cardioversion is contraindicated*: Rapid pharmacological rate control (target rate <110 bpm). Choose from one of the following drugs:
    - *Metoprolol*:
      - Intravenous metoprolol 2.5–5 mg over 2 minutes. Repeat every 5 minutes up to a maximum of 15 mg, if the patient tolerates the drug (no hypotension)
      - Oral metoprolol XL 25 mg stat and bd may be started in asymptomatic patients with mild tachycardia.
    - *Diltiazem*:
      - Intravenous diltiazem 20 mg over 2 minutes. If heart rate (HR) still >110 bpm, give a 35 mg bolus over 2 minutes. This regimen usually controls the ventricular rate within 4–5 minutes if the patient tolerates the drug (no hypotension)
      - Oral diltiazem 30 mg stat and q6h may be started in asymptomatic patients with mild tachycardia.
    - *Verapamil*:
      - Intravenous verapamil 5–10 mg over 2 minutes. Repeat dose every 15–30 minutes, if the patient tolerates the drug (no hypotension)
      - Oral verapamil 40 mg stat and tid may be started in asymptomatic patients with mild tachycardia.

- *Digoxin*:
    - Intravenous digoxin 0.5 mg in 50 mL normal saline (NS)/5% dextrose over 30 minutes. Repeat a 0.25 mg IV dose twice if needed (only in patients with AF due to RHD)
    - Oral digoxin 0.125 mg stat and od may be started in asymptomatic patients with mild tachycardia with pre-existent heart failure.
  - *Amiodarone*:
    - Can prevent recurrences in paroxysmal AF. Only used for rate control in chronic/persistent AF.
- *Assess the need for anticoagulation*:
  - All patients with AF due to RHD need to be anticoagulated
  - Use CHADSVasc score for all nonrheumatic AF to decide the need for anticoagulation (**Table 1**).
  - If indicated, start oral anticoagulation: Warfarin 5 mg od or sintrom 2 mg od
  - If anticoagulation not indicated, start aspirin 75 mg od
  - For chronic AF, oral anticoagulation needs to be given for 4 weeks prior and 3 weeks post-DC cardioversion.

TABLE 1: CHADSVasc score.

Condition	Points
• Congestive heart failure (or LV systolic dysfunction)	1
• *Hypertension*: BP >140/90 mm Hg (or treated hypertension on medication)	1
• Age 65–74 years	1
• Age ≥75 years	2
• Diabetes mellitus	1
• Sex category (i.e., female sex)	1
• Stroke in the past or TIA or thromboembolism	2
• Vascular disease (e.g., peripheral artery disease, MI, and aortic plaque)	1

Interpretation		
Score	Risk	Anticoagulation therapy
• 0 (male) or 1 (female)	Low	No anticoagulant therapy
• 1 (male)	Moderate	Oral anticoagulant should be considered
• 2 or greater	High	Oral anticoagulant is recommended

(BP: blood pressure; LV: left ventricular; MI: myocardial infarction; TIA: transient ischemic attack)

Source: Lip GY, Nieuwlaat R, Pisters R, Lane DA, Crijns HJ. Refining clinical risk stratification for predicting stroke and thromboembolism in atrial fibrillation using a novel risk factor-based approach: the euro heart survey on atrial fibrillation. Chest. 2010;137(2): 263-72.

Atrial Flutter

CHAPTER 40

INTRODUCTION

Atrial flutter is an abnormal cardiac rhythm characterized by rapid, regular atrial depolarization at a characteristic rate of approximately 300 beats per minute (bpm) and a regular ventricular rate of about 150 bpm [2:1 atrioventricular (AV) conduction] (**Fig. 1**).

CLINICAL MANIFESTATIONS

Palpitations, fatigue, lightheadedness, dyspnea, angina, hypotension, anxiety, presyncope, or infrequently syncope.

ELECTROCARDIOGRAM CHARACTERISTICS

- Atrial rate of about 300 bpm.
- Typical P waves are absent, and the atrial activity is seen as a saw-tooth pattern (also called F waves) in leads II, III, and aVF (**Table 1**).
- There is typically a 2:1 conduction across the AV node; as a result, the ventricular rate is usually one-half the flutter rate in the absence of AV node dysfunction.

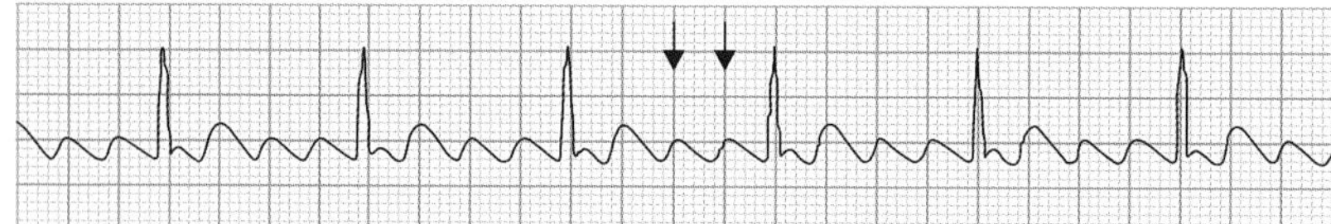

FIG. 1: Atrial flutter showing 4:1 conduction.

TABLE 1: Electrocardiogram characteristics of atrial flutter.

Heart rate	Rhythm	Baseline	QRS	Diagnosis
>100 bpm	Irregular/regular	Saw-tooth nature	<0.12 ms	Atrial flutter

MANAGEMENT

- *Hemodynamically stable patient*: Amiodarone 5 mg/kg in 5% dextrose over 30 minutes followed by 10 mg/kg over 23 hours.
  As in atrial fibrillation (AF), the major issues that must be addressed in atrial flutter are:
  - *Control of the ventricular rate*: Same as in AF
  - *Reversion to normal sinus rhythm*: Pharmacological or radiofrequency ablation
  - *Prevention of systemic embolization*: Same as in AF.
- *Patient with signs of unstable rhythm (hypotension/signs of shock/acutely altered sensorium/ischemic chest pain/acute heart failure):* Synchronized cardioversion starting at 50 J, if no response, increase to 100 J, then 200 J, with adequate sedation (midazolam 2 mg IV or ketamine 1–2 mg/kg IV).

Paroxysmal Supraventricular Tachycardia

INTRODUCTION

The term paroxysmal supraventricular tachycardia (PSVT) is applied to intermittent SVTs with abrupt onset and offset other than atrial fibrillation (AF), atrial flutter, and multifocal atrial tachycardia (MAT). PSVTs are often due to reentry, although the sites of reentry vary.

The major causes are:
- *Atrioventricular nodal reentrant tachycardia*: 60%
- *Atrioventricular reentrant (or reciprocating) tachycardia*: 30%
- *Atrial tachycardia or sinoatrial nodal reentrant tachycardia*: 10%.

The typical pattern of PSVT is shown in **Figure 1** and characteristics are shown in **Table 1**.

MANAGEMENT

Acute management of PSVT includes controlling the rate and preventing hemodynamic collapse.
- *Patient with signs of unstable rhythm (hypotension/signs of shock/acutely altered sensorium/ischemic chest pain/acute heart failure)*: Synchronized cardioversion starting at 25 J, if no response, increase to 100 J, then 150 J, with adequate sedation (midazolam 2 mg IV or ketamine 1–2 mg/kg IV).
- *Hemodynamically stable patient*:
   - Vagal maneuvers like breath-holding and the Valsalva maneuver (slow conduction in the atrioventricular (AV) node and can potentially interrupt the reentrant circuit).

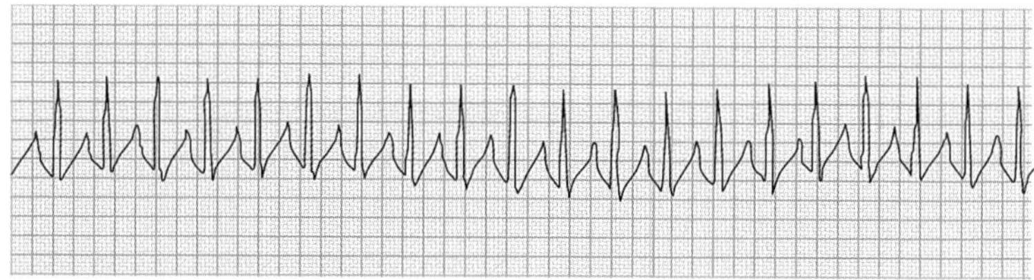

FIG. 1: Paroxysmal supraventricular tachycardia.

TABLE 1: Electrocardiogram characteristics of PSVT.				
Heart rate	*Rhythm*	*P wave*	*QRS*	*Diagnosis*
>100 bpm	Regular	Absent	<0.12 ms	Supraventricular tachycardia (SVT)

Carotid Massage

- External pressure on the carotid bulb stimulates baroreceptors in the carotid sinus, which triggers a reflex increase in vagus nerve activity and sympathetic withdrawal. The result is a temporary slowing of sinoatrial (SA) nodal activity and AV nodal conduction.
- The carotid sinus is usually located inferior to the angle of the mandible at the level of the thyroid cartilage. Apply steady pressure over one carotid sinus for 5–10 seconds.
- If there is no response, the procedure may be repeated on the other side after 1–2 minutes.
- This is generally safe and well-tolerated, but potential complications include profound hypotension, bradycardia, transient ischemic attack (TIA)/stroke, and arrhythmias.
- Do not perform the procedure if a carotid bruit is heard.

Adenosine

- Adenosine is a purine nucleoside base that markedly decreases heart rate and prolongs atrioventricular (AV)—nodal conduction.
- This drug is administered by rapid intravenous (IV) injection over 1–2 seconds through a peripheral line (preferably brachial) followed by a normal saline flush using a three-way stopcock.
- The patient should be supine and should have electrocardiogram (ECG) and blood pressure (BP) monitoring.
- The half-life of adenosine is very short (10–20 s) as it is rapidly cleared from plasma by rapid intracellular metabolism. Hence the need for a normal saline flush after administration to reach the heart faster.
- Dose of adenosine:
  - The usual initial dose in adults is 6 mg (100 µg/kg in children)
  - If not successful, administer a second dose of 12 mg (200 µg/kg in children) after 1–2-minutes
  - If not successful, administer a third dose of 12 mg (300 µg/kg in children) after 1–2 minutes

  Note: If a central IV access site is used, the initial dose should not exceed 3 mg.
- *Contraindications*: Sinus node disease, second- or third-degree heart blocks, long QT syndrome, hypotension, bronchial asthma/COPD
- *Side effects*: Mild side effects include flushing, chest discomfort, dyspnea, metallic taste, and a sense of "impending doom"
  - *Magnesium* may also be given both to correct a deficiency and also as a therapeutic agent for cardiac arrhythmias. Dose is 2 g IV over 5–10 minutes.
  - Alternatives to adenosine for the acute treatment of SVT include calcium channel blockers (CCBs) (verapamil/diltiazem) and beta-blockers (metoprolol or esmolol).
    - In cases of recurrent PSVT—attempt radiofrequency ablation (high success rates).

Wide Complex Tachycardias

42

CHAPTER

INTRODUCTION

Wide complex tachycardias (WCT) refer to dysrhythmias at a ventricular rate >100/min and are characterized by QRS >0.12 seconds. WCT are usually associated with ischemic heart disease or acute myocardial infarction and include ventricular tachycardia (VT) and ventricular fibrillation (VF) (**Table 1**). These WCT originate in the ventricles, but a supra-ventricular tachycardia (SVT) can also produce a WCT if associated with a conduction abnormality/aberrancy.

Ventricular Tachycardia

Ventricular tachycardia may be classified as monomorphic or polymorphic.

- *Monomorphic VT*: The QRS complexes are regular in pattern and at a rate of 150–200/min. Monomorphic VT can be classified as sustained and non-sustained.
  - *Sustained VT*: Defined as WCT lasting >30 seconds in duration or causing hemodynamic instability
  - *Non-sustained VT*: Defined as WCT >3 beats and lasting <30 seconds in duration
- Polymorphic VT: The QRS complexes vary in shape and structure in the same lead.
  - *Torsades de pointes*: This is a specific variant of polymorphic VT in which the QRS axis swings from a positive to negative direction in a single lead. Drugs that prolong repolarization (prolong QT interval) such as quinidine, disopyramide, procainamide, phenothiazines, and tricyclic antidepressants can trigger this arrhythmia.

Ventricular Fibrillation

Ventricular fibrillation refers to a totally disorganized depolarization and contraction of a small area of the ventricular myocardium. ECG shows a fine or

TABLE 1: Characteristics of wide complex tachycardias.

Condition	Heart rate (HR)	Baseline	P wave	QRS
Ventricular tachycardia	>100 bpm	Regular	Lost in QRS complex	>0.12 ms
Ventricular fibrillation	No pulse	Wavers unevenly	Absent	Absent
Torsades de pointes	>100 bpm	Varying amplitude and axis	Lost in QRS complex	>0.12 ms

a coarse zigzag pattern without distinguishable P waves or QRS complexes. It is never associated with a pulse or blood pressure.

MANAGEMENT

Ventricular Tachycardia (Fig. 1)

- *Patient with signs of unstable rhythm (hypotension signs of shock/acutely altered sensorium/ischemic chest pain/acute heart failure)*: Synchronized cardioversion starting at 100 J, if no response, increase to 150 J, then 200 J, with adequate sedation (midazolam 2 mg IV or ketamine 1–2 mg/kg IV).
- *Hemodynamically stable patient*:
  - *Monomorphic VT*:
    - Adenosine 6 mg intravenous (IV) rapid bolus followed by 12 mg IV bolus. Consider Adenosine ONLY if regular and monomorphic.
    - If no response, give Amiodarone 150 mg over10 minutes followed by 1 mg/min infusion for 6 hours.
    - If no response, give Magnesium sulfate ($MgSO_4$) 2 g IV over 3–5 minutes.
    - If no response, give Lignocaine 100 mg IV push.
    - If no response to the earlier drugs, try Synchronized cardioversion with 100 J, with adequate sedation (midazolam 2 mg IV or ketamine 1–2 mg/kg IV).
  - Polymorphic VT with long QT (Torsades de pointes) (**Fig. 2**):
    - Magnesium sulfate 2 g IV over 3–5 minutes
    - Amiodarone 150 mg over 10 minutes followed by 1 mg/min infusion for 6 hours.
    - If no response, give Lidocaine 1–1.5 mg/kg IV.

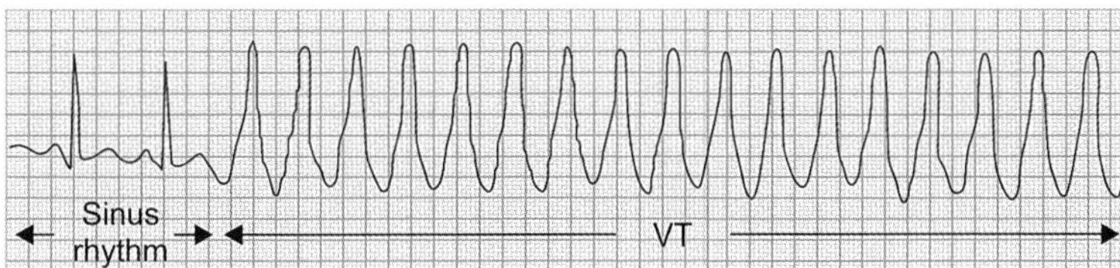

FIG. 1: Ventricular tachycardia.

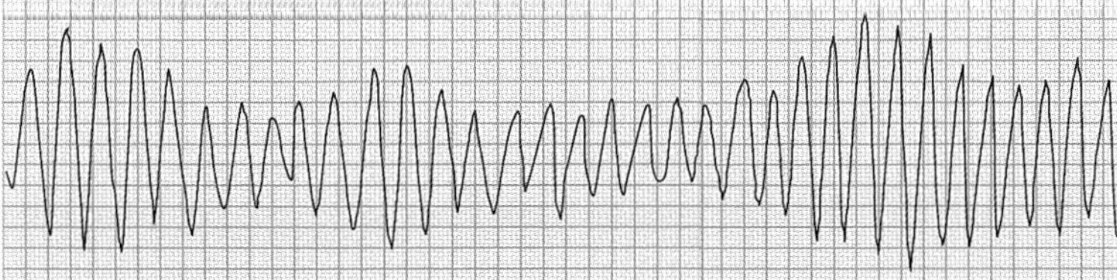

FIG. 2: Torsades de pointes.

- If no response to the earlier drugs, give Unsynchronized cardioversion with 200 J, with adequate sedation (midazolam 2 mg IV or ketamine 1–2 mg/kg IV).
- Other drugs that may be tried in refractory cases are beta blockers, calcium channel blockers, and phenytoin.

Ventricular Fibrillation (Fig. 3)

- Follow ACLS protocol for cardiac arrest and, defibrillate with 200 J
- Amiodarone 300 mg IV bolus after the third shock (refer ACLS guidelines)

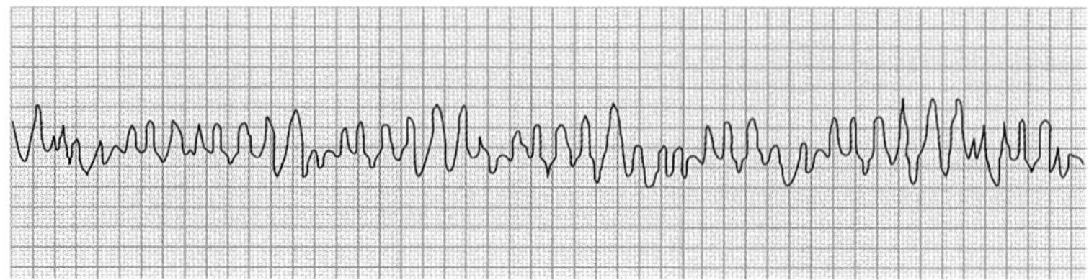

FIG. 3: Ventricular fibrillation.

A summary of electrical energy dosage required for cardioversion of different arrhythmias is shown in **Table 2**.

TABLE 2: Summary of electrical energy dosage.			
Rhythm	*Monophasic*	*Biphasic*	*Synchronized*
Initial energy (escalate if needed)			
Narrow complex regular (SVT, atrial flutter)	50–100 J	50–100 J	Yes
Narrow complex irregular (AF)	200 J	120–200 J	Yes
Wide regular (VT)	100 J	100 J	Yes
Wide irregular (VF)	360 J	200 J	No

(AF: atrial fibrillation; SVT: supraventricular tachycardia; VF: ventricular fibrillation; VT: ventricular tachycardia)

Valvular Emergencies

INTRODUCTION

Acute valvular emergencies can be divided into two primary categories:
1. Native valve emergencies
2. Prosthetic valve emergencies.

NATIVE VALVE EMERGENCIES

Native acute onset valvular emergencies are almost always regurgitant in nature. However, patients with inadequately treated chronic mitral stenosis (MS) may present to the ED with worsening of congestive cardiac failure.

- *Acute aortic regurgitation*:
  - *Causes*: Infective endocarditis, rupture of sinus of Valsalva, aortic dissection involving the root of the aorta
  - *Clinical features*: Features of cardiac failure, loud P2, and left ventricular (LV) third heart sound (S3). No cardiomegaly.
- *Acute mitral regurgitation*:
  - *Causes*: Chordal rupture, papillary muscle rupture, acute endocarditis, and blunt chest trauma
  - *Clinical features*: Pulmonary edema, hypotension, and LV S3. No cardiomegaly.

Investigations

Electrocardiogram (ECG), ECHO, chest X-ray (CXR), cardiac enzymes to rule out acute coronary syndrome (ACS), electrolytes, creatinine, and complete blood count (CBC).

Management

Regurgitant Lesions

- Manage cardiogenic shock and cardiac failure
- An intra-aortic balloon pump can be used in acute mitral regurgitation (MR) to decrease aortic impedance and regurgitant fraction.
- Beta-blockers contraindicated in acute regurgitant lesions as the slower heart rate increases the duration of diastole during which the regurgitation happens.
- Take blood cultures and empirically start treatment for infective endocarditis (IE) if patient has fever with peripheral features suggestive of IE
- Definitive treatment is surgery and replacing the valve.

Mitral Stenosis

Medical management of MS includes diuretic therapy to alleviate pulmonary congestion, control of atrial fibrillation and anticoagulation for patients at risk of arterial embolic events. Primary treatment for symptomatic MS is mechanical intervention by balloon mitral valvotomy (BMV), valve repair or valve replacement.

PROSTHETIC VALVE EMERGENCIES

Mechanical and biologic prostheses in any location are vulnerable to acute paravalvular regurgitant disease as a result of either suture failure or valve dehiscence related to endocarditis. Mechanical prostheses can have acute stenosis due to either pannus or acute thrombosis.

- *Acute valvular thrombus and embolism*: High-risk period is up to 3 months postoperative. Stroke or pulmonary embolism may occur and is usually seen in those who are noncompliant with anticoagulation.
  - *Treatment*: Optimize anticoagulation to attain a therapeutic international normalized ratio (INR) of 3–4.
- *Acute obstructive valve thrombus*: This is also seen in those with subtherapeutic anticoagulation. The onset may be gradual or sudden onset with dyspnea and fatigue. Embolic events may occur.
  - *Clinical diagnosis*: Auscultate for absence of prosthetic valve click, a strong indicator of prosthetic valve stenosis/occlusion.
  - *Diagnosis*: Urgent ECHO, to look for gradient across the prosthetic valve
  - *Treatment*: Surgery if obstructive, thrombosed, left-sided prosthetic heart valve causing New York Heart Association (NYHA) class III to IV symptoms. Urgency of the surgical intervention depends on how acute and how severe the presentation is.
    - Fibrinolytic therapy if obstructive, thrombosed, left-sided prosthetic valve caused recent onset (<14 days) NYHA class I to II symptoms, and a small thrombus (<0.8 cm^2).
    - Emergency surgery if thrombosed, left-sided prosthetic heart valve with a mobile or large thrombus ($\geq$0.8 cm^2).
    - Fibrinolytic therapy for obstructive thrombosed, right-sided prosthetic heart valves.
- *Valve regurgitation or paravalvular regurgitation*: This may be seen early postoperative period or due to infective endocarditis. Presents with a change in prosthetic sounds, dyspnea, or other signs of heart failure. Treatment includes managing the failure and surgical correction.

Basics of Electrocardiogram

HOW TO CALCULATE HEART RATE?

- *For regular rhythms*: In Lead II
    - 300/number of big squares between RR or
    - 1,500/number of small squares between RR.
- *For irregular rhythms*: In Lead II, number of R waves in 30 consecutive big squares × 10

WHAT IS A NORMAL SINUS RHYTHM?

The following are the characteristics of a normal sinus rhythm
- Regular rhythm at a rate of 60–100 bpm in adults
- Each QRS complex is preceded by a normal P wave.
- P waves should be upright in leads I and II and inverted in aVR (Normal P wave axis)
- PR interval remains constant.
- QRS complexes are <100 ms wide

HOW TO INTERPRET THE AXIS?

Look at QRS in lead I and aVF and see if it is predominantly positive or negative.
- *Lead I positive plus aVF positive*: Normal axis (0° to +90°)
- *Lead I negative plus aVF positive*: Right axis deviation (+90° to +180°)
- *Lead I positive plus aVF negative*: Left axis deviation (0° to –90°)
- *Lead I negative plus aVF negative*: Extreme right axis deviation (–90° to +180°) (**Figs. 1A** and **B**).

NORMAL DURATIONS

- **P wave duration**: <120 ms; It represents atrial depolarization
- **PR interval:** 120–200 ms; It represents the time taken for the electrical impulse to be conducted through the AV node
- **QRS complex:** 70–100 ms; It represents ventricular depolarization
- **QT interval:** Up to 440 ms; It represents the duration of time taken for the ventricles to depolarize and repolarize

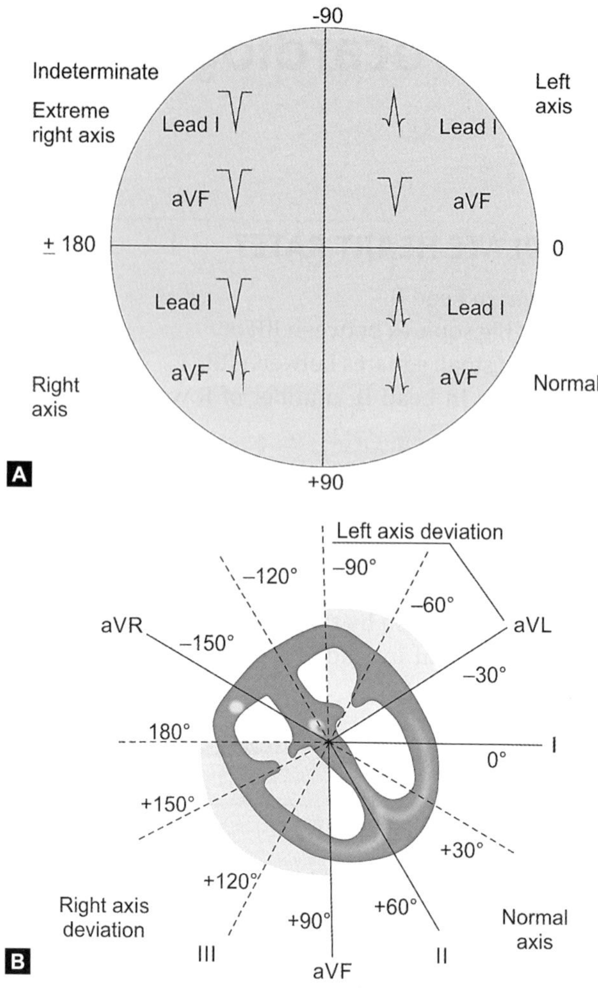

FIGS. 1A AND B: (A) Electrocardiogram (ECG) axis deviation diagram; (B) ECG axis.

P Wave

A P wave, by convention is the first positive deflection in the ECG complex. It represents atrial depolarization. A normal P wave, P pulmonale and P mitrale are shown in **Figure 2**.

A normal P wave shows the following characteristics:
- <120 ms in duration (3 small squares)
- <2.5 mm amplitude in the limb leads
- <1.5 mm amplitude in the chest leads
- Positive in lead II and negative in lead AVR

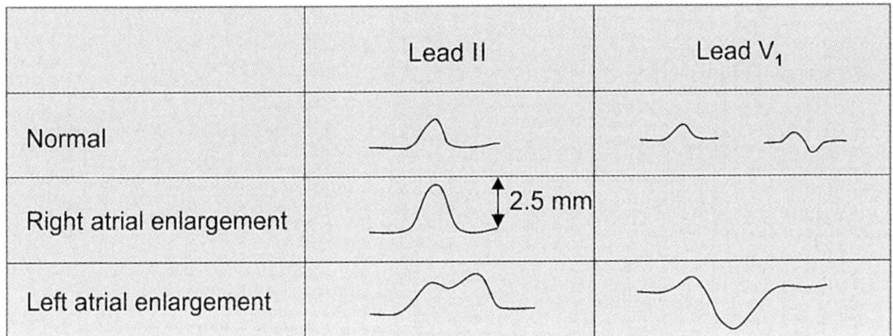

FIG. 2: Right and left atrial enlargements in lead II and lead V_1.

P pulmonale: This is a typical finding of right atrial enlargement (e.g., COPD, pulmonary hypertension, tricuspid stenosis) and is characterized by:
- P wave amplitude in inferior leads (II, III and AVF) >2.5 mm; or
- P wave amplitude in lead V_1 and V_2 >1.5 mm

P mitrale: This is a typical finding of left atrial enlargement (e.g., mitral stenosis) and is characterized by:
- P wave duration in lead II >120 ms; or
- Biphasic P wave in lead V_1

Q Wave

A Q wave, by convention is the first negative deflection in the ECG complex. It represents the normal left-to-right depolarization of the interventricular septum. A normal Q wave shows the following characteristics:
- <40 ms wide (1 small square)
- <2 mm in amplitude
- <25% of the depth of the QRS complex

Q waves can normally be present in leads III and aVR. They are considered to be pathological, if they are >0.04 seconds (1 small square) in duration or >1/4 of the height of the subsequent R wave.

R Wave

The first positive deflection in the QRS complex is called an R wave. It represents depolarization of the thick ventricular walls and is the largest wave of the QRS complex.

S Wave

A negative deflection after an R wave is called an S wave.
It represents depolarization of the Purkinje fibers and is usually a small wave.

T Wave

T wave is a positive deflection after a QRS complex. It represents ventricular repolarization.

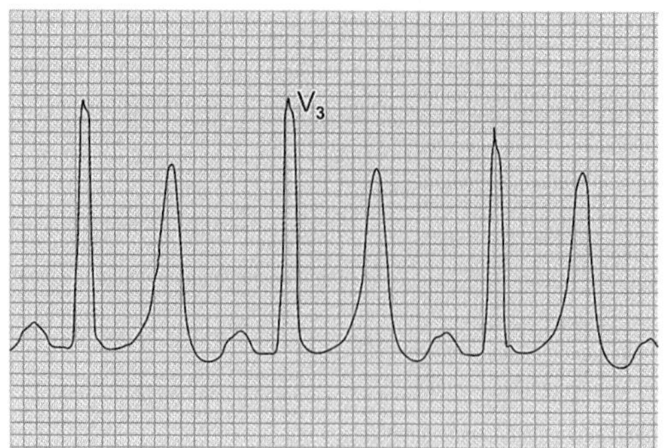

FIG. 3: Peaked T waves.

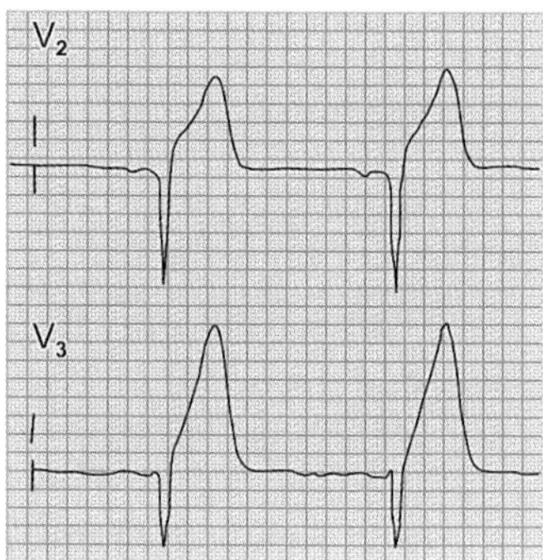

FIG. 4: Hyperacute T waves.

T waves are upright in all leads except aVR and V_1. T wave amplitude is normally <5 mm in limb leads and <10 mm in precordial leads.

Peaked T waves: Tall, narrow and symmetrically peaked T waves are seen in hyperkalemia (**Fig. 3**).

Hyperacute T waves: Broad, asymmetrically peaked T waves are seen in early STEMI (**Fig. 4**).

LEFT VENTRICULAR HYPERTROPHY(LVH) DIAGNOSTIC CRITERIA

Any of the following voltage criteria must be met to diagnose LVH.
- S wave in V_1 + R wave in V_5 or V_6 >35 mm (Sokolov Lyon criteria)
- S wave in V_3 + R wave in aVL >28 mm in men or >20 mm in women (Cornell voltage criteria)
- R wave in aVL >11 mm

Additional ECG findings usually seen in LVH are left atrial enlargement and left axis deviation.

LEFT BUNDLE BRANCH BLOCK (LBBB) DIAGNOSTIC CRITERIA

- Broad QRS complex (>120 ms)
- Dominant S wave in lead V_1
- Broad, monophasic 'M' shaped R wave in lateral leads (I, AVL, V_5, and V_6)
- Prolonged R wave peak time >60 ms in left precordial leads (V_5–V_6)
- Absence of Q waves in lateral leads (I, V_5, and V_6)

LBBB is almost always pathological, common causes being ischemic heart disease, anterior wall MI, aortic stenosis, hypertension, dilated cardiomyopathy, hyperkalemia, and digoxin toxicity.

RIGHT BUNDLE BRANCH BLOCK (RBBB) DIAGNOSTIC CRITERIA

- Broad QRS complex (>120 ms)
- RSR' pattern in leads V_1–V_3 ('M' shaped QRS complex)
- Wide, slurred S wave in the lateral leads – I, AVL, V_5 and V_6 ('W'-shaped QRS complex)

RBBB can be a normal finding in young, healthy people. Pathological causes include ischemic heart disease, rheumatic heart disease, corpulmonale, pulmonary embolism, myocarditis, and atrial septal disease.

BRUGADA SYNDROME

Brugada syndrome is a rhythm abnormality with a high incidence of sudden cardiac arrest in people with structurally normal hearts. This syndrome results from an inherited disorder of sodium channels and is usually seen in middle aged people. The typical ECG pattern is a coved ST segment elevation >2 mm in >1 of V_1–V_3 followed by a negative T wave (Brugada sign) (**Fig. 5**). Syncope and sudden cardiac arrest due to Brugada syndrome can often be triggered by fever, hypokalemia, hypothermia or drugs such as flecainide, propafenone, beta blockers, alpha blockers, calcium channel blockers, nitrates, cocaine and alcohol. The only definitive treatment is an implantable cardioverter defibrillator (ICD).

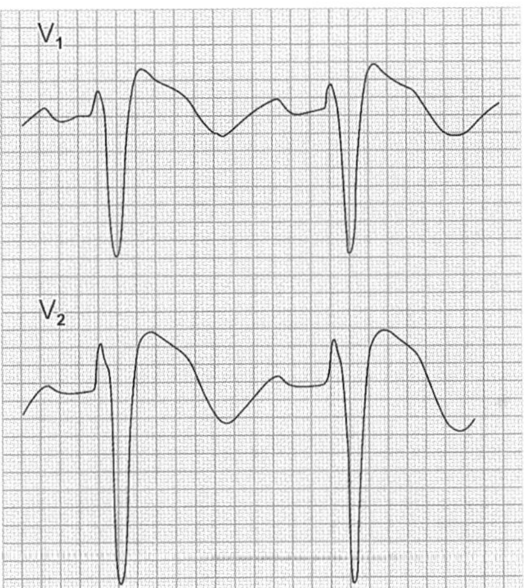

FIG. 5: Brugada sign.

Respiratory Emergencies

Bronchial Asthma

45
CHAPTER

INTRODUCTION

Asthma is a chronic inflammatory disorder characterized by airway hyperresponsiveness, variable airflow obstruction, and reversibility with bronchodilators.

CLINICAL FEATURES

Clinical features include recurrent episodes of chest tightness, breathless- ness, wheezing, and cough.

The following are the differences between asthma and chronic obstructive pulmonary disease (COPD) (**Table 1**).

TABLE 1: Differences between asthma and COPD.		
	Asthma	*COPD*
Age of onset	Children and young adults	Older age (>40 years)
Allergy/Atopy	Common	Uncommon
Family history	Common	Uncommon
Smoking association	Not causal, but may exacerbate	Yes, usually >10 pack years
Chronic productive sputum	Uncommon	Common
Airway inflammation	Eosinophilic	Neutrophilic
Airflow obstruction on spirometry	Reversible	Minimal or no reversibility
Disease course	Stable with exacerbations	Progressive worsening with exacerbations
Role of bronchodilators	Needed for immediate relief, can be taken as required	Regular therapy warranted
Response to steroids	Essential for disease control	Helpful in moderate to severe disease, and for acute exacerbations

CLASSIFICATION OF ACUTE ASTHMA

- *Life-threatening asthma*:
  - Peak expiratory flow rate (PEFR) less than 33% of best or predicted
  - Peripheral capillary oxygen saturation (SpO_2) <92%, normocapnic
  - Silent chest, cyanosis, and poor respiratory effort
  - Bradycardia, arrhythmia, and hypotension
  - Exhaustion, confusion, and coma.
- *Near-fatal*:
  - Raised partial pressure of arterial carbon dioxide ($PaCO_2$) requiring mechanical ventilation.
- *Acute severe asthma*:
  - Peak expiratory flow 33–50% of best or predicted
  - Respiratory rate >25 breaths/min
  - Pulse rate >110 beats/min
  - Not able to talk in sentences (cannot complete sentence in one breath).
- *Moderate exacerbation*:
  - PEFR 50–75% of best or predicted
  - Talks in phrases
  - Respiratory rate <25 breaths/min
  - Pulse rate <110 beats/min.

All that wheezes is not asthma!! Think of:
- Upper airway obstruction
- Foreign body aspiration
- Endobronchial malignancy
- Pulmonary edema: Cardiac asthma
- Chronic obstructive pulmonary disease.

The interpretation of spirometry used to confirm the diagnosis of asthma is shown in **Flowchart 1**.

INVESTIGATIONS

- Complete blood count (CBC)
- Creatinine
- Electrolytes
- Chest X-ray
- Electrocardiogram
- Arterial blood gas (ABG) only for moderate-to-severe asthma
- Do not do an ABG for mild cases of asthma.

MANAGEMENT OF ACUTE ASTHMA

- Stabilize airway, breath, and circulation (ABC)
- High-flow oxygen: Maintain $SpO_2 > 94\%$

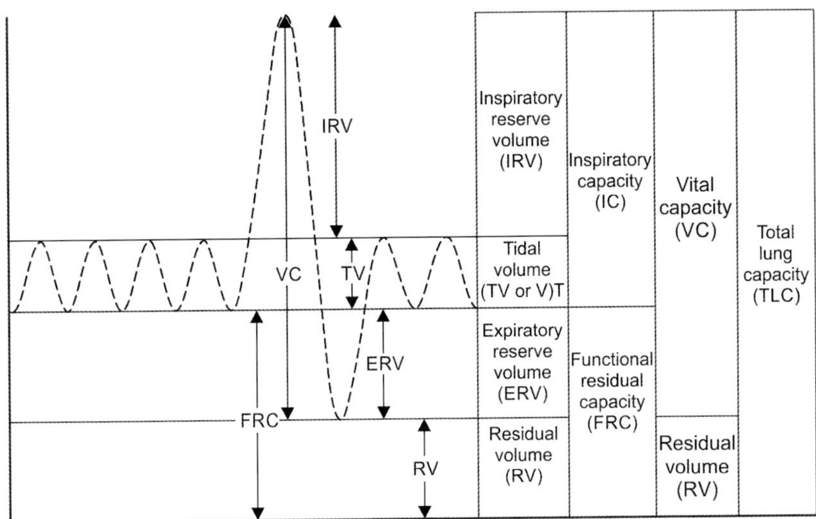

FIG. 1: Lung volumes on spirometry.

Source: Wikimedia Commons. (2011). LungVolume.jpg. [Online]. Available from: http://creativecommons. org/licenses/by-sa/3.0. [Last Accessed April, 2021].

Tidal Volume (TV): Refers to the volume of air drawn into and out of the lungs during normal breathing. Typically, 500 mL in a 70 kg man.

Inspiratory reserve volume (IRV): Refers to the additional volume of air that can be inspired at the end of a normal inspiration. Typically, 3,300 mL in a 70 kg man.

Expiratory reserve volume (ERV): Refers to the additional volume of air that can be expelled at the end of a normal expiration. Typically, 1,700 mL in a 70 kg man.

Residual volume (RV): Refers to the volume of air remaining in the lungs after a maximal expiration. Typically, 1,800 mL in a 70 kg man.

Vital capacity (VC): Refers to the maximum tidal volume when an individual breathes in and out as far as possible. Typically, 5,500 mL in a 70 kg man. VC = IRV + TV + ERV.

Total lung capacity (TLC): Refers to the volume of air in the lungs after a maximum inspiration. Typically, 7,500 mL in a 70 kg man. TLC = VC + RV.

Pulmonary Embolism

INTRODUCTION

Acute pulmonary embolism (PE) is a form of venous thromboembolism to the pulmonary artery or one of its branches and can be fatal. The source of the embolus is usually a thrombus originating in the deep veins of the lower limbs or pelvic veins. These emboli may lodge at the bifurcation of the main pulmonary artery or in the smaller lobar branches.

CLINICAL PRESENTATION

The most common presenting symptom is dyspnea, followed by pleuritic pain, cough, hemoptysis, and symptoms of deep venous thrombosis.

A high index of suspicion is needed in patients with risk factors and unexplained hypoxia. Use the modified Wells scoring system to assess the probability of pulmonary embolism (**Table 1**).

TABLE 1: Modified Wells scoring system for clinical assessment of suspected pulmonary embolism (PE).

Parameter	Points
Clinical symptoms of deep venous thrombosis (DVT) (leg swelling, pain on palpation)	3
Other diagnosis less likely than pulmonary embolism	3
Heart rate >100 beats/min	1.5
Immobilization (≥3 days) or surgery in the previous 4 weeks	1.5
Previous DVT/PE	1.5
Hemoptysis	1
Malignancy	1
Probability	**Score**
PE likely	> 4.0
PE unlikely	≤ 4.0

- *Immunologic lung diseases*: Goodpasture syndrome, Wegener's granulomatosis, systemic lupus erythematosus (SLE), and microscopic polyangiitis.
- *Cardiac and vascular diseases*: Pulmonary arteriovenous (AV) malformation, pulmonary embolism, mitral stenosis (MS), and aortic dissection.

MANAGEMENT

Airway

The most lethal sequelae of hemoptysis is hypoxia due to ventilation-perfusion match that occurs due to small airways and alveoli getting flooded with blood.

Administer supplemental oxygen to maintain SpO_2 >94%.

If hemoptysis is life threatening, secure the airway by a large-diameter endotracheal tube (ETT), 8 mm or larger to allow for bronchoscopy. If the bleeding persists and the bleeding side can be localized, advance the ETT into the main stem bronchus of the non-bleeding side to improve ventilation. The right main stem bronchus is easier to enter than the left bronchus.

Breathing

In patients with a known lateralizing source of bleeding, a mitigating 'lung down' approach can be employed in which the patient is positioned with the bleeding lung in the dependant position. This promotes and protects the unaffected lung and improves oxygenation.

Circulation

Massive hemorrhage can result in hemodynamic instability.
- Secure an IV access with a large bore cannula and administer crystalloids.
- Consider blood transfusions in patients with massive hemoptysis. Correct any coagulopathy, if present
- Administer injection tranexamic acid 1 g intravenous (IV) bolus followed by oral tranexamic acid 500 mg q6h

Antibiotics

Consider antibiotics for mild haemoptysis due to bronchitis or bronchiectasis if there is any evidence of a bacterial infection

Bronchoscopy

Early bronchoscopy performed at the bedside facilitates direct visualization of the central airways and allows therapeutic intervention. These include injection of vasoactive agents, balloon and topical haemostatic tamponade and thermocoagulation.

CT Chest

If the patient is hemodynamically stable, CT chest gives valuable information in localizing the site of bleeding and can guide bronchial artery embolization, if required.

Interventional Angiography

Bronchial artery embolization is the first line therapy for patients unable to tolerate bronchoscopy or surgery. Massive bleeding due to tuberculosis and bronchiectasis respond well. Rare complications include dissection and arterial perforation.

Neurological Emergencies

Cerebrovascular Accidents

INTRODUCTION

Cerebrovascular accidents include ischemic stroke and hemorrhagic stroke.
- *Ischemic stroke*: 80% of all strokes
- *Hemorrhagic stroke*: 20% of all strokes.

Transient ischemic attack (TIA) is a brief episode of neurologic dysfunction resulting from focal temporary cerebral ischemia not associated with cerebral infarction. In patients presenting with a TIA or stroke, use the ABCD2 score to prognosticate and predict the recurrence of stroke within the next 2 days (**Table 1**).

INVESTIGATIONS

A magnetic resonance imaging (MRI) stroke protocol or plain (computed tomography) CT brain may be done to confirm the diagnosis (**Flowchart 1**).

TABLE 1: ABCD2 score.

Age older than 60 years	1 point
BP: Systolic blood pressure ≥140 mm Hg or Diastolic blood pressure ≥90 mm Hg	1 point
• **C**linical unilateral weakness	2 points
• Speech impairment without weakness	1 point
Duration of TIA	
• ≥60 minutes	2 points
• 10–59 minutes	1 point
• <10 minutes	0 point
Diabetes	1 point

Stroke risk (In the next 48 h):
Scores 0–3: Low risk 1%
Scores 4–5: Moderate risk 4%
Scores 6–7: High risk 8%

(TIA: transient ischemic attack; BP: blood pressure).

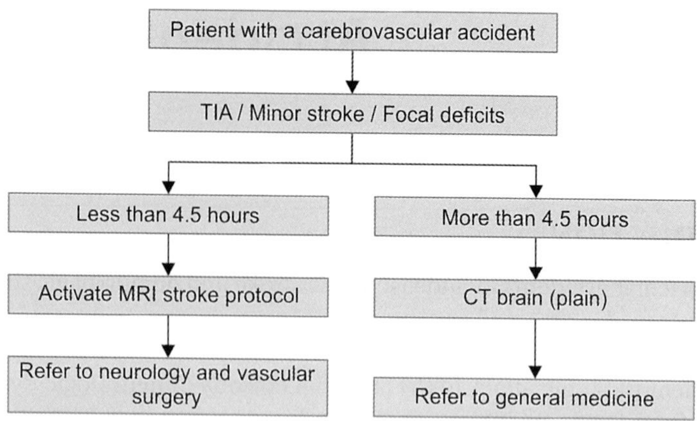

FLOWCHART 1: Stroke protocol in the emergency department.

MANAGEMENT OF HEMORRHAGIC STROKE

- *Antihypertensives*: Lower the blood pressure aggressively to target SBP of 140–160 mm Hg. Injection Labetalol 20 mg IV bolus and repeat if needed or tablet Nifedipine Retard 10–20 mg PO
- Start anticonvulsants (phenytoin or levetiracetam) if the bleed is in the cerebral cortex or has extended into the ventricles.
- Consider antiedema measures if there is a significant midline shift. Use either hypertonic saline or mannitol
  - 3% NaCl 100 mL over 30 minutes, then 100 mL infusion over 4 hours
  - 20% Mannitol 100–200 mL over 10 minutes followed by 100 mL every 8 hours
- Indications to refer neurosurgery for possibility of decompression surgery
  - Large bleed with midline shift
  - Cerebellar bleed greater than 3 cm
  - Intraventricular extension.

MANAGEMENT OF ISCHEMIC STROKE

Antihypertensives: Do not lower the BP aggressively unless the BP ≥185/110 mm Hg (for patients eligible for reperfusion therapy) or ≥220/120 mm Hg (for patients not eligible for reperfusion therapy).

Administer tablet Nifedipine Retard 10–20 mg PO or Injection Labetalol 10–20 mg IV over 1–2 min and repeat once if needed. However, remember that a very rapid reduction in BP may worsen the deficits by extending the infarct into the surrounding ischemic penumbra.

If not eligible for reperfusion therapy or >4.5 h from onset of symptoms:
- Tablet Aspirin (chewable) 150 mg PO stat followed by 75 mg od
- Tablet Atorvastatin 40 mg PO stat followed by 20 mg HSOD

If eligible for reperfusion therapy (<4.5 h from onset of symptoms):

Fibrinolytic therapy: Intravenous thrombolysis with recombinant tissue plasminogen activator (rtPA) at a doose of 0.9 mg/kg (10% as bolus and rest as infusion over 1 h) remains the first choice therapy.

Endovascular therapy: Intra-arterial rtPA, percutaneous angiographic clot removal (mechanical thrombectomy) and sonothrombolysis have all shown to have clinical benefit and can be used when expertise is available.

Contraindications for thrombolysis:
- Coma with complete hemiplegia
- Systolic blood pressure (SBP) >180 mm Hg or diastolic blood pressure (DBP) >110 mm Hg (consider thrombolysis if BP decreases)
- Clinical presentation suggestive of subarachnoid hemorrhage (SAH) even if the CT scan is normal
- Presumed septic embolus
- Heparin medication within the last 48 hours and has an elevated activated partial thromboplastin time aPTT
- International normalized ratio (INR) >1.7
- Known advanced liver disease and advanced right heart failure
- Platelet count <100,000 cells/mm^3
- Serum glucose <2.8 mmol/L or >22.0 mmol/L.

Malignant middle cerebral artery (MCA) infarct: This denotes a large MCA infarction, with or without involvement of the ipsilateral anterior cerebral artery (ACA) or posterior cerebral artery (PCA) territories that results in cerebral edema in the first 48 hours after a CVA, resulting in elevated intracranial pressure (ICP) or brain herniation. An infarct larger than two thirds of the MCA territory usually results in a malignant infarct.

If the patient has a malignant MCA infarct, do not give aspirin/clopidogrel. Approximately, 10% of ischemic strokes are classified as malignant or massive because of the presence of space-occupying cerebral edema that is severe enough to produce elevated intracranial pressure and brain herniation. Refer to neurosurgeon for decompressive craniotomy.

POSTERIOR CIRCULATION STROKE

Posterior circulation strokes are less common than anterior and middle cerebral artery strokes. Because of the variation in presentation and frequent transient nature of symptoms, posterior circulation strokes are often missed in the emergency department (ED). Hence, a high index of suspicion is needed in patients presenting with vertigo, cranial nerve deficits, especially sudden onset visual field deficits, etc.

Areas Supplied by the Posterior Circulation

Areas supplied by the posterior circulation are brainstem (medulla, pons, and midbrain), cerebellum, occipital cortex, inferior temporal lobe, and thalamus.

Symptoms

- Vertigo and nystagmus
- Ataxia and unsteadiness
- *Crossed syndromes*: Ipsilateral cranial nerve lesions with contralateral pyramidal or sensory tract lesions
- Sensory deficits (numbness, paresthesia) in the limbs or face
- *Visual field deficits*: Homonymous hemianopia, gun barrel vision
- Cranial nerve deficits.

Management

Treatment of a posterior circulation stroke is the same as that of any ischemic or hemorrhagic stroke. The important fact to remember is that the posterior fossa is a very tight space. Hence, a large infarct or bleed in the cerebellum may result in a significant increase in the intracranial pressure (ICP). Hence, a decompressive craniectomy may be required. Refer to neurosurgeon.

When to Refer

- Activate stroke protocol (neurology, radiology, and vascular surgery) for any patient presenting within 4.5 hours with a stroke or TIA
- In case of intracranial bleeds (parenchymal) inform both neurosurgery and medicine. If surgical intervention is required, neurosurgery will be the primary unit. If no surgical intervention is needed, medicine will be the primary unit.

Cerebral Venous Thrombosis

INTRODUCTION

- Cerebral venous thrombosis (CVT) refers to thrombosis of the dural sinus and/or cerebral veins. It is a very challenging condition to diagnose in the emergency department.
- Cerebral blood is drained by the superficial and deep venous systems into the major dural sinuses (superior sagittal sinus, inferior sagittal sinus, lateral sinus, cavernous sinus and straight sinus) and eventually into the internal jugular vein (IJV).
- Symptoms of CVT depend on the location and acuity of thrombus formation in the cerebral veins or dural sinuses.

RISK FACTORS

- Prothrombotic conditions (antithrombin III, protein C, and protein deficiency, antiphospholipid and anticardiolipin antibodies, factor V Leiden gene mutation, prothrombin G20210A mutation, hyperhomocysteinemia)
- Oral contraceptives pills (OCP)
- Pregnancy and the puerperium
- Malignancy
- Infections such as meningitis, sinusitis, otitis media, cellulitis of the face
- Head injury and mechanical precipitants

CLINICAL FEATURES

Symptoms and signs of CVT can be grouped in three major syndromes:

1. *Isolated intracranial hypertension syndrome*: Headache with or without vomiting, papilledema, and visual problems
2. *Focal syndrome*: Focal deficits, seizures, or both
3. *Encephalopathy*: Multifocal signs, mental status changes, stupor, or coma.

   Headache is the most common and prominent symptom of CVT and can vary from a sudden onset severe headache to a gradual onset progressively worsening type.

When to Suspect a CVT?

- Young/middle-aged women on OCP or in the peripartum period with severe headache not relieved with regular painkillers

- Patients with known malignancy who develop severe throbbing headache
- An infarct or a bleed seen in an atypical location on computed tomography (CT) brain.

DIAGNOSIS

Different techniques used for diagnosis are CT brain or magnetic resonance imaging (MRI) with magnetic resonance venography (MRV) (**Fig. 1**).

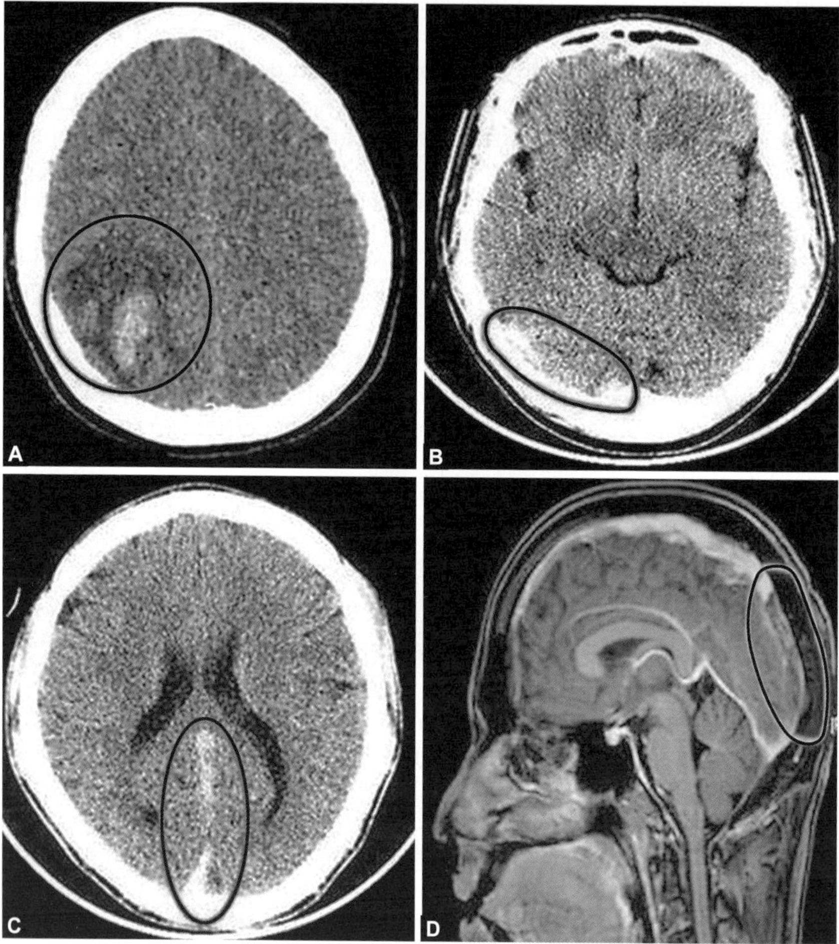

FIGS. 1A TO D: CT and MRI findings of cerebral venous thrombosis. (A) CT brain non-contrast: Hemorrhagic infarct in the right parietal region. (B) CT brain non-contrast: Hyperintensity in the right transverse sinus. (C) CT brain non-contrast: Hyperintensity in the straight sinus (cord sing). (D) MRI brain T1 weighted with gadolinium (sagittal): filling defect in superior sagittal sinus.

CT Brain

- May be normal in up to 30% of CVT cases
- Direct signs of CVT seen in one-third of cases are:
  - *Dense triangle sign (noncontrast CT)*: A hyperdensity with a triangular or round shape in the posterior part of the superior sagittal sinus caused by the venous thrombus
  - *Empty delta sign (contrast CT)*: A triangular pattern of contrast enhancement surrounding a central region lacking contrast enhancement in the posterior part of the superior sagittal sinus
  - *Cord sign (contrast CT)*: A curvilinear or linear hyperdensity over the cerebral cortex caused by a thrombosed cortical vein.
- Indirect signs of CVT are more common
  - Hemorrhagic lesions include intracerebral hemorrhage and hemorrhagic infarcts
  - Nonhemorrhagic lesions include focal areas of hypodensity caused by edema or venous infarction, usually not respecting the arterial boundaries, as well as diffuse brain edema.

MRI Brain with Venography

MRV is the most sensitive imaging method for demonstrating the thrombus and the occluded dural sinus or vein. MRV features include nonvisualization of the vessel (indicates absent flow), flow defect, and presence of collateral veins at the site of occlusion.

MANAGEMENT

- Lower the intracranial pressure (ICP) with 3% NaCl infusion (0.5–1 mL/kg/h)
- Seizure control with phenytoin 10–20 mg/kg IV loading dose and 100 mg IV q8h
- *Anticoagulation*: Give unfractionated heparin 5000 U IV stat and q6h or low-molecular-weight heparin (LMWH) (Enoxaparin 1 mg/kg s/c stat and q12h)
- *Endovascular treatment*: Direct endovascular interventions have been used as an alternative treatment in those who worsen despite adequate anticoagulation.

Intracranial Hemorrhage

Intracranial hemorrhage encompasses four types of intracranial bleeds: extradural hematoma (EDH), subdural hematoma (SDH), subarachnoid hemorrhage (SAH), and intraparenchymal hemorrhage.

EXTRADURAL HEMATOMA

- Extradural/epidural hematomas are rare, but may form as a result of blunt injury to the head associated with a skull fracture. Damage to the middle meningeal artery results in blood collecting in the epidural space. Venous epidural hematomas are common in children.
- These hematomas are biconvex/lenticular (**Fig. 1**) and are most often located in the temporal or temporoparietal regions.
- Clinical features include loss of consciousness, headache, nausea, vomiting or seizures. A lucid interval between the time of injury and neurological deterioration is characteristic of an EDH.
- *Management:*
  - Stabilize airway, breathing, and circulation (ABC)
  - Antiepileptics: To prevent seizures. Administer phenytoin 10–20 mg/kg IV or other antiepileptics
  - Refer to neurosurgery for urgent surgical evacuation of the hematoma and stopping the bleeding source.

SUBDURAL HEMATOMA

- These are more common after a blunt injury to the head and result from the shearing of small bridging vessels of the cerebral cortex.
- On a CT brain, SDH appears to adhere to the contours of the brain (**Fig. 1**). An acute SDH is typically hyperdense while a chronic SDH appears hypodense.
- Parenchymal damage due to pressure effect is much more severe than that caused by an EDH.
- An acute SDH usually presents with recent trauma, headache, nausea, vomiting, altered sensorium, seizures or focal neurological deficits.
- *Management:*
  - Stabilize ABC
  - Antiepileptics: To prevent seizures (phenytoin 10–20 mg/kg IV or other antiepileptics
  - Refer to neurosurgery for burr hole evacuation of the hematoma or a craniotomy if required.

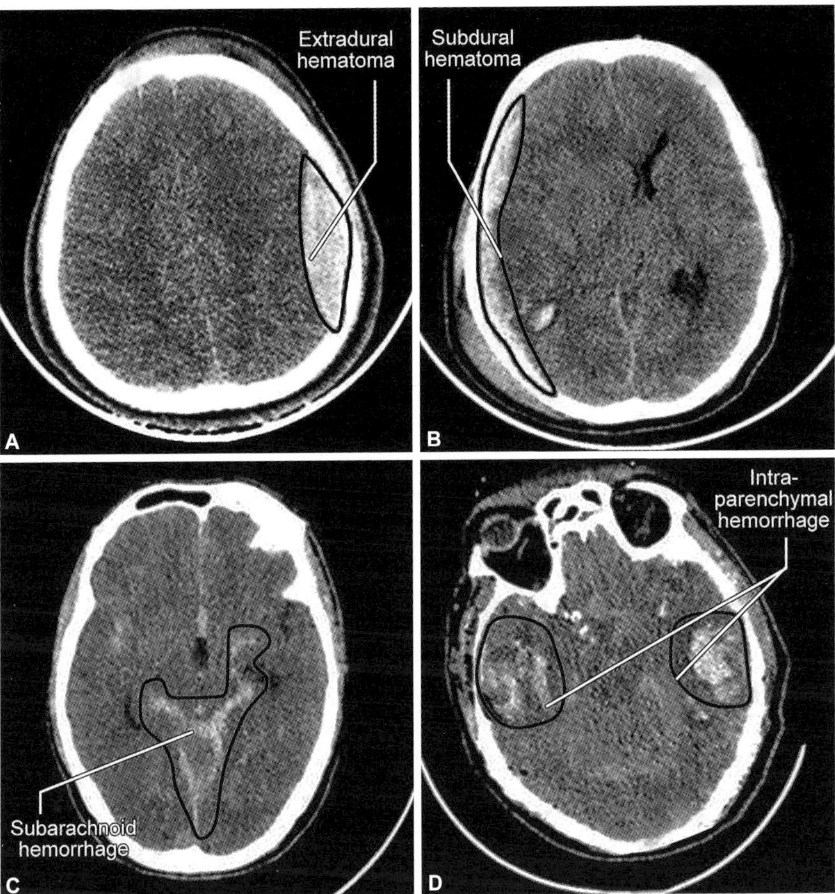

(EDH: extradural hematoma; SAH: subarachnoid hemorrhage; SDH: subdural hematoma)

FIGS. 1A TO D: Intracranial hemorrhage showing EDH, SDH, SAH, and intraparenchymal hemorrhage.

SUBARACHNOID HEMORRHAGE

Subarachnoid hemorrhage (SAH) refers to bleeding into the subarachnoid space. Most are caused by a ruptured saccular aneurysm. These aneurysms form at bifurcations of large or medium-sized intracranial arteries and 85% of them are in the anterior circulation, mostly in the circle of Willis.

Clinical Presentation

- Sudden onset severe headache, typically described as a thunderclap headache with or without focal neurological deficits is the most consistent symptom.
- Many patients describe it as "the worst headache of my life". Other symptoms include dizziness, loss of consciousness, seizures, diplopia or visual loss.

- Rebleeding and vasospasm are the two major complications of SAH and must be addressed immediately. The risk of rebleed is highest in the first 24 hours.
- The mortality rate of SAH in the first month is almost 50%.

Diagnosis

- Noncontrast CT scan of the brain typically shows hyperdense material filling the subarachnoid spaces around the brain, commonly around the circle of Willis (**Fig. 1**). A contrast CT may obscure the SAH.
- In patients with a strong suspicion of SAH and a normal CT brain, a lumbar puncture is mandatory. Look for an elevated opening pressure and an increased cerebrospinal fluid (CSF) red blood cell (RBC) count.
- Once the diagnosis of SAH is made, the site of bleeding can be confirmed by a digital subtraction angiography (DSA).

Management

- Stabilize ABC
- *Blood pressure (BP) control*: Target BP is SBP <160 mm Hg. Give Nifedipine R 10 mg stat or IV antihypertensives depending on the BP at arrival
- *Antiepileptics*: To prevent seizures. Administer phenytoin 10–20 mg/kg IV or other antiepileptics
- *Antifibrinolytic therapy*: Oral tranexamic acid 500–1,000 mg q8h or IV tranexamic acid 1,000 mg over 10 minutes, followed by 1,000 mg infusion over 8 hours has been shown to decrease the rate of rebleed in some studies
- *Prevention of vasospasm and delayed cerebral edema*: Give Nimodipine 60 mg PO q4h
- Refer to Neurosurgeon for surgical management of an aneurysm or an arterio-venous malformation.
- An external ventricular drain (EVD) may be required to prevent hydrocephalus

INTRAPARENCHYMAL HEMORRHAGE

- Intraparenchymal hemorrhage refers to bleeding into the brain parenchyma usually as a result of a cerebrovascular accident, aneurysm rupture, trauma, tumor, etc. The incidence increases with increasing age.
- Majority of the contusions occur in the frontal and temporal lobes.
- Patients typically present with focal neurological deficits, headache, altered sensorium, or seizures.
- CT brain shows hyperdense lesions within the brain parenchyma (**Fig. 1**)
- *Management:*
  - Stabilize ABC
  - *Antiepileptics*: To prevent seizures. Administer phenytoin 10–20 mg/kg IV or other antiepileptics
  - Lower the intracranial pressure (ICP) with 3% NaCl infusion (0.5-1 mL/kg/h)
  - Management depends on the etiology of the hemorrhage and could range from aggressive surgical evacuation, craniectomy or just observation and conservative management.

Guillain–Barré Syndrome

INTRODUCTION

Guillain–Barré syndrome (GBS) is an acute autoimmune polyradiculoneuropathy that is usually provoked by a preceding acute infection (*Campylobacter jejuni,* human herpes virus, *mycoplasma pneumonia,* etc.).

CLINICAL FEATURES

- GBS manifests as a rapidly progressive, symmetric ascending paralysis of both the lower limbs with or without sensory involvement. The disease course is <4 weeks.
- The usual presentation is an ascending paralysis first noticed in the legs and evolving over hours to a few days to the upper limbs and eventually the diaphragm
- Almost 30% of patients require ventilatory support due to diaphragmatic weakness.
- The lower cranial nerves are also frequently involved resulting in bulbar weakness, difficulty in maintaining airway and handling secretions
- Deep tendon reflexes are typically absent. Bowel and bladder functions are usually spared.

GBS Variants

- Acute inflammatory demyelinating polyradiculoneuropathy (AIDP)
- Acute motor axonal neuropathy (AMAN)
- Acute sensorimotor axonal neuropathy (AMSAN)
- Miller Fisher syndrome (MFS), characterized by ophthalmoplegia, ataxia and areflexia.

DIAGNOSIS

Diagnosis of GBS is made by a combination of typical clinical features, examination findings, and supportive laboratory evidence.

Electrodiagnostic Tests

Electromyography (EMG) and nerve conduction velocity (NCV) studies typically show acute polyneuropathy with demyelinating features (prolonged distal latencies, conduction velocity slowing and evidence of conduction block) in AIDP. A predominantly axonal pattern is seen in AMAN and AMSAN.

Cerebrospinal Fluid (CSF) Analysis

By the end of the first week of illness, cerebrospinal fluid (CSF) analysis typically shows an elevated protein (100-1000 mg/dL) with a normal sugar and cell count (albumin-cytologic dissociation). Sustained presence of leucocytes in CSF suggests an alternate diagnosis.

Differential Diagnosis

- *Acute myelopathy*: Usually associated with back pain and sphincter disturbances
- *Diphtheria*: Ascending paralysis with early oropharyngeal disturbances
- *Lyme disease*: distinguished by CSF pleocytosis, history of tick bite and presence of CSF lyme antibodies
- *Hypokalemic periodic paralysis*: recurrent episodes of acute paralysis with severe hypokalemia. Deep tendon reflexes typically intact.
- *Tick borne paralysis*: Mimics GBS; carefully examine for ticks. It is a non-infectious condition caused by neurotoxins in the saliva of certain ticks
- *Botulism*: Caused by botulism neurotoxin secreted by *Clostridium botulinum*. Starts with cranial nerve palsies and progresses to descending flaccid paralysis.
- *Acute intermittent porphyria*: Characterized by a triad of weakness, psychosis and abdominal pain with or without seizures.
- *Acute poisoning*: Arsenic or thallium

MANAGEMENT

- The first step in the management of a patient with suspected GBS is assessment of respiratory function in order to support the work of breathing if needed. This can be best assessed by a single breath count at the best side. Secure airway and stabilize breathing.
- *Close respiratory monitoring*: Up to 30% of patients develop neuromuscular respiratory failure requiring invasive mechanical ventilation.
- *Disease-modifying treatment*: The main modalities of therapy for GBS include plasma exchange (plasmapheresis) and administration of intravenous immunoglobulin (IVIG).
  - IVIG is administered at a dose of 2 g/kg over 2 days.
  - In plasmapharesis, 200–250 mL/kg of plasma is exchanged during 5 sessions over 1–2 weeks.

INTRODUCTION

Hanging is a form of strangulation that is caused by the victim being suspended from the neck.

- *Complete hanging*: When the whole body hangs off the ground and the entire weight of the victim is suspended at the neck, the hanging is said to be complete.
- Significant cervical spinal cord injuries usually result from hangings that involve a fall from a height greater than the victim's height.
- *Incomplete hanging*: This implies that some part of the body is touching the ground and that the weight of the victim is not fully supported by the neck.

PATHOPHYSIOLOGY

In judicial hanging, the head is effectively decapitated from the neck and torso due to fracture of the upper cervical spine.

In other mechanisms of strangulation injuries (nonjudicial hanging, incomplete hanging, and strangulation), the following mechanisms are postulated as the cause of death:

- Venous obstruction, leading to cerebral congestion, hypoxia, and unconsciousness
- Arterial obstruction due to carotid pressure, leading to low cerebral blood flow and collapse
- Vagal collapse due to pressure to the carotid sinuses resulting in increased parasympathetic tone
- Airway obstruction due to compression on the trachea resulting in hypoxia and death.

HISTORY

Victims are generally brought to the emergency department by friends, or family members or strangers. Ask them about the height of the drop as the extent of injury to the cervical spine increases in severity with increasing height.

EXAMINATION

- Look for any ligature mark, lacerations, abrasions, contusions or edema on the neck
- Look for subconjunctival and skin petechiae above the site of choking

- If gentle palpation of the larynx causes severe pain, it may indicate laryngeal fracture
- Look for features of stridor and respiratory distress
- Mental changes may be a sign of hypoxic damage to the brain.

INVESTIGATIONS

- In nonjudicial hangings, cervical spine injury is rare. Therefore, X-ray of the cervical spine is not needed in most cases
- Soft-tissue X-ray of the neck anteroposterior (AP) and lateral should be obtained in all strangulation victims. Look for hyoid bone fracture
- Noncontrast computed tomography (CT) scan of the brain is indicated when the neurologic status is compromised
- Routine blood investigations and arterial blood gas (ABG).

MANAGEMENT

- Assess airway and breathing
- Remember the possibility of an unstable cervical spine while securing airway. If in doubt, apply a cervical collar and avoid head tilt during intubation
- Secure the airway. Consider early endotracheal intubation if sensorium is low, as this could be due to hypoxia. Early intubation and ventilation improve neurological outcome. If endotracheal intubation is unsuccessful, consider cricothyroidotomy.
- Keep the patient on continuous cardiac monitoring to identify and manage dysrhythmias.
- Cerebral edema and raised intracranial pressure may require strategies like hyperventilation, diuretics an fluid restriction.

INTRODUCTION

Seizure is defined as an abnormal neurological activity caused by excessive electrical activity in the brain.

Epilepsy is defined as recurrent unprovoked seizures due to a genetically determined or acquired brain disorder.

Less than one-half of epilepsy cases have an identifiable cause. Patient may present to the emergency department with a new onset, recurrent or a breakthrough seizure.

- *New-onset seizures*: First episode of a seizure
- *Breakthrough seizures*: Occurs if patient is noncompliant with antiepileptics or if the serum drug levels are below the therapeutic range.

MANAGEMENT (TABLES 1 AND 2)

- Assess airway, breathing and circulation. Maintain and protect the airway, including the use of a oropharyngeal airway if needed. Protect the patient from self injury during this time.
- Identify and correct rapidly reversible ictal insults like hypoxia and hypoglycemia.
- Hypoglycemia is a common reversible metabolic causes of seizures. Check RBS for all patients and correct with 50% dextrose solution if indicated.
- If patient is noncompliant with antiepileptic medications:
  - Loading dose oral/IV of phenytoin or sodium valproate or levetiracetam
  - Do not send serum levels of antiepileptics
  - Restart regular dose of antiepileptics
  - Discharge and advice the patient to followup in epilepsy clinic.

TABLE 1: Summary of evaluation and management of seizures.		
	New-onset seizures	*Breakthrough seizures*
Investigations to be sent	CBC, electrolytes, creatinine, LFT CT brain (plain)	Hb, TC, DC, electrolytes, creatinine. Drug levels if patient is compliant with medications
Management	Loading dose of antiepileptics Refer to neurologist	Discharge if sensorium normal. Refer to neurologist/medicine if drowsy or in status epilepticus

(CBC: complete blood count; LFT: liver function test; CT: computed tomography; Hb: hemoglobin; TC: total count; DC: differential count)

TABLE 2: Doses of antiepileptic drugs.

Drug	Loading dose	Maintenance dose	Side effects
Phenytoin	IV: 10–20 mg/kg Oral: 10–20 mg/kg	300–400 mg/day in 2–3 divided doses	Ataxia, nystagmus, rashes, nausea, vomiting, blood dyscrasias, gum hyperplasia, hirsutism, vitamin K and folate deficiency
Phenobarbitone	IV: 10–20 mg/kg Oral: 10–20 mg/kg	30–180 mg/day in 2–3 divided doses	Drowsiness, sedation, lethargy, ataxia, dystonia and respiratory depression
Carbamazepine	No loading dose. Causes severe giddiness	800–2000 mg in 2 divided doses	Dizziness, diplopia, nausea, vomiting, ataxia, blurred vision, aplastic anemia and Steven–Johnson syndrome
Oxcarbazepine	No loading dose	600–2400 mg/day in 2 divided doses	Somnolence, headache, dizziness, rash and hyponatremia
Sodium valproate	Oral: 30 mg/kg IV: 30 mg/kg	Valproate SR/Chrono 500–1,000 mg in 2 divided doses	Nausea, vomiting, tremors, sedation and irritability
Levetiracetam	IV: 10–20 mg/kg (higher dose for status epilepticus) Oral: 500–1,000 mg	500 mg twice daily	Somnolence, asthenia, and dizziness
Clobazam (Frisium)	No loading dose	10–20 mg in 1 or 2 divided doses	Sedation, dizziness, ataxia, blurred vision, diplopia, irritability, and depression

- If patient is compliant with antiepileptic medications:
  - Loading dose oral/IV of phenytoin or carbamazepine or sodium valproate or levetiracetam
  - Look for a precipitating factor (e.g., hypoglycemia, hyponatremia)
  - Send trough serum levels of the regular antiepileptic
    - *If serum levels are low*: Increase the dose of the regular antiepileptics. If already on a maximum dose, add on a new antiepileptic before discharge
    - *If serum levels are normal*: Add on a new antiepileptic and advice the patient to followup in epilepsy clinic.
- Phenytoin loading should be monitored for electrocardiogram (ECG) changes, bradycardia, and hypotension
- Avoid phenytoin and valproate in the first trimester of pregnancy. The drugs of choice in pregnancy are levetiracetam or phenobarbitone

- Advice the patient to return to the emergency department if he/she notices new onset of rash or discoloration at the injection site. Extravasation of phenytoin can cause severe tissue necrosis.

STATUS EPILEPTICUS

Historically, status epilepticus was defined as a single episode of seizure lasting more than 30 minutes or a series of episodes of seizures during which neurological function is not regained between the episodes in a 30-minutes period.

Currently, the accepted operational definition of status epilepticus is:

- ≥5 minutes of continuous seizures, or
- ≥2 episodes of seizures between which there is incomplete recovery of consciousness.

Etiology

- Acute structural brain injury (stroke, trauma, SAH, cerebral ischemia)
- Nonadherence to antiepileptic medications
- *Metabolic abnormalities*: Hypoglycemia, hepatic encephalopathy, uremia, hyponatremia, hyperglycemia, hypocalcemia and hypomagnesemia
- Withdrawal syndromes associated with the discontinuation of alcohol, barbiturates, or benzodiazepines.

Management of Status Epilepticus

- The steps in the management of status epilepticus are shown in **Flowchart 1**.
- Go to the next step only if seizures are not controlled after loading dose of first antiepileptic
- At any stage, if the airway is compromised, or when midazolam infusion is started, consider rapid sequence intubation
- Avoid propofol, if the patient is hypotensive.

FOSPHENYTOIN

Fosphenytoin is a water-soluble prodrug of phenytoin that can be used instead of phenytoin for treatment of seizures in the ED.

- **1 mg Phenytoin = 1.5 mg; Fosphenytoin = 1 mg Phenytoin equivalent (PE)**
- *Loading Dose:*
  Adult: 18–20 mg PE/kg iv
  Children: 10–20 mg PE/kg iv
- *Maintenance Dose*:
  Adult: 4–6 mg PE/Kg iv twice a day
  Children: 2–3 mg PE/Kg iv twice a day
- *Infusion rate:* 150 mg PE/min

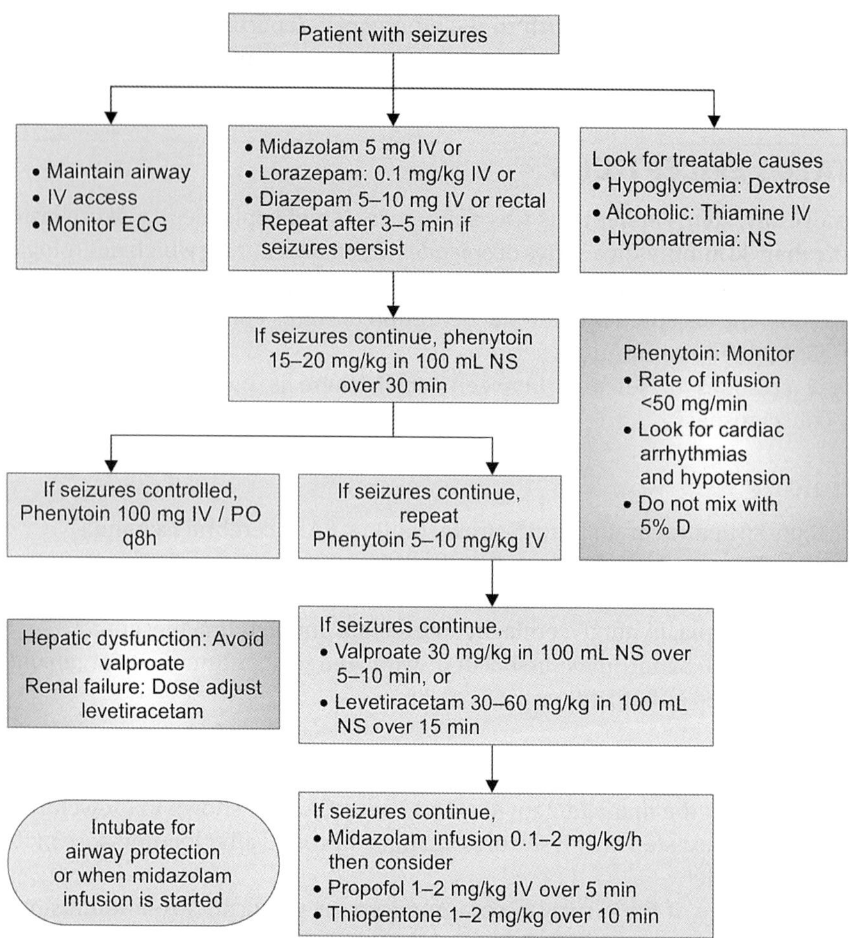

FLOWCHART 1: Management of a patient with status epilepticus.

- *Dilution:* 100 mL normal saline or 100 mL 5% dextrose
- *Advantages:* Less hypotension, less pruritus, less arrhythmia as preservative propylene glycol is not used
- *Monitoring:* Monitoring to be continued for half an hour post-infusion as Maximum phenytoin dose reached after 20 minutes of infusion

APPROACH TO A PATIENT WITH HEADACHE

- Take a detailed history on the onset, type, duration, aggravating, and relieving factors, associated stressors and symptoms.
- Determine the need for a computed tomography (CT) scan of the brain. History of projectile vomiting, diplopia, nystagmus, early morning increase in headache and severe throbbing headache strongly suggests raised intracranial pressure (ICP) and would warrant neuroimaging.
- If there is a strong suspicion of cerebral venous thrombosis (CVT), request for a CT brain/magnetic resonance imaging (MRI) brain with magnetic resonance venography (MRV).
- If any obvious stressor is identified, treat like a tension headache and prescribe paracetamol and a low dose of tricyclic antidepressants (TCA) (tablet Amitriptyline 10 mg hs od for 1 week). Refer the patient to psychiatrist for counseling.

The following clinical situations may warrant neuroimaging:

- The worst headache ever
- Recent significant increase in the pattern, frequency, or severity of headaches
- New or unexplained neurologic symptoms or signs
- Headache always on the same side
- Headaches not responding to treatment
- New-onset headaches after age 50 years
- New-onset headaches in patients with cancer or human immunodeficiency virus (HIV) infection.

MIGRAINE

Migraine is an episodic disorder characterized by severe headache generally associated with nausea and/or light and sound sensitivity. A prodrome of blurred vision, visual aura, malaise, anorexia, vomiting may be seen in one-third of patients. This usually lasts for 5–30 minutes. The headache may last for 4–72 hours and is usually throbbing and unilateral but may be generalized.

Treatment of Acute Attacks

- *Mild-to-moderate attacks*: Simple analgesics like Paracetamol 1 g stat and prn with an anti-emetic (Metoclopramide 10 mg PO tid). Nonsteroidal anti-inflammatory drugs (NSAIDs) also are effective for most episodes of migraine.

- *Moderate-to-severe attacks*:
  - Sumatriptan (5HT1 antagonist) dose of 25–50 mg PO prn or 6 mg s/c is effective but can cause vasoconstriction and is contraindicated in ischemic heart disease (IHD) and uncontrolled hypertension
  - NSAIDs may be added to Sumatriptan for severe attacks
  - Tablet Metoclopramide 10 mg PO tid for associated nausea and vomiting.

When to Start Prophylaxis for Migraine?

More than four headaches per month or headaches that last longer than 12 hours are generally considered reasonable thresholds for starting preventive therapy. The usual drugs are:
- Tablet Flunarizine10 mg hs od
- Tablet Amitriptyline 10–25 mg hs od
- Tablet Propranolol 10–20 mg bd.

CLUSTER HEADACHE

This distinctive vascular headache syndrome is characterized by 1–3 short lived attacks of peri-orbital pain daily over a 1–2-month period followed by pain-free interval of up to 1 year. Pain is strictly unilateral, affects the same side, typically lasts 30 min–2 hours and is explosive in nature. Associated symptoms include homolateral lacrimation, redness, nasal stuffiness, and nausea. Usually seen in men aged 20–50 years, this episodic pattern may become established in the chronic form.

Treatment is mainly prevention of attacks by drugs like prednisolone (60 mg daily × 7 days and rapidly taper), lithium (600–900 mg daily), ergotamine and sodium valproate.

TRIGEMINAL NEURALGIA

Also known as tic douloureux, it is a chronic pain syndrome characterized by recurrent brief episodes of unilateral neuralgic pain in the sensory distribution of the trigeminal nerve. The pain is often accompanied by facial spasms or tics. The number of episodes may vary from 1 to 100 per day.

Etiology

Most cases (80–90%) are caused by compression of the trigeminal nerve root by an aberrant loop of an artery or vein. Other causes include vestibular schwannoma, meningioma, epidermoid or other cyst, saccular aneurysm or arteriovenous malformation (AVM).

Neuroimaging

CT or MRI brain with contrast is used to look for structural lesions.

Treatment

Start with tablet Carbamazepine 100–200 mg bd and increase to 600–800 mg daily. Other drugs like baclofen (15 mg tid), lamotrigine (50–100 mg od) or gabapentin (300 mg od/bd) may be added for refractory pain.

Refer to neurosurgeon for microvascular decompression or ablative procedures.

TEMPORAL ARTERITIS

Temporal arteritis (TA) also known as giant cells arteritis is a chronic systemic vasculitis mainly involving large to medium vessels, especially branches of the internal carotid artery and is seen exclusively in patients over 50 years of age.

Clinical features: The characteristic headache of TA is described as severe and throbbing felt over the frontotemporal region with or without jaw claudication. The involved temporal artery may be tender with a feeble pulse. Ischemic optic neuritis with loss of vision is a dreaded complication.

Diagnosis: Diagnosis requires histopathological confirmation and is confirmed if three of the following criteria are fulfilled:
- Age >50 years
- New-onset localized headache
- Temporal artery tenderness/decreased pulse
- Erythrocyte sedimentation rate (ESR) >50 mm/h
- Temporal artery biopsy finding of granulomatous inflammation with multinucleated giant cells

Management: Corticosteroids are the mainstay of therapy and must be started immediately on high clinical suspicion, especially if vision is compromised.

Start oral prednisolone 40–60 mg PO od and refer to neurology for confirmation of diagnosis.

Bell's Palsy 57
CHAPTER

INTRODUCTION

Bell's palsy is the most common cause of sudden-onset lower motor neuron (LMN) facial nerve palsy. It usually results from a viral infection [herpes simplex virus (HSV), varicella zoster virus (VZV), human herpesvirus 6 (HHV-6), and Lyme disease] that causes swelling of the facial nerve within the temporal bone.

EXAMINATION FINDINGS

LMN Facial Nerve Palsy

Deviation of the angle of the mouth to the opposite side, absence of forehead wrinkling and inability to close the eye on the same side, hyperacusis on the affected side (due to stapedius muscle paralysis), decreased lacrimation (greater petrosal nerve involvement) and metallic taste (chorda tympani nerve).

Attempting to close the eye on the affected side results in upward gaze, known as the Bells phenomenon.

DIFFERENTIAL DIAGNOSIS FOR BELL'S PALSY

Other Causes of LMN Facial Palsy

- *Ramsay Hunt syndrome*: Due to herpes zoster virus (HZV) infection of the geniculate ganglion. In addition to LMN facial palsy, a painful herpetiform vesicular eruption in the external auditory meatus and vestibulocochlear dysfunction are characteristic findings. The pain is considerably mire severe than that of Bells palsy with a poorer rate of recovery of facial nerve palsy. Treatment is similar: Prednisolone and antiviral therapy for 7–10 days.
- *Pontine tumors or vascular events*: Other cranial nerves are also usually involved.
- *Middle ear infection and cholesteatoma*: Acute otitis media can be treated with antibiotics and may require myringotomy for decompression. Malignant otitis externa, caused by *Pseudomonas aeroginosa* may cause facial nerve palsy and requires prolonged anti-pseudomonal antibiotic therapy with or without surgical debridement.
- Trauma
- Parotid gland tumors
- Sarcoidosis.

MANAGEMENT

- If patient presents within 72 hours of onset of symptoms:
  - Tablet prednisolone 1 mg/kg in 2 divided doses × 5 days. Then decrease by 10 mg each day and stop by the 10th day.
  - Antivirals have not proven to be of much added benefit. If herpetic vesicles are seen on the skin or inner ear, give tablet Valacyclovir 1,000 mg bd × 5 days.
  - *Refer to ophthalmologist*: Artificial tears and an eye patch at night are needed to prevent corneal ulceration.
  - *Refer to ENT specialist*: To assess the inner ear and to rule out other local causes. In rare cases, surgical decompression of the facial nerve may be indicated.
  - *Refer to physiotherapist*: Transcutaneous electrical nerve stimulation (TENS) exercises have been used to try to promote motor recovery in patients with Bell's palsy, but strong evidence for its benefits is lacking.
- If patient presents after 72 hours of onset of symptoms:
  - *Refer to ophthalmologist*: Artificial tears and an eye patch at night are needed to prevent corneal ulceration.
  - *Refer to ENT specialist*: To assess the inner ear and to rule out other local causes.
  - Steroids are less effective if started after 72 hours of onset of symptoms. May be given if the patient complains of ear pain suggestive of facial nerve swelling in the temporal bone.
  - Antivirals are not beneficial if started late. Therefore, not indicated.
  - *Refer to physiotherapist*: TENS have been used to try to promote motor recovery in patients with Bell's palsy, but strong evidence for its benefits is lacking.

Long-term outcome after 6 months for most patients with Bell's palsy is good. Many patients, especially those treated early have good functional recovery.

INTRODUCTION

Drug-induced dystonia (tardive dystonia; tardive dyskinesia; acute dystonic reaction): A number of drugs are capable of causing dystonia. Most people develop an acute dystonic reaction after a one-time exposure to the drug.

Drugs causing dystonic reactions are typical antipsychotics (chlorpromazine, fluphenazine, haloperidol, perphenazine, prochlorperazine, thioridazine, trifluoperazine), metoclopramide (perinorm).

CLINICAL PRESENTATION

- Symptoms may include intermittent spasmodic or sustained involuntary contractions of muscles of the face, neck, trunk, pelvis, and extremities. The symptoms are usually transient
- Painful forced extension of the neck is a common presentation and can be quite distressing to the patient and relatives.

TREATMENT

For the treatment, any of the following drugs may be given:
- *Diphenhydramine (Benadryl)*: Given for its anticholinergic effect
  - Can be given as a syrup (10–20 mL stat and repeat, if needed) or
  - Injection Diphenhydramine 25–50 mg IV over 2 minutes or 50 mg IM stat
  - Continue oral dosage (10 mL tid) for 3–4 days to prevent recurrence of symptoms.
- Promethazine (Phenergan) 25–50 mg IV stat.
- *Benztropine*: Blocks striatal cholinergic receptors. Dosage: 1–2 mg IV, then 1–2 mg PO q12h to prevent recurrence.
- *Benzodiazepines*: Lorazepam or diazepam can be given intravenously.
- *Trihexyphenidyl (pacitane)*: Dose of 2 mg PO stat; increase as necessary to usual range: 5–15 mg/day in 3–4 divided doses.

Stop the drug precipitating dystonia and refer to neurology.

Gastrointestinal and Hepatic Emergencies

Gastrointestinal Bleeding

INTRODUCTION

Blood loss from the gastrointestinal (GI) tract may occur in four ways: (1) hematemesis, (2) hematochezia, (3) melena, and (4) occult loss.

Upper GI bleed is defined as bleeding originating proximal to the ligament of Treitz, while lower GI bleed originates distal to it.

UPPER GASTROINTESTINAL BLEED

Causes of upper GI bleed: Peptic ulcer, esophagogastric varices, arteriovenous malformation, GI tumor, Mallory-Weiss tear, etc.

History

- Ask for history of alcohol consumption and smoking.
- *Drug history*: Use of nonsteroidal anti-inflammatory drugs (NSAIDs), aspirin, anticoagulants, antiplatelet agents.
- Ask for previous GI bleed and other sites of bleeding.

Symptoms

- Abdominal pain, hematemesis, and melena.
- Melena is the usual presentation, but stool may be frankly bloody or maroon with massive or brisk upper GI bleeding.

Examination

- Tachycardia or orthostatic hypotension changes suggest moderate-to-severe blood loss; hypotension suggests life-threatening blood loss.
- Perform a rectal examination to assess stool color (black/red/normal) to differentiate between melena and hematochezia.
- Look for features of chronic liver disease (ascites, jaundice) that could suggest a variceal bleed.
- Significant abdominal tenderness accompanied by signs of peritoneal irritation (e.g., involuntary guarding) suggests perforation.

Investigations to be sent:
- Complete blood count, electrolytes, creatinine, liver function test, rapid blood borne virus screen, chest X-ray, electrocardiogram, prothrombin time, activated partial thromboplastin time.
- Arrange cross-match for blood if hemoglobin (Hb) is less than 7 g%.

Management

- Assess and stabilize airway, breathing, and circulation.
- Start two large bore intravenous (IV) cannulae and commence IV fluid resuscitation.
- If the GI bleed is severe, arrange for cross-matched blood for transfusion.
- *Acid suppression with proton-pump inhibitor (PPI)*: Injection pantoprazole 80 mg/omeprazole 40 mg IV stat.
- *Prokinetics*: Metoclopramide 10 mg IV stat and q8h.
- *If a variceal bleed is suspected*: Octreotide IV bolus of 100 µg followed by 100 µg IV q6h.
- Administer antibiotics (injection ceftriaxone 1 g IV stat) 2 hours prior to the upper GI endoscopy.
- Initiate blood transfusions if the Hb is <7 g% (**Box 1**).
- Transfuse fresh frozen plasma for coagulopathy.
- Transfuse platelets for thrombocytopenia (platelets <50,000) or platelet dysfunction (e.g., chronic aspirin therapy).
- Refer to gastroenterology for upper GI endoscopy.

BOX 1	Blood transfusion protocols for upper gastrointestinal bleed.

- If Hb is <6 g%, cross-match and transfuse two pints packed cells over 6 h
- If Hb is between 6 and 7 g%, cross-match and transfuse one-pint packed cells over 4 h
- If Hb >7 g% upper GI endoscopy can be done immediately
- Target Hb >8 g% for patients with ischemic heart disease

(Hb: Hemoglobin)

LOWER GASTROINTESTINAL BLEED

Causes of lower GI bleed: Diverticulosis, angiodysplasia, hemorrhoids, GI malignancies, inflammatory bowel disease:

- Anal hemorrhoids are the most common cause of lower GI bleed. Proctoscopy is often diagnostic. Refer to Chapter 102 for details of management.
- Other conditions like diverticulosis or angiodysplasia can be diagnosed by colonoscopy.
- Primary treatment includes fluid resuscitation and blood product transfusion for severe bleeding.

INTRODUCTION

It is critical to diagnose acute severe pancreatitis as soon as possible in the emergency department (ED) as it can be associated with significant mortality.

According to the revised Atlanta classification (**Table 1**), the diagnosis of acute pancreatitis is confirmed if two of the following three criteria are fulfilled:

1. Abdominal pain consistent with acute pancreatitis (acute onset of a persistent, severe, epigastric pain often radiating to the back).
2. Serum lipase or amylase at least three times greater than the upper limit of normal.
3. Characteristic findings of acute pancreatitis on ultrasonography (USG) or computed tomography (CT) abdomen.

CLINICAL FEATURES

Patients typically present with epigastric abdominal pain but may also be diffuse. The onset of pain is relatively rapid, increasing in severity over a few hours. The constant and severe pain may radiate to the back, with patients wriggling to try a position of comfort and is often relieved by leaning forward. Hypotension, tachycardia, and shock indicate severe disease with complications.

ETIOLOGY OF ACUTE PANCREATITIS

- Gallstones (60%)
- Alcohol (20%)
- *Others*: Hypertriglyceridemia, hypercalcemia, trauma, iatrogenic, systemic vasculitis, drugs [thiazides, nonsteroidal anti-inflammatory drugs (NSAIDs), sulfonamides, azathioprine, tetracyclines, valproate], infections [mumps, rubella, coxsackie B, Epstein–Barr virus (EBV), cytomegalovirus (CMV), ascaris, *Clonorchis sinensis*].

TABLE 1: Modified Atlanta Grading (2012) of severity of acute pancreatitis.

Mild acute pancreatitis	No organ failure, no local, or systemic complications
Moderately severe acute pancreatitis	Organ failure that resolves within 48 h (transient organ failure) and/or local or systemic complications without persistent organ failure
Severe acute pancreatitis	Persistent organ failure (>48 h) that may involve one or multiple organs

INVESTIGATIONS

- Complete blood count (CBC), electrolytes, creatinine, liver function test (LFT), calcium, amylase, lipase, chest X-ray (CXR), electrocardiogram (ECG).
- *USG abdomen*: The only indication of an USG abdomen during the acute stage is to identify an impacted gallstone that may be relieved by endoscopic retrograde cholangiopancreaticography (ERCP). The presence of an impacted gallstone would reflect as an abnormal LFT (elevated ALP or transaminitis). Urgent USG in the ED is indicated only in patients with a deranged LFT suggestive of choledocholithiasis.

MANAGEMENT

- *Fluid replacement*: Establish intravenous (IV) access and start fluid replacement. Patients are usually volume depleted and hence aggressive fluid resuscitation is essential.
- *Pain control*:
  - Injection paracetamol 1,000 mg in 100 mL normal saline (NS) IV stat plus
  - Injection morphine 5 mg IV stat (reassess and repeat dose after 30 minutes, if needed), or
  - Injection tramadol 50 mg IV stat
  - If pain persists after 4 hours, morphine 5 mg IV can be repeated every 4 hours.
- Administer injection pantoprazole 40 mg IV and ondansetron 8 mg IV.
- If evidence of infection/sepsis, administer empiric broad spectrum antibiotics (ertapenem/meropenem).
- Keep the patient nil per oral (NPO) till pain relief is achieved. The benefit of nasogastric (NG) tube placement is unproven. Oral feeds can slowly be started in mild pancreatitis once pain subsides (usually after 12 h).
- *Biliary pancreatitis*: In patients with gallstone-induced pancreatitis, urgent ERCP within 72 hours reduces complications and mortality.

Spontaneous Bacterial Peritonitis

INTRODUCTION

Spontaneous (primary) bacterial peritonitis (SBP) refers to ascitic fluid infection as a result of bacteremic seeding without an obvious surgically treatable intra-abdominal focus of infection. It almost always occurs in patients with cirrhosis and ascites.

The diagnosis of SBP is confirmed by:
- Positive ascitic fluid bacterial culture
- Elevated ascitic fluid absolute neutrophil count ($\geq$250 cells/mm^3)
- Exclusion of secondary causes of bacterial peritonitis.

SBP must be differentiated from secondary peritonitis, where bacteria spread into the peritoneum from an intra-abdominal focus or perforation of a viscus. The diagnosis of SBP can be made only after ruling out a primary intra-abdominal source of infection.

CLINICAL FEATURES

- Fever, diffuse abdominal pain/tenderness, altered mental status, diarrhea, paralytic ileus, and hypotension.
- Renal failure develops in 30–40% of patients with SBP and is a major cause of death.

ETIOLOGY

Gut bacteria such as *Escherichia coli* and *Klebsiella*, but entero-bacteriaceae are the usual causes but streptococcal and staphylococcal infections can also cause SBP.

INVESTIGATIONS

- Perform a diagnostic ascitic tap and send for ascitic fluid TC, DC and culture sensitivity
- Complete blood count (CBC), electrolytes, creatinine, blood c/s.

INDICATIONS FOR ANTIBIOTIC THERAPY

- Empiric therapy for SBP should be started in a patient with ascites who has any of the following findings:
  - Temperature >37.8°C (100°F)
  - Abdominal pain and/or tenderness
  - Altered sensorium
  - Ascitic fluid absolute neutrophil count ≥250 cells/mm^3.

MANAGEMENT

- Stabilize airway, breathing, and circulation (ABC).
- *Start broad spectrum antibiotics*: Cefoperazone-sulbactam 1 g IV stat or meropenem 1 g in 100 mL normal saline (NS) IV stat if the patient is in shock. Most patients require a 5-day course of antibiotics.
- Refer to gastroenterology for further management.

HEPATO-RENAL SYNDROME

Hepato-renal syndrome is a potentially fatal complication in a patient with cirrhosis and ascites. It is characterized by worsening uremia with oliguria and sodium retention in the absence of a potentially identifiable cause of renal failure. This condition may be precipitated by severe GI bleed, sepsis or aggressive attempts at diuresis or paracentesis.

Diagnosis is confirmed by worsening renal failure and demonstration of avid urinary sodium retention (urine spot sodium is typically <5 mmol/L).

Treatment is usually unsuccessful. Early albumin infusion may be tried, but liver transplantation remains the only option.

Hepatic Encephalopathy

Hepatic encephalopathy is a reversible impairment of neuropsychiatric function associated with impaired hepatic function characterized by altered sensorium and behavior, personality changes, asterixis and distinctive electroencephalographic (EEG) changes.

It is a recurring complication of cirrhosis of the liver and may be acute and reversible or chronic and progressive. Elevated ammonia levels have been implicated as the pathogenesis of this condition.

CLINICAL FEATURES

The clinical manifestations vary in severity from mild cognitive dysfunction, irritability, confusion and profound coma.

Examination Findings

- *Asterixis*: Seen in mild-to-moderate encephalopathy. Asterixis is a low amplitude, alternating flexion and extension of the wrist that occurs when the hand is held in extension.
- *Other features of cirrhosis*: Palmar erythema, spider naevi, testicular atrophy, loss of axillary and pubic hair, ecchymotic patches and ascites
- *Fetor hepaticus*: Seen in severe cases, it refers to a musty breath odour, presumably due to ammonia and ketones in the breath.

Hepatic encephalopathy can be graded in severity as:
- *Grade I*: Changes in behavior, mild confusion, slurred speech, disordered sleep.
- *Grade II*: Lethargy, moderate confusion.
- *Grade III*: Marked confusion (stupor), incoherent speech, sleeping but arousable.
- *Grade IV*: Coma, unresponsive to pain.

INVESTIGATIONS

- Complete blood count (CBC), electrolytes (look for hypokalemia), creatinine, LFT, RBS
- Perform a diagnostic ascitic tap and send for ascitic fluid TC, DC, and culture sensitivity to rule out spontaneous bacterial peritonitis (SBP).

MANAGEMENT

The initial management of acute hepatic encephalopathy in patients with cirrhosis involves two steps.

1. *Identification and correction of precipitating causes*: These include
   - *Gastrointestinal (GI) bleeding*: Consider blood transfusion and urgent UGI scopy for therapeutic interventions
   - *Infection*: Commonly SBP/UTI. Administer broad spectrum antibiotics
   - *Hypokalemia and/or metabolic alkalosis*: KCl supplementation
   - Renal failure
   - *Hypovolemia*: Careful administration of fluids
   - *Hypoxia*: Administer supplemental oxygen
   - *Sedative or tranquilizer use*: Consider naloxone for opioid use
   - *Hypoglycemia*: Intravenous dextrose administration
   - *Constipation*: Laxatives like Syrup lactulose
2. *Measures to lower the blood ammonia concentration*:
   - Syrup lactulose 30 mL (mixed in a glass of water or fruit juice) PO stat and q4h till two to three well-formed stools are passed per day. Lactulose, a disachharide (galactose + fructose) is minimally absorbed and is degraded into lactic acid in the colon. By acidifying the GI tract, ammonia is trapped and excreted in the stools. It can be given orally or rectally.
   - *Oral antibiotics*: These may be used as second line therapy among patients who do not respond to a 48-hour therapy with disaccharides. Neomycin (1 g PO bd), rifaximin (400 mg PO tid) or Ampicillin (500 mg PO bd) may be effective in lowering blood ammonia.
   - Bowel wash at the earliest. This decreases the absorption of protein and nitrogenous products from the intestines.
   Refer to gastroenterology for further management.

Acute Cholangitis

CHAPTER 64

INTRODUCTION

Acute cholangitis refers to bacterial infection of the biliary system (biliary ducts). It requires the presence of 2 factors; biliary obstruction (usually by a stone) and bacterial growth in the bile, resulting in inflammation and often dilatation of the biliary ducts. It is often caused by choledocholithiasis, which refers to the presence of one or more gall stones in the common bile duct (CBD) resulting in obstruction of the flow of bile.

Cholangitis must be differentiated clinically from cholecystitis, which refers to inflammation of the gall bladder, usually due to gall stones with or without bacterial infection or involvement of the rest of the biliary system.

- The organisms causing cholangitis usually ascend from the duodenum.
- If the biliary tract obstruction persists, intraluminal pressure increases, resulting in reflux of the bacteria into the hepatic veins and lymphatic vessels and eventually into the systemic circulation, resulting in sepsis.
- The common causes of biliary obstruction are biliary calculi (30–70%), benign stenosis (5–30%), malignancy (10–30%) and bile duct stent blocks.

BACTERIOLOGY (USUALLY POLYMICROBIAL)

- *Escherichia coli* (most common), *Klebsiella* species, Enterobacter, Enterococcus, Streptococcus, *Pseudomonas aeruginosa*.
- Anaerobes (*Bacteroides*/Clostridia) are usually present as part of a mixed infection.

CLINICAL FEATURES

- The classic presentation is fever, jaundice, and right upper quadrant abdominal pain (Charcot's triad). Approximately 25% of patients with cholangitis may not have all three symptoms.
- Suppurative cholangitis may cause hypotension and altered sensorium in addition to the Charcot's triad (Reynolds' pentad).

INVESTIGATIONS

- Complete blood count (CBC), electrolytes, creatinine, liver function test (LFT), blood culture/sensitivity (C/S), blood borne virus screen (BBVS), chest X-ray (CXR), electrocardiogram (ECG), prothrombin time (PT), activated partial thromboplastin time (aPTT) are needed, if intervention likely.

- Liver function test shows features of cholestasis [hyperbilirubinemia, elevated alkaline phosphatase (ALP)].
- Ultrasonography (USG) abdomen: Look for:
  - Common bile duct (CBD) dilatation with or without intrahepatic biliary radicle dilatation (IHBRD)
  - Evidence of an etiology for bile obstruction (stone, tumor, or stent).

DIAGNOSIS

The closest differential for a cholangitis is cholecystitis which also presents with right upper quadrant pain. Patients with cholangitis have high fever and appear more ill than those with cholecystitis. Another important feature is the presence of jaundice and elevated bilirubin in cholangitis, which are uncommon in cholecystitis. Ultrasonography evidence of dilated common and intrahepatic ducts is required to distinguish cholangitis from cholecystitis.

MANAGEMENT

- Monitor and stabilize airway, breathing, and circulation (ABC).
- Obtain a blood culture and administer broad-spectrum parenteral antibiotics (piperacillin-tazobactam/meropenem).
- Analgesics as needed (paracetamol/tramadol/morphine)
- The key to successful treatment is early decompression of the biliary tract which can be achieved by the following:
  - Endoscopic sphincterotomy with stone extraction and/or stent insertion (depending on the cause of the obstruction) is the treatment of choice for restoring biliary drainage.
  - Percutaneous transhepatic cholangiography (PTC) can be considered when endoscopic retrograde cholangiopancreatography (ERCP) is unavailable, unsuccessful, or contraindicated.

Section **10**

Hematological Emergencies

Anemia   65

INTRODUCTION

Anemia can be defined as a reduced absolute number of circulating red blood cells (RBCs). The criteria for anemia in men and women are less than 14 g/dL and less than 12 g/dL, respectively. Two general approaches can be used to identify the cause of anemia: (1) kinetic approach and (2) morphologic approach.

1. *Kinetic approach:* According to this approach, anemia can be caused by three independent mechanisms (**Table 1**).
2. *Morphologic approach:* In this approach, the causes of anemia are classified according to measurement of RBC size, as seen on the blood smear. The normal RBC has a volume [mean corpuscular volume (MCV)] of 80–96 femtoliters (fL) (**Table 2**).

RETICULOCYTE COUNT

- Anemia with a high reticulocyte count reflects an increased erythropoietic response to continued hemolysis or blood loss.

TABLE 1: Kinetic approach of the cause of anemia.

Cause	Examples
Decreased RBC production	- *Lack of nutrients:* Iron, vitamin B_{12}, folic acid deficiency - *Bone marrow disorders:* Aplastic anemia, pure RBC aplasia, marrow infiltration - *Bone marrow suppression:* Drugs, chemotherapy, irradiation - *Ineffective erythropoiesis:* Alpha- and beta-thalassemia, myelodysplastic syndrome, sideroblastic anemias - *Others:* Chronic renal failure, hypogonadism, hypothyroidism
Increased RBC destruction	- *Inherited hemolytic anemias:* Hereditary spherocytosis, sickle cell disease, thalassemia major - *Acquired hemolytic anemias:* Coombs-positive autoimmune hemolytic anemia, thrombotic thrombocytopenic purpura, hemolytic uremic syndrome, malaria, paroxysmal nocturnal hemoglobinuria - Hypersplenism
Blood loss	- *Obvious bleeding:* Trauma, melena, hematemesis, menometrorrhagia - *Occult bleeding:* Slowly bleeding ulcer or carcinoma

(RBC: red blood cell)

Type	Examples
Macrocytic anemia MCV >100 fL	• *Abnormalities of DNA metabolism:* Vitamin B_{12} deficiency, folate deficiency, drugs (hydroxyurea, zidovudine, methotrexate, azathioprine) • *Shift to immature or stressed red cells:* Aplastic anemia/Fanconi anemia, pure red cell aplasia • *Primary bone marrow disorders:* Myelodysplastic syndromes • *Others:* Alcohol abuse, liver disease, hypothyroidism
Microcytic anemia MCV <80 fL	• *Reduced iron availability:* Iron deficiency, anemia of inflammation, copper deficiency • *Acquired disorders of heme synthesis:* Lead poisoning, acquired sideroblastic anemias • *Reduced globin production:* Thalassemia, other hemoglobinopathies • *Rare congenital disorders:* Sideroblastic anemias, porphyria, and defects in iron absorption, transport, utilization, and recycling
Normocytic anemia MCV = 80–100 fL	• Systemic disorders • Cancer-associated anemia • Anemia of chronic renal disease

TABLE 2: Morphologic approach of the cause of anemia.

(MCV: mean corpuscular volume)

- A stable anemia with a low reticulocyte count is strong evidence for deficient production of RBCs.
- Normal range is 0.5–2.0%.
- *Investigations to be sent*: Complete blood count profile, reticulocyte count, electrolytes, creatinine.
- *If hemolysis is suspected*: Liver function test, lactate dehydrogenase, urea, uric acid, calcium, phosphate, urinalysis, chest X-ray (CXR).
- *If patient is a pure vegetarian (get this history from all patients)*: Vitamin B_{12} and folate levels.

MANAGEMENT

- If the patient has signs of failure, transfuse one to two packed red cells urgently; target hemoglobin (Hb) >7 g%.
- Identify and treat the underlying cause.

For Iron Deficiency Anemia

- *Dietary*: Advice increased dietary iron intake
- *Deworm*:
  - Tablet mebendazole 100 mg bd × 3 days. Repeat after 2 weeks (safe in pregnancy), or
  - Tablet albendazole 400 mg stat. Repeat after 2 weeks, or
  - Tablet tinidazole 2 g stat.

- *Oral iron therapy:*
  - Tablet ferrous sulfate 200 mg (60 mg elemental iron) tid × 6 months, or
  - Tablet ferrous fumarate 152 mg + folic acid 1,500 µg (Livogen) bd × 6 months, or
  - Tablet ferrous fumarate 350 mg + folic acid 2,000 µg + vitamin B_{12} 15 µg (Autrin) od × 6 months.

  After 6 months, if the Hb is normal, iron supplementation should be continued for a further 6 months till iron stores are replenished.
- Parenteral iron therapy.

For Suspected B_{12}/Folate Deficiency

- *For pernicious anemia:* Injection vitamin B_{12} 1,000 µg intramuscular (IM)/ subcutaneous (SC) once daily for 1 week, followed by 1,000 µg every week for 4 weeks and then 1,000 µg every month for 6 months. Supplement this with tablet folate 5 mg OD till complete hematological recovery.
- *In pure vegetarians:* Oral B_{12} and folate supplementation with neurobion/ multivitamin tablets may be tried. However, if the degree of anemia is severe, initial 1 week of IM/SC vitamin B_{12} injections may be necessary.

  The evaluation of a patient with anemia is shown in **Flowchart 1**.

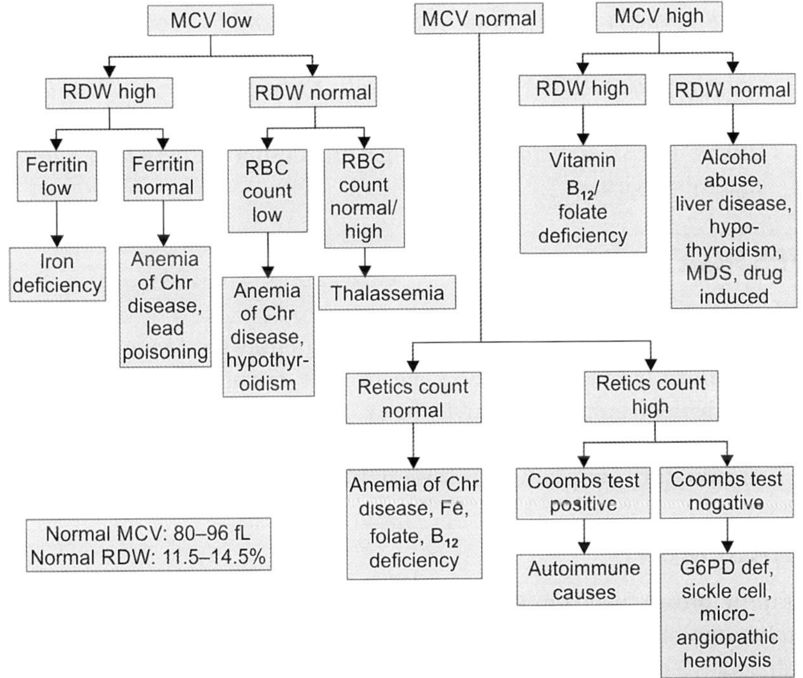

(G6PD: glucose-6-phosphate dehydrogenase; MDS: myelodysplastic syndrome; MCV: mean corpuscular volume; RBC: red blood cell; RDW: red blood distribution width; Chr: Chronic)

FLOWCHART 1: Evaluation of anemia.

Febrile Neutropenia

INTRODUCTION

Patients with malignancies on cytotoxic chemotherapy that affects hemopoiesis and integrity of gastrointestinal mucosa, frequently develop fever due to colonizing bacteria or fungus. It is critical to recognize neutropenic fever early and to initiate empiric antibiotics promptly to prevent progression to a sepsis syndrome and possibly death.

Neutropenia is usually defined as an absolute neutrophil count (ANC) <1,500 cells/µL, and severe neutropenia is usually defined as an ANC <500 cells/µL or an ANC that is expected to decrease to <500 cells/µL over the next 48 hours.

MICROBIOLOGY

- Bacteremia is documented in only 10–25% of neutropenic fever episodes.
- Common organisms are:
  - *Gram-positive*: (60%) *Staphylococcus epidermidis*, coagulase negative staphylococci, *Staphylococcus aureus*, *Streptococcus viridans*
  - *Gram-negative*: (30%) *Escherichia coli*, *Klebsiella* species, *Pseudomonas aeruginosa*
  - *Others*: (10%) *Acinetobacter*, fungal infections (*Aspergillus*, *Candida*), anaerobes, viruses.

INVESTIGATIONS

Investigations to be sent:
- Perform a thorough physical examination to identify any focus of infection:
  - Complete blood count (CBC), electrolytes, creatinine, liver function test (LFT), blood culture/sensitivity (c/s)
  - *If urinary symptoms are present*: Urinalysis and urine c/s
  - If respiratory symptoms are present: Chest X-ray (CXR).

MANAGEMENT

- Empiric broad-spectrum antibacterial therapy should be initiated immediately after blood cultures have been obtained. Administer cefoperazone-sulbactam 3 g intravenous (IV) stat plus amikacin 15 mg/kg IV stat.
- Refer to hematology immediately for further management.

Acute Leukemia

CHAPTER 67

INTRODUCTION

Acute leukemia may occur de novo or may transform from chronic myeloid leukemia (CML) [70% to acute myeloid leukemia (AML) and 30% to acute lymphoid leukemia (ALL)] or from myelodysplastic syndrome (MDS).

TYPES OF ACUTE LEUKEMIA

Types of acute leukemia have been shown in **Table 1**.

TABLE 1: Types of acute leukemia.	
Acute lymphoid leukemia (ALL)	*Acute myeloid leukemia (AML)*
World Health Organization (WHO) classification:	French–American–British (FAB) classification:
• B-lymphoblastic leukemia/ lymphoblastic lymphoma	• M0: Undifferentiated acute myeloblastic leukemia
• B-lymphoblastic leukemia/lymphoma, not otherwise specified	• M1: Acute myeloblastic leukemia with minimal maturation
• B-lymphoblastic leukemia/lymphoma with maturation	• M2: Acute myeloblastic leukemia with maturation
• T-lymphoblastic leukemia/lymphoma	• M3: Acute promyelocytic leukemia
	• M4: Acute myelomonocytic leukemia
	• M5: Acute monocytic leukemia
	• M6: Acute erythroid leukemia
	• M7: Acute megakaryocytic leukemia

CLINICAL PRESENTATION

Patients with acute leukemia may present with problems due to:
- *Red cells*: Anemia, fatigue
  - *White cells*: Leukopenia may cause fever, while leukostasis due to high blast count may result in myocardial infarction (MI), respiratory impairment, renal failure, stroke or acute confusional state.
  - *Platelets*: Bleeding manifestations
  - *Coagulopathy*: Disseminated intravascular coagulation (DIC) and shock due to sepsis is frequently seen in AML M3.

MANAGEMENT

- Assess and stabilize airway, breathing, and circulation (ABC).
- Treat anemia/bleeding with appropriate blood product transfusion.
- If the patient has fever or neutropenia, consult hematology immediately and start antibiotics.

CHRONIC MYELOID LEUKEMIA

- Chronic myeloid leukemia is a myeloproliferative disorder associated with the Philadelphia chromosome t(9;22)(q34;q11) and/or the *BCR- ABL* fusion gene.
- The course of CML has three phases:
  1. *Chronic phase*: Approximately 85% of patients are in this phase at the time of diagnosis. Blast cells comprise less than 10%
  2. *Accelerated phase*: Blast cells in blood and marrow between 10% and 19%
  3. *Blast phase*: Blast crisis, occasionally of sudden onset, is an ominous clinical event that is difficult to treat. Peripheral blood or bone marrow blasts comprise ≥20%.
- Transformation may be suggested clinically by the development of signs and symptoms more typical of acute leukemia (e.g., night sweats, weight loss, fever, bone pain, symptoms of anemia). The blast crisis may be lymphoid in 30% (to ALL) or myeloid in 70% (to AML).
- Patient with blast crisis may develop complications like fever, tumor lysis and renal failure.

Treatment

- Treat fever and tumor lysis, if present.
- Treat anemia/bleeding with appropriate blood product transfusion.
- Tyrosine kinase inhibitors (imatinib, dasatinib, nilotinib). Imatinib is generally well-tolerated with side effects being nausea, vomiting, edema, neutropenia, and thrombocytopenia.

Tumor Lysis Syndrome

INTRODUCTION

Tumor lysis syndrome (TLS) is an oncologic emergency that is caused by massive tumor cell lysis with the release of large amounts of potassium, phosphate, and nucleic acids into the systemic circulation.

Catabolism of the nucleic acids to uric acid leads to hyperuricemia, and the marked increase in uric acid excretion can result in the precipitation of uric acid in the renal tubules. This can also induce renal vasoconstriction, impaired autoregulation, decreased renal blood flow, and inflammation, resulting in acute kidney injury. Hyperphosphatemia with calcium phosphate deposition in the renal tubules can also cause acute kidney injury.

Tumor lysis syndrome most often occurs after the initiation of cytotoxic therapy in patients with high-grade lymphomas (particularly the Burkitt subtype) and acute lymphoid leukemia (ALL). However, TLS can occur spontaneously and with other tumor types.

CLINICAL MANIFESTATIONS

- The symptoms associated with TLS largely reflect the associated metabolic abnormalities (hyperkalemia, hyperphosphatemia, and hypocalcemia).
- They include nausea, vomiting, diarrhea, anorexia, lethargy, hematuria, heart failure, cardiac dysrhythmias, seizures, muscle cramps, tetany, syncope, and possible sudden death.

CAIRO-BISHOP DEFINITION

- Laboratory TLS (LTLS) is defined as any two or more abnormal serum values present within 3 days before or 7 days after instituting chemotherapy in the setting of adequate hydration (with or without alkalinization) and use of a hypouricemic agent.
- Clinical TLS (CTLS) is defined as LTLS plus one or more of the following that was not directly or probably attributable to a therapeutic agent: Increased serum creatinine concentration ($\geq$1.5 times the upper limit of normal), cardiac arrhythmia/sudden death or a seizure.

INVESTIGATIONS

Complete blood count (CBC), electrolytes, creatinine, urea, liver function test (LFT), blood culture/sensitivity, calcium (Ca), phosphate (PO_4), uric acid, lactate dehydrogenase (LDH), urinalysis, arterial blood gas (ABG).

PREVENTION

Aggressive hydration [intravenous (IV) and oral] is the cornerstone of preventing TLS.

MANAGEMENT OF ESTABLISHED TUMOR LYSIS SYNDROME

- Aggressive hydration to induce high urine output to minimize the likelihood of uric acid or calcium phosphate precipitation in the tubules. Administer crystalloids (NS/RL) and monitor urine output to maintain a target of 2 mL/kg/h. About 4–6 L of IV fluids may be required per day. Closely monitor cardiovascular status to avoid fluid overload. Loop diuretics like furosemide may be used to maintain target urine output but generally not required in those with normal renal and cardiac function.
- *Alkalinization of urine*: Sodium bicarbonate ($NaHCO_3$), 100 mL IV stat, is only indicated in patients with metabolic acidosis. The aim is to keep urine pH >7.
- Management of electrolyte abnormalities associated with TLS:
  - *Hyperuricemia*: Allopurinol 300 mg PO stat and 100–200 mg q8h, or Febuxostat 40–80 mg PO stat, or Rasburicase 0.2 mg/kg IV over 30 minutes and od for 5 days
  - *Hyperkalemia*: Correct hyperkalemia (Refer Chapter 10)
  - *Hypocalcemia*: Administer 10 mL of 10% calcium gluconate IV over 4 minutes. Treat hyperphosphatemia first before correcting calcium.
  - *Hyperphosphatemia*: Oral phosphate binders containing aluminum hydroxide (Syrup Digene gel 10 mL stat and q2h) can be given.
- In refractory cases *Renal replacement therapy*/hemodialysis can be considered. Indications are:
  - Severe oliguria or anuria
  - Persistent hyperkalemia
  - Hyperphosphatemia-induced symptomatic hypocalcemia
  - A calcium-phosphate product ≥70 mg/dL^2.

Sickle Cell Crisis

69

INTRODUCTION

Hemoglobinopathies are disorders affecting the production, structure or function of hemoglobin. Sickle cell syndromes are caused by a mutation of the β-globin gene, resulting in HbS, which when deoxygenated results in the characteristic sickle-shaped RBC. Sickled cells lose the pliability to traverse small capillaries, and thus get sequestered in the spleen and other organs, causing acute complications.

Acute complications of sickle cell disease include:

- *Infections:* Common infections include bacteremia and meningitis due to encapsulated organisms (*Streptococcus pneumoniae and Haemophilus influenzae*), pneumonia due to *Mycoplasma pneumoniae, Chlamydia pneumoniae,* and viruses (parvovirus, H1N1 influenza, Zika virus, SARS-CoV-2).
- *Severe anemia:* Hemolytic anemia occurs as a result of splenic sequestration, aplastic crisis, or hyperhemolysis.
- *Vaso-occlusive phenomena:* Vaso-occlusive phenomena and hemolysis are the clinical hallmarks of sickle cell disease. Vaso-occlusion results in recurrent painful episodes and a variety of serious organ system complications. Hemolysis of red blood cell (RBC) causes chronic anemia and pigment gallstones.

CLINICAL PRESENTATION OF SICKLE CELL CRISIS

- *Painful (vaso-occlusive) crisis*: Excruciating pain usually in long bone, ribs, sternum, and vertebra.
- *Chest crisis*: The most common cause of mortality. Vaso-occlusion of pulmonary microvasculature results in reduced perfusion and infarction. Precipitated by pneumonia, pregnancy, and smoking.
- *Cerebral infarction*: Usually in children. High risk of recurrence.
- *Splenic and hepatic sequestration*: RBC trapped in spleen/liver may cause organomegaly, severe anemia, and circulatory collapse.
- *Aplastic crisis*: It is caused by parvovirus infection, exacerbated by folate deficiency.
- *Hemolytic crisis*: Can cause chronic anemia and pigment crisis
- *Priapism*: Prolonged, painful erection due to local vaso-occlusion. Major crisis are often preceded by "stuttering" priapism episodes.

MANAGEMENT

- Give adequate analgesia. Oral NSAIDs may be sufficient for minor crises. Administer parenteral opiates (injection morphine 5 mg IV) for moderate or severe pain and titrate to response.
- Adequate hydration should be ensured (oral or IV).
- Administer oxygen, especially in severe chest crisis.
- Give tablet folic acid 5 mg PO od.
- If an infective etiology is suspected, start broad-spectrum antibiotics.
- *Give thromboprophylaxis for deep vein thrombosis (DVT)*: Low-molecular-weight heparin (LMWH)/unfractionated heparin (UFH)
- *Exchange transfusion*: This can be performed either by manual phlebotomy or by automated red cell exchange. Indications include chest crisis, cerebral infarction, severe persisting painful crisis, and priapism.
- Hydroxyurea is the drug of choice in the overall management of sickle cell disease as it reduces the incidence of acute vaso-occlusive events.
- Hematopoietic stem cell transplantation remains the only life long cure for sickle cell disease.

Anticoagulants

INTRODUCTION

Anticoagulants include heparin, warfarin, direct thrombin inhibitors (DTIs), direct factor Xa inhibitors, and fondaparinux.

ORAL ANTICOAGULANTS

- The commonly used oral anticoagulants are warfarin and acenocoumarol (Sintrom).
  - *Warfarin*: "WARF"—Wisconsin Alumni Research Foundation; "ARIN"—coumarin.
    - It is a synthetic derivative of dicoumarol.
    - It has a longer half-life (36 h), cheaper but has significant drug interactions.
    - *Starting dose for anticoagulation:* 5 mg od and increase by 2.5 mg after 3 days, if needed based on PT with INR.
  - *Sintrom/Acenocoumarol*:
    - It is also a derivative of coumarin (generic).
    - It has a shorter half-life (10 h), costlier and has lesser drug interactions.
    - *Starting dose for anticoagulation:* 2 mg od and increase by 1 mg after 3 days, if needed based on PT with INR.
- They inhibit reduction of vitamin K to its active form and lead to depletion of vitamin K-dependent clotting factors (II, VII, IX, X, and proteins C, S, Z).
- Therapeutic goals of anticoagulation have been shown in **Table 1**.

TABLE 1: Therapeutic goals of anticoagulation.

Indication	International normalized ratio (INR) goal for anticoagulation	Duration
Proximal deep vein thrombosis	2–3	6 months
Calf deep vein thrombosis	2–3	3 months
Pulmonary embolism	2–3	6 months
Atrial fibrillation	2–3	Lifelong
Mechanical heart valve	2.5–3.5	Lifelong
Antiphospholipid antibodies (APLA) with thrombosis	2.5–3.5	Lifelong

TABLE 2: Management of supratherapeutic international normalized ratio (INR).

INR	Bleeding	Recommended action
>Therapeutic range—5	No/minor bleeding	• Withhold one dose and restart warfarin at a lower dose • Check INR after 2 days and follow-up with primary unit
>5–9	No/minor bleeding	• Withhold one dose and restart warfarin at a lower dose • Administer 10 mg vitamin K_1 IV stat • Check INR after 1 day and follow-up with primary unit (monitor INR more frequently to achieve therapeutic range)
>9	No/minor bleeding	• Withhold warfarin for at least 3 days • Administer 10 mg vitamin K_1 IV od for 3 days • Resume warfarin at a lower dose when INR is in therapeutic range (monitor INR more frequently to achieve therapeutic range)
Any INR	Severe bleeding	• Withhold warfarin • Administer 10 mg vitamin K_1 IV over 30 minutes, repeat at 12-hour intervals if the INR remains elevated • Supplement FFP (15 mg/kg), depending on clinical urgency • Monitor and repeat INR as needed

- Oral anticoagulant overdose (accidental or deliberate) results in prolongation of prothrombin time (PT) with international normalized ratio (INR). Risk factors for significant bleeding include local lesions (peptic ulcer, colon angiodysplasia), higher levels of anticoagulation (INR >2.5) and coexistent hematological abnormalities.
- Management of supratherapeutic INR has been shown in **Table 2**.

PARENTERAL ANTICOAGULANTS

- Heparins including unfractionated and low-molecular-weight heparin (LMWH) products:
  - *Unfractionated heparin:*
    - Unfractionated heparin (UFH) comes from porcine intestinal mucosa and it directly inactivates thrombin and factor Xa, via antithrombin.
    - UFH prolongs the thrombin time (TT) and activated partial thromboplastin time (aPTT).
    - The dose for prophylaxis is 5,000 U intravenous (IV)/subcutaneous (SC) q6h. aPTT monitoring is not necessary.
    - For therapeutic anticoagulation, UFH is administered as 80 U/kg IV bolus, followed by 18 U/kg/h infusion. The rate of infusion is titrated based on aPTT monitoring 6 hours later.
    - Protamine sulfate is used as an antidote to reverse bleeding caused by UFH. Approximately 1 mg protamine sulfate IV neutralizes 100 U of

heparin, up to a maximum dose of 250 mg, the dose can be given as 25–50 mg IV over 10 minutes and the rest of the calculated dose as IV infusion over 8–16 hours.

○ *Low-molecular-weight heparins*:
   – LMWHs are produced by enzymatic cleavage of UFH, and they indirectly inactivate thrombin and factor Xa via antithrombin.
   – aPTT monitoring is not needed during treatment with LMWH.
   – Peak factor Xa levels measured 4 hours after a SC dose may be used for monitoring.
   – Contraindicated in patients with a creatinine clearance <10 mL/min. Patients with creatinine clearance <30 mL/min need renal dose adjustment ("od" instead of "bd").
   – Protamine sulfate does not fully reverse the anticoagulant effect of LMWH.
   – *Dose and indications of LMWH:*
     Enoxaparin: 1 mg/kg SC bd daily [unstable angina, non-ST segment elevation myocardial infarction (NSTEMI), deep vein thrombosis (DVT), pulmonary embolism (PE)]
     Dalteparin: 200 IU/kg SC bd daily (DVT, PE).

○ *Fondaparinux*:
   – It is a synthetic pentasaccharide factor Xa inhibitor.
   – As it does not inhibit thrombin, it does not prolong the aPTT.
   – Factor Xa level monitoring is not recommended, but may be necessary in patients with renal failure, obesity, and cachexia.
   – Dose of fondaparinux has been shown in **Table 3**.

○ *Direct factor Xa inhibitors*: Apixaban, rivaroxaban, and edoxaban.
○ *Direct thrombin inhibitors*: Argatroban and bivalirudin are synthetic DTI used in patients with heparin-induced thrombocytopenia (HIT). These are administered as IV infusions.

TABLE 3: Dose of fondaparinux.

Non-ST segment elevation myocardial infarction (NSTEMI)	2.5 mg SC od
Deep vein thrombosis (DVT), pulmonary embolism (PE)	
50 kg	5 mg SC od
50–100 kg	7.5 mg SC od
>100 kg	10 mg SC od

INTRODUCTION

Normal regulation of bleeding is a complex process involving platelets and the coagulation system.

- Bleeding related to platelets usually presents as petechial and mucosal bleeding.
- Bleeding related to coagulation defects presents as spontaneous or deep bleeds.

CONGENITAL PLATELET DISORDERS

- *Glanzmann's thrombasthenia*: Defect in the platelet integrin $\alpha IIb\beta 3$.
- *Bernard-Soulier syndrome*: Giant platelet disorder.

   Treatment: Platelet transfusion [10 platelet rich concentrate (PRCs) for intracranial bleed/4 PRCs for other bleeds].

ACQUIRED PLATELET DEFECTS

- *Decreased platelet production*: Due to marrow infiltration (tumor, infection), viral infections [rubella, human immunodeficiency virus (HIV)], drugs (heparin, sulfa antibiotics), radiation, vitamin B_{12}/folate deficiency.
- *Increased platelet destruction*:
  - *Idiopathic thrombocytopenic purpura (ITP)*: Platelet destruction is mediated by production of autoantibodies that attach to circulating platelets. The presence of lymphadenopathy, hepatosplenomegaly or hyperbilirubinemia should suggest an alternate diagnosis like leukemia, lymphoma, systemic lupus erythematosus (SLE), etc.
    - Initial therapy for ITP is usually steroids (prednisolone 1 mg/kg/day).
    - Platelets should be transfused only if needed, following the first dose of steroids.
    - Transfuse patients only if the bleeding is life-threatening.
    - Avoid using antiplatelet medications such as aspirin or nonsteroidal anti-inflammatory drugs (NSAIDs).
  - *Thrombotic thrombocytopenic purpura (TTP) and hemolytic–uremic syndrome (HUS)*: These are thrombotic microangiopathies caused by platelet—von Willebrand factor (vWF) aggregates and platelet-fibrin aggregates respectively, resulting in thrombocytopenia, microangiopathic hemolytic anemia and organ ischemia. The typical pentad of TTP is seen in <30% of patients and includes thrombocytopenia, hemolytic anemia, fever, renal dysfunction and fluctuating neurological deficits.

Laboratory investigations show presence of schistocytes, normal prothrombin time (PT) and activated partial thromboplastin time (aPTT), elevated lactate dehydrogenase (LDH) and thrombocytopenia.
Mainstay of treatment is plasma exchange. If not available, transfusion of fresh-frozen plasma (FFP) or high-dose glucocorticoids may be tried.

- ○ *Viral infections*: HIV, mumps, varicella, Epstein–Barr virus (EBV).
- *Platelet loss*: Due to excessive hemorrhage or hemodialysis.
- *Splenic sequestration*: Due to sickle cell crisis or cirrhosis.
- *Qualitative platelet abnormalities*: Certain disorders can cause qualitative or functional disorders of platelet function. These include uremia, liver disease, disseminated intravascular coagulation (DIC), multiple myeloma, etc.

ACQUIRED COAGULATION DISORDERS

- *Liver disease*: Mainly due to decreased synthesis of clotting factors, including vitamin K-dependent carboxylation of factors, II, VII, IX and X. FFP may be required to correct the bleeding. If fibrinogen levels are less than 100 mg/dL, cryoprecipitate may be used. Desmopressin may also be used.
- *Renal disease*: Hemostatic abnormalities are commonly present in patients with renal failure due to abnormalities in clotting factors and quantitative and qualitative platelet dysfunction. Retention of uremic toxins causes inhibition of platelet aggregation. In uremic patients with prolonged bleeding times and active bleeding, desmopressin (0.3 mg/kg, max 20 mg, SC or IV or 3 mg/kg, max 300 mg, intranasal spray every 12 h up to three doses) may be given.
- *Disseminated intravascular coagulation*: DIC is an acquired syndrome, characterized by inappropriate and widespread activation of the coagulation system resulting in intravascular fibrin formation. Concomitant activation of the fibrinolytic system also occurs, resulting in breakdown of fibrin clots, consumption of coagulation factors, and bleeding.
  - ○ DIC usually results in multiple organ dysfunction. Although bleeding and thrombosis may occur simultaneously, one usually predominates.
  - ○ Laboratory findings include thrombocytopenia, low fibrinogen level, elevated D-dimer, prolonged PT and aPTT.
  - ○ Treatment includes supportive measures and treatment of the underlying illness.
  - ○ The differences between DIC, TTP/HUS are shown in **Box 1**.

BOX 1 **Diagnosis of DIC, TTP/HUS.**

- The presence of schistocytes on peripheral smear suggests DIC, TTP or HUS
- How to differentiate DIC from TTP/HUS:
  - ○ In DIC, PT and aPTT will be prolonged
  - ○ In TTP/HUS, PT and aPTT will be normal

CLOTTING DISORDERS

- *Inherited clotting disorders*: These disorders cause a hypercoagulable state.
  - *Protein C and S deficiency*: Autosomal dominant. These patients are at a higher risk of developing skin necrosis.
  - *Factor V Leiden mutation*: Also called activated protein C resistance, it is the most prevalent inherited hypercoagulable disorder. Usually presents with venous thromboembolism and pregnancy-related complications (preeclampsia, abruption, stillbirth).
  - *Prothrombin gene mutation 20210A*: Presents with venous thromboembolism and pregnancy-related complications.
  - *Antithrombin deficiency*: Presents with venous thromboembolism and pregnancy-related complications.
  - *Hyperhomocysteinemia*: Associated with both arterial and venous thrombosis. Treatment is with folic acid 5 mg od, along with pyridoxine and vitamin B_{12}.
- *Acquired clotting disorders*:
  - *Antiphospholipid syndrome*: APS is an autoimmune condition that may be associated with complications during pregnancy such as preeclampsia and fetal loss or stroke.
  - *Pregnancy and estrogen use*: There is increased risk of venous thromboembolism and cerebral venous thrombosis.
  - *Malignancy*: Many malignancies are associated with an increased risk of venous thromboembolism.

Hemophilia and von Willebrand Disease

72

HEMOPHILIA

Hemophilia A and B are hereditary X-linked recessive disorders of bleeding that present in male children. As these are X linked disorders, men are overwhelmingly affected with women being asymptomatic carriers. These bleeding disorders typically present early in life with spontaneous deep bruises, hemarthrosis, retroperitoneal or intracranial bleeding.

- *Hemophilia A*: Deficiency of factor VIII.
- *Hemophilia B*: Deficiency of factor IX.

Clinical presentation depends on degree of factor deficiency:

- *Mild*: >5% factor activity. Bleeding is rare.
- *Moderate*: 1–5% activity. Spontaneous bleeding is rare.
- *Severe*: <1% activity. Serious bleeding diathesis may be seen. Acute hemarthrosis, intramuscular bleeds, intracranial bleeding, hematuria, post-trauma bleeding may be severe.

Investigations

- Complete blood count (CBC) profile, ultrasonography (USG) scan for muscle hematomas, computed tomography (CT) scan for headache/focal deficits.
- Coagulation workup typically shows a prolonged activated partial thrombo-plastin time (aPTT) with all other tests normal.

Management

- *Mild-to-moderate hemophilia with minor bleeding*: Desmopressin—DDAVP (0.3 µg/kg IV in 50 mL NS over 30 min, or 300 µg intranasally q12h). Increases factor VIII activity three to five times. DDAVP has no effect on factor IX activity.
- *Mild-to-moderate hemophilia with major bleeding or severe hemophilia with any bleeding*: Factor VIII replacement is the mainstay of therapy. Every 1 U/kg infused increases activity by 2%. A 50 U/L IV bolus increases factor VIII activity by about 100% over baseline.
- Superficial mucosal bleeding may be controlled with anti-fibrinolytic therapy. Administer oral tranexamic acid 500–1,000 mg q8h or IV tranexamic acid 10 mg/kg q8h.
- If factor VIII concentrate is not available, cryoprecipitate or FFP may be used to control acute bleeding.

  Hemophilia B is treated with factor IX replacement. Each 1 IU/kg of factor IX replacement increases plasma factor IX activity by 1%.

VON WILLEBRAND DISEASE

von Willebrand disease (vWD) is the most common inherited bleeding disorder in the world. vWD is characterized by reduced levels or abnormal function of von Willebrand factor (vWF), which normally promotes platelet adhesion and protects factor VIII from destruction. Hence, there is reduced factor VIII level in severe disease.

Clinical Features

- The clinical presentation is less severe than hemophilia with hemarthroses and muscle bleeds being rare.
- Epistaxis, prolonged bleeding from trivial wounds, oral cavity bleeding, excessive menstrual bleeding.

Diagnosis

Diagnosis is confirmed by an assay of vWF activity by measurement of ristocetin cofactor (RCoF) activity. Normal RCoF values are 50–200 IU/dL. Levels of <30 IU/dL are considered definitive for vWD.

Management

- Desmopressin induces the release of vWF from storage sites in the endothelium and is the mainstay of therapy. The dose is 0.3 µg/kg (max 20 µg) SC/IV every 12–24 h for 3–4 doses.
- Plasma derivatives like cryoprecipitate that contains vWF and factor VIII can also be used to control acute bleeding.
- Intermediate purity factor VIII concentrate or vWF plasma derived concentrate transfusions, if available, may be used.

CHAPTER 73

Blood Products and Transfusion

BLOOD COMPONENTS

Blood components are those products derived from whole blood:
- *Packed red cells*: Each pack is from a single donor. A transfusion of 4 mL/kg will increase circulating hemoglobin (Hb) by 1 g/dL.
- *Platelets*: They may be either pooled or derived from a single donor by plateletpheresis. Crossmatching is not necessary before transfusion.
- *Fresh frozen plasma*: FFP is plasma obtained after separation of whole blood from RBC s and platelets and then frozen within 8 hours of collection. It contains coagulation factors (fibrinogen, albumin, protein C, protein S, antithrombin, tissue factor pathway inhibitor). It is free of erythrocytes, leucocytes and platelets. 10–20 mL/kg (4–6 units in adults) will increase factor levels by approximately 20%. FFP must be ABO compatible with the recipient's red cells.

FFP is indicated in patients with the following:
- Congenital or acquired deficiency of clotting factors with active bleeding
- For planned surgeries or invasive procedures in the presence of abnormal coagulation tests
- For reversal of warfarin induced coagulopathy in the presence of active bleeding
- *Cryoprecipitate*: Cryoprecipitate is the cold insoluble protein fraction of FFP. One unit of cyoprecipitate (20–50 mL) contains fibrinogen (factor I), antihemophilic factor (factor VIII), fibrin stabilizing factor (factor XIII) and von Willebrand factor (vWF). Cryoprecipitate is indicated in bleeding due to hemophilia, von Willebrand disease, hypofibrinogenemia (disseminated intravascular coagulation). Crossmatching is not necessary before transfusion.

COMPLICATIONS OF BLOOD TRANSFUSION

- *Immune-mediated reactions*:
  - *Febrile transfusion reaction*: Most common reaction, presents with fever, chills, and malaise. Usually caused by cytokines from leukocytes in transfused red cell or platelet components.
  - *Acute hemolytic reaction*: Most serious reaction, presents with fever, chills, pain at transfusion site, nausea, vomiting, and dark urine. Often a result of ABO/Rh incompatibility due to administration error.
  - *Allergic reaction*: Presents with urticaria, pruritis, hives which may progress to laryngeal oedema or bronchospasm. Anaphylaxis is rare.

- *Transfusion Related Acute Lung Injury (TRALI)*: Presents with sudden onset of non-cardiogenic pulmonary oedema within 6 hours of transfusion. Associated with the presence of antibodies in the donor blood to recipient leukocyte antigens and may be fatal.
    - *Graft-vs-Host Disease (GVHD)*: Presents with rash, fever, diarrhea, and hepatic dysfunction 1–4 weeks after transfusion. There is no effective treatment for GVHD.
- *Nonimmune reactions*:
    - *Transfusion associated circulatory overload (TACO)*: Presents with acute respiratory distress within 6 hours of transfusion of large volume of blood, especially in the elderly. Slow the transfusion and administer diuretics.
    - *Hypothermia*: When large volume of freshly thawed fresh frozen plasma (FFP) is transfused
    - *Electrolyte toxicity*: Hyperkalemia due to red blood cell (RBC) leakage during storage. Citrate, commonly used to anticoagulate blood components chelates calcium and may cause hypocalcemia
    - Iron overload
    - *Infections*: Hepatitis C, B, human immunodeficiency virus (HIV), cytomegalovirus (CMV), human T-cell lymphotropic virus (HTLV), parvovirus B_{19}, malaria.

MANAGEMENT OF SUSPECTED TRANSFUSION REACTION

- Immediately discontinue the transfusion.
- Check and monitor vital signs.
- Check if the right blood product has been given to the right patient.
- Treat the patient symptomatically:
    - *For mild febrile reaction*: Injection/tablet paracetamol
    - *For mild allergic reaction*: Injection chlorpheniramine (Avil) 1 amp IV stat
    - For severe anaphylactic reaction with stridor/wheeze/hypotension:
        - Injection chlorpheniramine (Avil) 1 amp (22.75 mg/mL: 2 mL) IV stat
        - Injection adrenaline 0.5 mg IM in the anterolateral thigh
        - Treat like anaphylaxis (refer chapter 3).
- *TRALI*: Stop the transfusion. Administer oxygen and aggressive respiratory support. Avoid diuretics.
- For mild reactions, discontinue transfusion for 30–60 minutes and restart slowly.
- For severe reactions, stop the transfusion and send the blood product to blood bank along with a patient's blood sample in a ethylenediaminetetraacetic acid (EDTA) tube and a urine sample.

Endocrine Emergencies

CHAPTER 74

Thyrotoxic Crisis

INTRODUCTION

Thyrotoxic crisis or thyroid storm is a rare but potentially life-threatening emergency induced by a sudden release of thyroid hormones in patients with thyrotoxicosis. It occurs in 1–2% of patients with thyrotoxicosis and is characterized by exaggerated symptoms, further distinguished by the presence of fever, marked tachycardia, central nervous system (CNS) dysfunction, and gastrointestinal symptoms.

CLINICAL FEATURES

The clinical presentation of a thyroid storm is quite dramatic with the common triggers being infection, diabetic ketoacidosis, hypoglycemia, radioactive iodine treatment, and thyroid hormone overdose.

Hyperthermia (104-106°C) and tachycardia (heart rate >150/min) are quite prominent.

CNS dysfunction is a hallmark of thyroid storm and presents with restlessness, agitation, delerium, seizures, and coma.

Gastrointestinal symptoms (nausea, vomiting, diarrhea, abdominal pain, and sometimes cholestatic jaundice) are also pronounced.

Other features of thyrotoxicosis are quite evident in patients with thyroid storm. These include fine tremors, muscle wasting, hyperreflexia, exophthalmos, ophthalmoplegia, wide pulse pressure, congestive heart failure, atrial fibrillation or flutter.

INVESTIGATIONS

Serum thyroid stimulating hormone (TSH): In primary hyperthyroidism, TSH levels are low due to negative feedback mechanism of high thyroid hormone levels, while TSH is increased in secondary hyperthyroidism because of increased production in the pituitary.

Free thyroxine (FT4) and triiodothyronine (T3): A low TSH with elevated FT4 or T3 confirms the diagnosis of thyrotoxicosis.

Thyroid antibody titers: Thyroid stimulating antibodies (to thyroglobulin or thyroid peroxidase) are detected in Graves disease.

MANAGEMENT

- Identify and treat the precipitating factor.
- Stop excessive thyroid hormone synthesis, action, and reduce enterohepatic circulation. Remember the mnemonic 5Bs provided in **Table 1**.

TABLE 1: Medical management of thyroid storm.

5Bs	Aim	Drug and dose
Block synthesis	Inhibit synthesis of thyroid hormones	• Propylthiouracil (PTU) 600 mg PO stat and 200 mg q4–6h or • Carbimazole: 20–30 mg PO q4–6h
Block T_4 into T_3 conversio	Reduce T_4 to T_3 conversion, promote vasomotor stability, and possibly treat an associated relative adrenal insufficiency	Hydrocortisone 100 mg IV q6h (PTU also blocks peripheral T_4 to T_3 conversion)
Block release[a]	Inhibit thyroid hormone release from the glands	• Iopanoic acid 1 g IV stat and q8h for 24 h, followed by 500 mg IV bd; *or* • Lugol's solution: 5–10 drops PO q6–8h; *or* • Potassium iodide: 5–10 drops PO q6–8h

Beta-blocker	Symptomatic relief and blocking peripheral effects of excess thyroid hormones	• *Propranolol*:
		  ○ 1–2 mg/min slow IV bolus, repeat q15 min till maximum dose of 10 mg/day is reached. Use IV route only in hemodynamically unstable patients
		  ○ Tablet propranolol 40–80 mg q4–8h
		• Metoprolol 100 mg PO q6h

Bile acid sequestrants	To decrease entero-hepatic recycling of thyroid hormones	Cholestyramine 4 g PO q6–12h

[a] To be given at least 1 hour after the administration of PTU.

Myxedema Coma

CHAPTER 75

INTRODUCTION

Myxedema coma is a state of severe hypothyroidism in which the functioning of every organ system in the body slows down significantly, resulting in altered sensorium, hypothermia, and other changes due to physiological decompensation. Common causes of hypothyroidism are given below

- *Primary hypothyroidism (intrinsic dysfunction of the thyroid gland)*: Autoimmune etiology (Hashimoto thyroiditis), post-ablation (surgical, radio-iodine), infiltrative diseases (lymphoma, sarcoidosis, amyloidosis, tuberculosis), and drugs (amiodarone, lithium).
- *Secondary hypothyroidism (disorders at hypothalamic-pituitary axis)*: Panhypopituitarism, pituitary adenoma, tumours impinging on hypothalamus, infiltrative causes (sarcoidosis, hemochromatosis).

CLINICAL PRESENTATION

- *Dermatological manifestations*: Manifestations are puffiness of the hands and face (due to deposition of mucopolysaccharides in the dermis), thickened nose, swollen lips, and enlarged tongue. Nonpitting pedal edema is a classical finding.
- *Neurologic manifestations*: These include decreased mental status with confusion, lethargy, obtundation, or coma. Focal or generalized seizures may occur. Atypical forms include myxedema madness (psychotic features).
- *Hyponatremia*: It is seen in 50% of cases and may cause seizures or worsen the sensorium.
- *Hypothermia*: It is due to decrease in thermogenesis as a result of decrease in metabolism.
- *Hypoventilation*: Contributing factors include central respiratory center depression, respiratory muscle weakness, mechanical obstruction due to the enlarged tongue, and sleep apnea.
- *Hypoglycemia*: It may be caused by hypothyroidism alone or, more often, by concurrent adrenal insufficiency.
- *Cardiovascular abnormalities*: These include bradycardia, decreased myocardial contractility, a low cardiac output, and sometimes hypotension.

DIAGNOSIS

Diagnosis is initially based upon the history, physical examination, and exclusion of other causes of coma.

- Primary hypothyroidism is confirmed by a high TSH and low FT4 or T3 levels.
- Secondary hypothyroidism is confirmed by a low TSH and low FT4 or T3 levels.

MANAGEMENT

General supportive care includes securing airway and breathing. Supplemental oxygen, respiratory support, cardiac monitoring for dysrhythmias, rewarming for hypothermia, dextrose containing fluids for hypoglycemia and correction of electrolyte abnormalities may be required.

Thyroid Hormone Replacement

- Tablet T_4 (thyronorm/eltroxin) in a loading dose of 200–400 μg followed by a daily dose of 1.6 μg/kg.
- Tablet T_3 (Cytomel) may also be given in a dose of 5–20 μg stat, followed by 2.5–10 μg q8h, depending upon the patient's age and coexistent cardiac risk factors.

  Note: The biologic activity of T_3 (triiodothyronine and liothyronine) is greater and its onset of action is more rapid than T_4 (levothyroxine).
- Hydrocortisone 100–200 mg IV q6h because of associated hypopituitarism and secondary adrenal insufficiency. Administer steroids before thyroid hormone replacement.
- Intravenous thyroxine can be prepared (by pharmacy) in severe cases, if requested during an emergency.

Intravenous Thyroxine Preparation Method

- 10 tablets of 100 μg thyroxine (LT4) crushed
- 14 mg of mannitol added
- Reconstituted to make 100 mL mixture with 7.4% $NaHCO_3$
- So 100 mL will contain 1,000 μg of thyroxine (1 mL = 10 μg). The entire content is filtered with 0.2 μg Vygon antibacterial filter.

ADRENAL HORMONES

- *Glucocorticoids*: Cortisol is the main glucocorticoid produced by the adrenal gland.
- *Mineralocorticoids*: Aldosterone helps to regulate the body's sodium and potassium levels, blood volume, and blood pressure.
- *Androgens*: Testosterone, dehydroepiandrosterone (DHEA), and DHEA sulfate.

Conversion formula for various steroids for glucocorticoid effect:

20 mg of hydrocortisone = 6 mg of deflazacortisone = 5 mg of prednisolone = 4 mg of methylprednisolone = 1 mg of dexamethasone/betamethasone

CAUSES

- *Primary adrenal insufficiency*: Also known as Addisons crisis, it is due to intrinsic adrenal gland dysfunction and results in decreased cortisol and aldosterone production.
  - *Immune-mediated*: Isolated or part of polyglandular syndrome
  - *Infection*: Tuberculosis, histoplasmosis, and cytomegalovirus
  - *Vascular*: Infarction or hemorrhage
  - *Infiltration*: Metastatic malignancy, hemochromatosis, sarcoidosis, and amyloidosis
  - *Iatrogenic*: Ketoconazole, etomidate, rifampicin, and anticonvulsants.
- *Secondary adrenal insufficiency*: It is due to hypothalamic-pituitary dysfunction leading to insufficient adrenocorticotropic hormone (ACTH) production by the pituitary. This results in cortisol deficiency only.
  - *Pituitary cause*: Tumor/apoplexy/infiltration/infection
  - *Chronic exogenous steroid intake (>2 weeks)*: This is the most common cause of adrenal insufficiency. The dose implicated is variable (even dose <10 mg Prednisolone equivalent over 2 weeks is sufficient to cause secondary adrenal insufficiency).

CLINICAL FEATURES

The symptoms are generalized fatigue, marked orthostatic hypotension, loss of appetite, weight loss, nausea, vomiting, and skin hyperpigmentation (skin creases, pressure areas, mucous membranes, and nipples seen only in primary insufficiency).

DIAGNOSIS

- A history of chronic steroid abuse may give a clue to the diagnosis of secondary adrenal insufficiency.
- Hyponatremia and hyperkalemia are the two major electrolyte abnormalities of primary adrenal insufficiency.

Demonstration of inappropriately low cortisol production is the first step in establishing the diagnosis. Send a random serum cortisol level. Plasma ACTH level should also be sent if suspicion of adrenal insufficiency is high. Both samples should be sent before initiating glucocorticoid therapy.

- If serum cortisol is low and plasma ACTH is high, the patient has primary adrenal insufficiency (i.e., primary adrenal disease).
- If both serum cortisol and plasma ACTH are low, the patient has secondary (i.e., pituitary disease) or tertiary (i.e., hypothalamic disease) adrenal insufficiency.

MANAGEMENT

The treatment is replacement of deficient hormones.

- Injection hydrocortisone 100–200 mg IV stat followed by 100 mg q6h or injection dexamethasone 8 mg IV q8h.
- Fluid resuscitation with crystalloids (NS/RL).
- Correct hypoglycemia and start 10% Dextrose infusion if necessary.
- Replace mineralocorticoids (fludrocortisone 100 µg PO od) after adequate hydration. Not required when hydrocortisone is used, because hydrocortisone has sufficient mineralocorticoid effect.
- *Look for an underlying infection*: If suspected, start broad-spectrum antibiotics.

Diabetic Emergencies

CHAPTER 77

HYPOGLYCEMIA

Patients are usually symptomatic at glucose levels of 50–55 mg/dL (hypoglycemic thresholds are variable).

Causes

- Most common cause is a relative imbalance of administered versus required insulin or oral hypoglycemic agents (OHAs).
- Alcohol
- Addison's disease
- Pituitary insufficiency
- Insulinoma
- Liver failure
- Postgastric surgery.

Symptoms

- *Neurogenic symptoms*:
  - Tremors, palpitations, and anxiety or arousal (catecholamine-mediated and adrenergic)
  - Sweating, hunger, and paresthesia (acetylcholine-mediated and cholinergic).
- *Neuroglycopenic symptoms*:
  - Cognitive impairment, behavioral changes, psychomotor abnormalities and at lower plasma glucose concentrations, seizure, and coma.

Management

- *Conscious patient*: Oral simple carbohydrates (sugar and glucose powder).
- *Unconscious patient*: Administer 50% Dextrose 100 mL intravenous (IV) stat followed by 10% dextrose 500 mL over 4 hours till hypoglycemia is corrected.
- In cases of OHA overdose or refractory hypoglycemia, continue 10% Dextrose infusion for 8–12 hours.
- Monitor general random blood sugar (GRBS) every 2 hours.
- Look for the etiology of hypoglycemia, evaluate and treat it.

Discharge Recommendation

- If due to OHA or insulin excess, stop OHA for 2 days or decrease the dose of insulin for the next 2 days
- Advice the patient to always keep simple sugars with them at all times and take it as soon as symptoms start
- Refer the patient to follow up in Medicine OPD with AC/PC and HbA1C.

DIABETIC KETOACIDOSIS

Diabetic ketoacidosis (DKA) is an acute, major, life-threatening complication of diabetes that mainly occurs in patients with type 1 diabetes mellitus (T1DM), but it is not uncommon in some patients with type 2 diabetes mellitus (T2DM). Three ketone bodies are produced and accumulate in DKA: Acetoacetic acid (true ketoacid), beta-hydroxybutyric acid and acetone. Nitroprusside test commonly used for urine ketones detects only acetoacetic acid; hence may be falsely negative in DKA and also can not be relied upon to quantify the severity of acidosis. Direct serum assays for beta-hydroxybutyrate have become the preferred diagnostic tests.

Clinical Features

- The most common early symptoms of DKA are insidious increase in polydipsia and polyuria.
- Malaise, generalized weakness, fatigability, altered sensorium, and associated symptoms of infections may be seen.
- Patients would be extremely dehydrated with a fluid deficit of at least 6 liters.

Examination: If the GRBS is high, look for dryness of tongue and start IV fluids immediately before performing any test. Fluid resuscitation is lifesaving.

Precipitating Cause

- Look for any precipitating cause and address it
- Common precipitating causes—The 5Is
  - Insulin—nonadherence
  - Infection or inflammation
  - Ischemia or infarction
  - Intra-abdominal process—pancreatitis, cholecystitis, appendicitis, splenic injury, and ischemic bowel
  - Iatrogenic—steroid use.

Diagnostic Triad

- High plasma sugar level (>250 mg%)

- *Ketosis*: Urine ketones positive (2+ or 3+. Remember that ketone 1+ positive is a common finding and does not mean ketosis). If available, serum ketones >3 mmol/L is more accurate and diagnostic of diabetic ketosis.
- *Acidosis*: Serum bicarbonate < 18 mEq/L or ABG pH < 7.30.

Management

The order of therapeutic priorities is fluids first, then potassium correction and then insulin administration.

Fluid Resuscitation

This is the most important step. Start normal saline (NS) at the following rate (Rule of diminishing of ½)

- NS 1,000 mL over 30 minutes
- NS 500 mL over 30 minutes
- NS 500 mL over 60 minutes
- NS 500 mL every 2 hours till fluid deficit is corrected.

Tailor the above rates with the patient's cardiopulmonary status. Reassess every 2 hour and look for fluid overload.

Restrict fluids in those with congestive cardiac failure or pulmonary edema.

Type of Fluid

- *Initial replacement*: NS
- If serum Na^+ >155 mEq/L, use ½ NS
- Once GRBS is <250 mg%, change the infusate to 5% Dextrose. Do not stop insulin infusion.

Insulin Administration

- Administer a bolus of 10 units IV regular insulin.
- Insulin infusion at 6 units/h and check the GRBS q1h.
- The expected decline of the glucose per hour is 50 mg/dL. If not, increase the infusion by 2 units/h (consider a bolus of 4 units insulin if the GRBS is persistently high and does not show a decreasing trend).
- If significant hypokalemia exists (K^+ <3 mEq/L), *do not* start insulin infusion or give the bolus dose until IV KCl supplementation is initiated urgently.
- When blood glucose levels reach 250 mg%, decrease insulin infusion to 4 units per hour and change infusate to 5% Dextrose. *Do not stop insulin infusion.* If blood sugars continue to drop, change infusate to 10% Dextrose.

Potassium Correction

- Metabolic acidosis results in pseudohyperkalemia and the actual K levels may be lower than the result shown.
- Start K^+ correction unless K level is >5 mEq/L.

- If K^+ is <5 mEq/L, add 1.5–4.5 g KCl in 1,000 mL NS over 4 hours as a parallel infusion.
- Decrease the amount of KCl supplementation in patients with renal failure.

Treat the Precipitating Cause

If there is any evidence of infection, start broad-spectrum antibiotics, i.e., carbapenems.

Correct Severe Metabolic Acidosis

- Administer $NaHCO_3$ only if the serum pH is less than 6.9. Give 100 mL bolus followed by 10 mL/h infusion.
- There is no role for dialysis in patients with DKA.

Correct Other Electrolyte Abnormalities

Serum phosphate usually falls during treatment as it moves intracellularly with potassium. Supplement with Syrup Neutral phosphate 30 mL stat and repeat dose based on serum phosphorus levels.

> Every patient with DKA should have at least three IV lines. One each for IV fluids, insulin infusion, and K correction. Additional lines for antibiotics or $NaHCO_3$ may be needed. Start a central line at the earliest.

HYPEROSMOTIC HYPERGLYCEMIC NONKETOTIC STATE (HHNK)

The HHNK is characterized by progressive hyperglycemia and hyperosmolarity typically in debilitated elderly patients with undiagnosed or poorly controlled diabetes mellitus, limited access to water and a precipitating illness. This condition, unlike DKA, evolves over days or weeks and the patient complaints of fatigue, anorexia, dyspnea, chest or abdominal pain or a neurological complaint. This condition is characterized by hyperglycemia, dehydration, and serum hyperosmolarity without ketosis or significant acidosis.

Diagnosis

- Very high plasma glucose levels
- *High plasma osmolality*: >350 mOsm/kg
- No metabolic acidosis.

Differences between DKA and HHNK

- The amount of fluid deficit is much higher in HHNK (average deficit 10–12 L).
- Glucose levels are usually very high in HHNK.

- Hypernatremia is common in HHNK. If present, use ½ NS or ¼ NS as the replacement fluid.
- Use lesser doses of insulin (typically half the dose used in DKA) in HHNK as these patients may be more sensitive to insulin action.

Management

Management is similar to DKA management, except the above-mentioned differences.

SLIDING SCALE FOR INSULIN ADMINISTRATION

Intravenous infusion of short-acting actrapid insulin, 1 mL (40 units) in 39 mL of NS, to be adjusted according to GRBS every 2 hours (**Table 1**).

TABLE 1: Sliding scale for insulin infusion.

GRBS (mg%)	Insulin infusion rate
<80	No insulin
81–150	0.5
151–200	1
201–250	1.5
251–300	2
301–350	2.5
351–400	3
401–450	4
451–500	5
>500	6.0

(GRBS: General random blood sugar)

Pheochromocytoma

INTRODUCTION

Catecholamine-secreting tumors that arise from chromaffin cells of the adrenal medulla and the sympathetic ganglia are referred to as "pheochromocytomas" and "catecholamine-secreting paragangliomas" (extra-adrenal pheochromocytomas), respectively.

The classic triad of symptoms in patients with a pheochromocytoma consists of episodic headache, sweating, and tachycardia. About 50% have paroxysmal hypertension. Patients are usually volume depleted at presentation and should be rehydrated prior to initiation of therapy.

LABORATORY INVESTIGATIONS

- 24 hours urine measurement of catecholamines (metanephrine and normetanephrine).
- If the biochemical results are abnormal, abdominal imaging with CT/MRI is needed to locate the tumor.

MANAGEMENT

- Adequate fluid replacement.
- *Acute hypertensive crisis*: Phentolamine 2–5 mg intravenous bolus and repeat every 15–20 minutes as necessary. Alternate drug is nitroprusside infusion (0.5–1.5 μg/kg/min and titrate).
- To prepare a patient for surgery, initiate alpha-blockade with prazosin XL 2.5 mg PO daily and increase to 10 mg PO over 1 week. Phenoxybenzamine 10 mg PO daily and increase gradually to 40 mg PO tid may also be tried. Once blood pressure is controlled with alpha-blockade, add propranolol 10–20 mg PO tid.
- *Do not administer beta-blocker without adequate alpha-blockade* as unopposed alpha receptor stimulation can precipitate a hypertensive crisis.

Obstetric and Gynecological Emergencies

- **High-dose oral contraceptive pills:** OCPs containing 30 mcg ethinyl estradiol given 8th hourly for 48–72 h until bleeding stops and can then be tapered by giving twice a day for 5 days followed by once a day for 2 weeks.
- **Blood products:** If the patient has severe anemia in failure, transfuse packed red cells. Correct any obvious coagulopathy or thrombocytopenia with fresh frozen plasma/cryoprecipitate/platelets as indicated.
- If the patient is hemodynamically stable and bleeding is mild, discharge on tranexamic acid with or without progestogens and advice to follow up in obstetrics OPD with an USG abdomen.
- Perform a pregnancy test for any patient with bleeding PV in the reproductive age group, if there is a recent history of sexual activity. If a threatened abortion is suspected, perform a vaginal examination and an ultrasound in order to decide plan of management.

REFERENCE

1. Munro MG, Critchley HO, Fraser IS, FIGO Menstrual Disorders Committee. The two FIGO systems for normal and abnormal uterine bleeding symptoms and classification of causes of abnormal uterine bleeding in the reproductive years: 2018 revisions. Int J Gynecol Obstet.2018;143:393-408.

CHAPTER 81

Hyperemesis Gravidarum

INTRODUCTION

Nausea with or without vomiting is a common symptom in the first trimester of pregnancy, seen in about 60–80% of all pregnancies. Hyperemesis gravidarum, seen in about 2% of all pregnancies, refers to severe nausea and vomiting resulting in dehydration, ketosis, weight loss, electrolytes and acid-base imbalances, nutritional deficiencies, and even death. These symptoms usually resolve spontaneously by mid-pregnancy. The presence of abdominal pain, however, is highly unusual and suggests an alternate diagnosis such as cholelithiasis or cholecystitis (more common in pregnancy), pancreatitis, gastroenteritis, pyelonephritis, hepatitis or ectopic pregnancy.

EVALUATION

Physical examination is usually normal except for signs of dehydration. Laboratory investigations include complete blood count (CBC), electrolytes, creatinine, urea, and urine ketone. The presence of ketonuria is an important finding as it an early sign of starvation. Serial measurements of urine ketones may be done to determine adequacy of rehydration therapy.

MANAGEMENT

- Assess hydration status and start intravenous (IV) fluids [normal saline/ Ringer's lactate (NS/RL)]. If ketones are positive, use 5% Dextrose or DNS instead of RL. Initially, keep the patient nil per oral till symptoms of nausea subsides.
- Proton pump inhibitor (pantoprazole) and antiemetic (metoclopramide/ ondansetron).
- If the patient is experiencing persistent vomiting, it is important to replenish low levels of vitamins like thiamine (100 mg IV stat and od for 2–3 days).
- If there is no dehydration and nausea resolves with symptomatic treatment, the patient can be discharged on antiemetics (doxylamine succinate + pyridoxine + folic acid twice daily: Commonly available as doxinate tablet) and to follow-up in OPD.

Pelvic Inflammatory Disease

INTRODUCTION

Pelvic inflammatory disease (PID) is primarily a disease of sexually active women.

It includes a spectrum of acute infections of the upper genital tract structures in women (salpingitis, endometritis, myometritis, parametritis, oophoritis, and tubo-ovarian abscess). Any one or all of the genital tract structures may be involved. The minimum criteria required to make a presumptive clinical diagnosis of PID in sexually active young women are:

- Lower abdominal tenderness
- Adnexal tenderness, and
- Cervical motion tenderness.

ETIOLOGY

Most common sexually transmitted organisms that cause the disease are *Chlamydia trachomatis* and *Neisseria gonorrhoeae*. These originate in the lower genital tract and ascend to the upper tract. Other organisms include herpes simplex virus, trichomonas vaginalis, mycoplasma genitalium, *Ureaplasma urealyticum*, *Gardanella vaginalis*, *Bacteroides* species, etc.

Complications include tubo-ovarian abscess, scarring and adhesions of the fallopian tubes, infertility, chronic pelvic pain, and dyspareunia.

MANAGEMENT

There is no single diagnostic test for PID. Evaluation of any woman in the reproductive age group in the ED should include a pregnancy test. Consider the possibility of an ectopic pregnancy or septic abortion.

- *Analgesics*: (Mefenamic acid 500 mg + dicyclomine 20 mg), NSAIDs and paracetamol if required for pain relief.
- *Antibiotics*: Empiric antibiotic therapy is recommended to patients with suspected PID. The regimen must be tailored to local antibiotic resistance pattern. Doxycycline 100 mg PO BD/azithromycin 500 mg PO od plus metronidazole 500 mg PO q8h × 5–10 days is the most commonly used regimen. Injection ceftriaxone 250 mg IM single dose plus doxycycline 100 mg PO BD × 14 days is an alternate option.
- Patients who do not respond to 72 hours of antibiotic therapy may require laparoscopic or surgical interventions like drainage of tubo-ovarian abscess or pus loculations
- If an intra-uterine device (IUD) is present, it should be removed after initiation of antibiotics.

INTRODUCTION

Ovarian torsion is a gynecological emergency where the ovary either partially or completely twists on its ligamentous supports. This often results in impedance of its blood supply.

When the fallopian tube twists along with the ovary, it is referred to as adnexal torsion.

CLINICAL PRESENTATION

- Torsion is commonly seen in young girls in the reproductive age group because of regular formation of a corpus luteal cyst during the menstrual cycle. Up to 80% of cases of ovarian torsion are associated with a benign ovarian malignancy.
- Acute onset of moderate to severe pelvic pain, adnexal mass, often with nausea, vomiting, and fever. A recent vigorous activity (often intercourse) may be an inciting event.
- Fever may be a marker of adnexal necrosis, particularly in the setting of leukocytosis.

INVESTIGATIONS

The investigations to be sent are complete blood count (CBC), electrolytes, creatinine, and urea.
- Urine Pregcolor test should carried out in the reproductive age group to rule out an ectopic pregnancy.
- *If surgical intervention is required:* Rapid blood borne virus screen (BBVS)
- Arrange for an USG of the abdomen and pelvis. USG findings include enlarged ovary with a heterogeneous stroma and small peripherally displaced follicles, ovarian mass or evidence of hemorrhage.
- Doppler ultrasound scan is inconsistent due to dual blood supply of the ovary from both ovarian and uterine arteries. Despite this limitation, doppler may still be useful if abnormal venous flow is demonstrated. Visualization of the twisting of the pedicle with coiled vessels, known as 'whirlpool sign' is an accurate sign of adnexal torsion.

DIFFERENTIAL DIAGNOSIS

- *Ectopic pregnancy*: A negative serum human chorionic gonadotropin (HCG) and a pregcolor test excludes ectopic pregnancy.
- *Ruptured ovarian cyst*: Pelvic pain is often at midcycle. May have a history of vigorous physical activity as an inciting agent. Can be differentiated by sonography.
- *Tubo-ovarian abscess*: The clinical course is usually indolent and associated with fever.
- *Appendicitis*: Can be difficult to differentiate clinically. Sonography required to confirm ovarian torsion.
- *Renal calculi*: Typical pain starts in either flank and is colicky in nature.
- *Pyelonephritis*: Associated with fever and dysuria. Urinalysis findings of leucocytes or pyuria in this setting can confirm the diagnosis of pyelonephritis.

MANAGEMENT

- Administer analgesics for pain relief. Administer morphine 5 mg IV/SC or tramadol 50 mg IV and repeat doses as required.
- The mainstay of treatment of ovarian torsion is swift operative evaluation to preserve ovarian function and prevent other adverse effects (e.g., hemorrhage, peritonitis, and adhesion formation).
- Most torsed ovaries are considered potentially viable, unless there is a clearly necrotic appearance. Ovaries are usually salvageable if the patient is taken up to the operating room within 8 hours of onset of symptoms.
- Refer to Obstetrician/Gynecologist.

Pregnancy Induced Hypertension (Preeclampsia and Eclampsia)

INTRODUCTION

Hypertensive disorders occur in 6–8% of pregnancies with various grades of severity.

- Gestational hypertension characterized by elevated blood pressure (BP) of >140/90 mm Hg that starts in pregnancy and usually resolves within 6 weeks of the postpartum period.
- Preeclampsia is a gestational hypertension associated with proteinuria (>300 mg/24 h).
- *Eclampsia* is a severe complication of preeclampsia characterized by the occurrence of new onset generalized tonic-clonic seizure (GTCS) or coma. It occurs after the 20th week of gestation or in the immediate postpartum period, for up to 3 weeks.
- HELLP syndrome (Hemolysis, Elevated liver enzymes and low platelets) is a variant of pre-eclampsia often seen in multi-gravid patients. It is characterized by epigastric or right upper quadrant pain and must be considered in any pregnant or postpartum patient presenting to the ED with abdominal pain as the chief complaint.

CLINICAL PRESENTATION

- Gestational hypertension presents with elevated systolic or diastolic blood pressure with no proteinuria or evidence of organ damage.
- Preeclampsia is associated with proteinuria and evidence of vasospastic effects in end organs. Symptoms include headache, right hyochondrial or epigastric pain, visual disturbances (scotoma, loss of vision, diplopia, visual field defects). Laboratory abnormalities include thrombocytopenia, elevated creatinine and LFT derangement.
- Eclapmsia is characterized by the occurrence of seizures (usually GTCS) or coma in the setting of preeclampsia. One third of eclampsia seizures occur in the 28 day postpartum period, but usually in the first 48 hours of delivery.

Complications of preeclampsia, eclampsia and HELLP syndrome include fetal death, abruptio placentae, neurological damage from recurrent seizures, intracranial bleeding, hepatic or splenic hemorrhages, and acute renal failure.

DIAGNOSIS

Eclampsia is a purely clinical diagnosis made in a patient with pre-eclampsia presenting with new onset GTCS with or without an elevated BP. All patients with a sustained BP of >140/90 mm Hg with any symptom secondary to hypertension need to considered for hospitalization and evaluation by an obstetrician.

MANAGEMENT

- *Prevention of maternal hypoxia and trauma*: Place the patient in left lateral position and administer supplemental oxygen (4–5 L/min).
- *Treatment of hypertension, if present*: Injection labetalol 20 mg intravenous (IV) is given over 2 minutes and the dose may be repeated at 10-minute intervals. If not available, tablet nifedipine R 10 mg may be given orally. The drug of choice for chronic hypertension is methyldopa (250 mg q6h and titrated higher) due to its safety profile to the fetus.
- *Active seizures*: The anticonvulsive drug of choice is magnesium sulfate.
  - *Loading dose*: 4 g IV over 15–20 minutes (20% solution)
  - *Maintenance dose*: 1 g/h as a continuous IV infusion.
- Recurrent seizures in patients on maintenance $MgSO_4$ therapy can be treated with an additional bolus of 2 g $MgSO_4$ over 5–10 minutes, with frequent monitoring for signs of Mg toxicity (e.g., loss of patellar reflex, respiratory rate <12/min and oliguria).
- If seizures persist, midazolam or lorazepam infusion may be started. If patient is in status, mechanically ventilate and treat like status epilepticus.
- *Evaluation for prompt delivery*: The treatment of pre-eclampsia is delivery of the fetus. This decision is more complicated in mild pre-eclampsia and when the fetus of <37 weeks of gestation.

Postpartum Hemorrhage

INTRODUCTION

Postpartum bleeding or hemorrhage is defined as the loss of >500 mL of blood within the first 24 hours postpartum in a woman who has had a normal vaginal delivery or >1,000 mL in a woman who has had a cesarean section.

It may also be defined as a decrease in hemoglobin of 10% from baseline within the first 24 hours postpartum. It is one of the leading causes of maternal mortality. Most cases are due to uterine atony, the remainder is due to traumatic causes.

CLINICAL FEATURES

Orthostatic hypotension, fatigue, and anemia result from moderate bleeding. In severe cases, the hypovolemic shock may cause anterior pituitary necrosis (Sheehan's syndrome). Myocardial ischemia and dilutional coagulopathy may also occur. The risk of postpartum depression is increased in these patients making the care of the newborn more difficult.

In patients with significant coagulopathy, consider other possibilities like abruptio placenta, HELLP (hemolysis, elevated liver enzyme levels, and low platelet levels) syndrome, and fatty liver of pregnancy or septicemia.

INVESTIGATIONS

The investigations to be sent are complete blood count (CBC), electrolytes, creatinine, cross-match for packed cells, and rapid blood borne virus screen (BBVS).

- *If coagulopathy is suspected:* Prothrombin time (PT), activated partial thromboplastin time (aPTT), and fibrinogen.

MANAGEMENT

- *Fluid resuscitation*: Secure IV access with 2 large bore peripheral IV cannulae and start fluid resuscitation with crystalloids (NS/RL)
- *Blood transfusion*:
  - Packed red blood cells depending on the degree of blood loss
  - Fresh frozen plasma and cryoprecipitate are required if the patient has dilutional coagulopathy.
  - Consider activating massive transfusion protocol for significant bleeding

- Determine if the cause of postpartum hemorrhage (PPH) is an atonic uterus or a traumatic cause. Uterine atony can be determined by placing the hand on the uterine fundus and finding a boggy, soft uterus.
  - If the uterus is atonic, medical management should be initiated immediately.
    - *Commence bimanual massage*: Place one hand on the fundus and the other hand anterior to the cervix in the vagina and massage.
    - Administer oxytocin 20 units IV in 500 mL RL/NS bolus followed by a 10 units IM dose. Then, add 40 units in 1 L NS and run as an infusion over 4 hours.
    - If bleeding continues, methylergometrine (methergine) 0.2 mg IM and repeat the dose every 30 minutes up to a maximum of three doses (contraindicated in hypertension and ischemic heart disease).
    - If bleeding continues, give prostaglandin F2 alpha. 250 µg IM q15 minutes up to a maximum of eight doses.
    - Misoprostol 800 µg rectally can be given in severe cases.
  - If the PPH is likely to be traumatic in origin:
    - Explore the uterine cavity and control bleeding by packing the uterine cavity rolled gauze to create a tamponade effect.
    - Look for any bleeding vessel in the cervix and vagina and ligate it.
    - After delivery, if pain and uterine bleeding is persistent despite the use of uterotonic agents, consider the possibility of uterine rupture with or without intra-abdominal bleeding. Palpation of the uterine cavity may reveal the opening which may be anterior, posterior, fundal or lateral. Consider uterine arterial embolization or surgical intervention, if the bleeding is uncontrolled.
    - If a mass is seen in the vaginal vault and the uterus cannot be palpated per abdominally, consider the possibility of an uterine inversion.
- Administer tranexamic acid for its anti-fibrinolytic activity in controlling hemorrhage. *Dose*: 1 g IV over 10 minutes, followed by IV infusion of 1 g over 8 hours.

ENT Emergencies

INTRODUCTION

Epistaxis is a common problem, occurring in up to 60% of the general population.

ANATOMY

Epistaxis may be classified as anterior or posterior, depending upon the source of bleeding.

Anterior Bleeds

Anterior bleeds are by far the most common source of bleeding. Up to 90% occur within the vascular watershed area of the nasal septum known as Kiesselbach's plexus (**Fig. 1**). Anastomosis of four primary vessels occurs in this area:

- Septal branch of the anterior ethmoidal artery
- Lateral nasal branch of the sphenopalatine artery
- Septal branch of the superior labial branch of the facial artery
- Greater palatine artery.

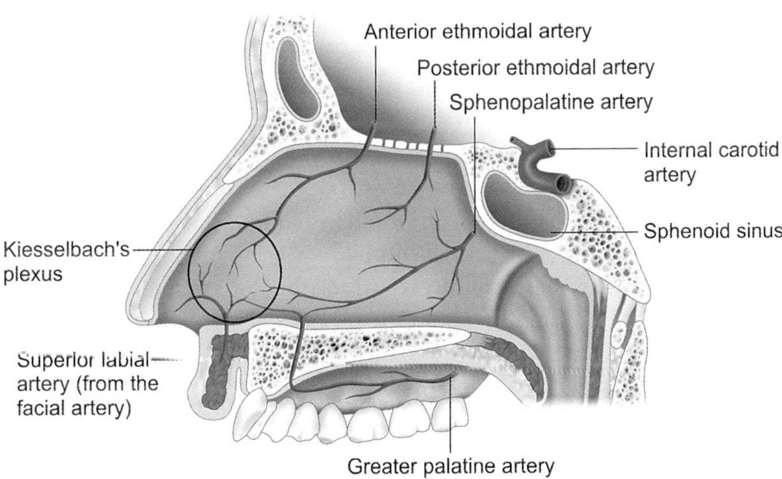

FIG. 1: Kiesselbach's plexus.

Posterior Bleeds

Posterior bleed arises most commonly from the posterolateral branches of the sphenopalatine artery and Woodruff's venous plexus in hypertensives, but may also arise from the carotid artery.

MANAGEMENT

- Grasp and pinch the nose and maintain continuous pressure.
- Apply a few cubes of ice wrapped in a cloth over the bridge of the nose.
- Maintain airway. If patient is conscious, maintain a propped up position leaning forward to prevent aspiration.
- Start IV line. Start crystalloids if there is evidence of hemodynamic shock.
- If the patient is a hypertensive, control blood pressure (BP) aggressively. However, patients frequently have elevated BP due to stress, adequate analgesia, and mild sedation helps to lower BP.
- If the patient is on anticoagulants, check prothrombin time/activated partial thromboplastin time and correct the coagulopathy.
- Refer to ENT for further management.

Nasal Packing

Nasal packing is most easily accomplished with a nasal tampon. These are usually made of Merocel, a synthetic open-cell foam polymer that appears to provide a less hospitable medium for *Staphylococcus aureus* than traditional gauze packing. It is inserted as follows:

- Ask the patient to sit and look directly ahead and attempt the sniffing position. Patients often try to tilt the head back to facilitate a nasal examination, but the nasopharynx lies in the anteroposterior plane and extension of the neck will obscure most of the cavity from view.
- After positioning the patient properly, pretreat with a topical anesthetic (e.g., 2% Lidocaine) and topical vasoconstrictor (e.g., Oxymetazoline).
- Coat the tampon with bacitracin ointment to facilitate placement, and possibly decrease the risk of toxic shock syndrome.
- Insert the tampon by sliding it directly along the floor of the nasal cavity until nearly the entire tampon lies within the nasal cavity.

INTRODUCTION

Stridor is an abnormal, high-pitched sound produced by turbulent airflow through a partially obstructed airway at the level of the supraglottis, glottis, subglottis, or trachea.

It can occur during inspiration, expiration, or both, although it most typically occurs with inspiration.

- Inspiratory stridor suggests a laryngeal obstruction
- Expiratory stridor implies tracheobronchial obstruction
- Biphasic stridor suggests a subglottic or glottic anomaly.

ETIOLOGY

In Children

Stridor occurs due to the following: Laryngotracheobronchitis, foreign body aspiration, bacterial tracheitis, retropharyngeal abscess, peritonsillar abscess, epiglottitis, and laryngomalacia.

In Adults

Stridor may be due to the following reasons:
- Malignancies of larynx, trachea, or esophagus.
- Superior vena cava (SVC) syndrome may cause stridor due to secondary interstitial edema of the head and neck, which may narrow the lumen of the nasal passages and larynx.
- Patients on radiotherapy for malignancies of the head and neck.
- Tracheal stricture due to previous endotracheal intubation or tracheostomy.
- Foreign body aspiration.

MANAGEMENT

- *Maintain airway*: If possible, perform endotracheal intubation. Tracheostomy may be required for laryngeal abnormalities.
- Start oxygen supplementation.
- *Corticosteroids*: Inj. Hydrocortisone 100–200 mg IV stat.
- *Adrenaline nebulizations*: 1 in 10,000 dilution (1 mL Adrenaline in 9 mL NS). Take 1 mL for nebulization every 10 minutes till definite treatment is done.
- *Antibiotics*: For epiglottitis, bacterial tracheitis, retropharyngeal abscess, and peritonsillar abscess (Amoxicillin-Clavulanate/Ceftriaxone).
- Refer to ENT urgently.

Vertigo and Benign Paroxysmal Positional Vertigo

VERTIGO

Vertigo is a symptom of illusory movement (feels as if the person or the objects around them are moving when they are not).

It arises because of asymmetry in the vestibular system due to damage to or dysfunction of the labyrinth, vestibular nerve, or central vestibular structures in the brainstem. The evaluation of a patient with vertigo is shown in **Flowchart 1**. The common causes of vertigo are shown in **Table 1** and the clinical features of the common causes are shown in **Table 2**.

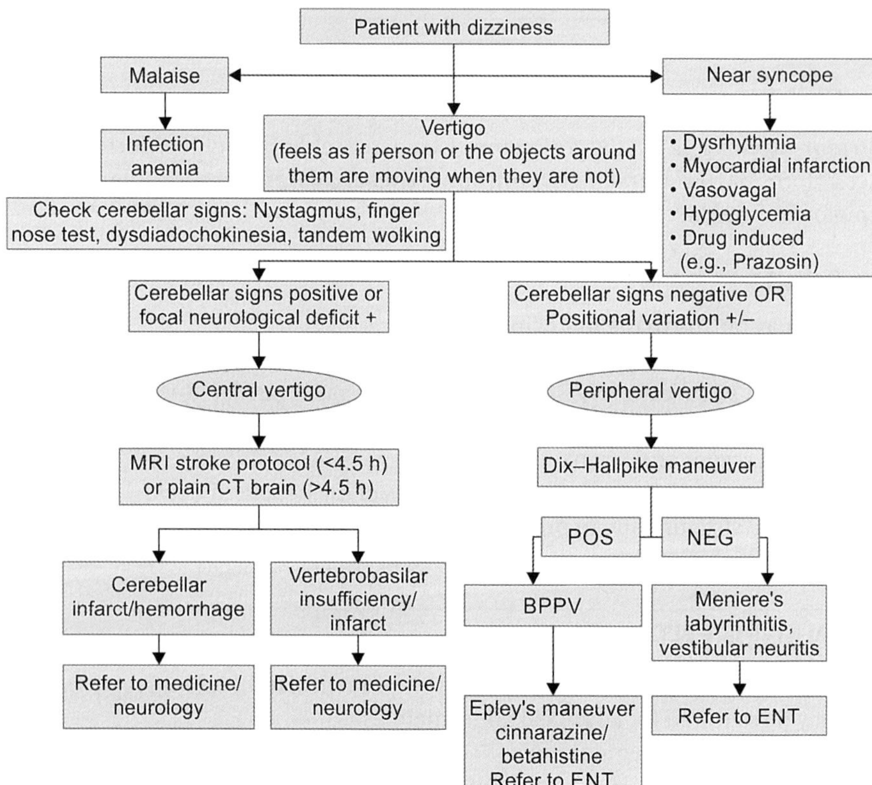

FLOWCHART 1: Evaluation of a patient with vertigo.

TABLE 1: Causes of vertigo.

Peripheral causes	Central causes
• Benign paroxysmal positional vertigo • Vestibular neuritis • Ménière's disease • Herpes zoster oticus • Labyrinthine concussion • Otitis media	• Vestibular migraine • Brainstem ischemia • Cerebellar infarction and hemorrhage

TABLE 2: Clinical features of common causes of vertigo.

	Time course	Suggestive clinical setting	Associated neurologic symptoms	Auditory symptoms	Other diagnostic features
Benign paroxysmal positional vertigo	Recurrent, brief	Predictable head movement/positions precipitate symptoms	None	None	Dix–Hallpike maneuver is diagnostic
Vestibular neuritis	Single episode, acute onset, may last days	Accompanying viral syndrome	Falls toward side of lesion and no brainstem signs	Usually none	Head thrust test usually abnormal
Ménière's disease	Recurrent episodes, last minutes to several hours	Spontaneous onset	None	May be preceded by ear pain, U/L hearing loss, and tinnitus	Audiometry shows U/L sensorineural hearing loss
Vestibular migraine (peripheral)/central nystagnus)	Recurrent episodes, last several minutes-to-hours	History of migraine	Migraine headache and/or other migrainous symptoms	Usually none	Between episodes, tests are usually normal

BENIGN PAROXYSMAL POSITIONAL VERTIGO (BPPV)

It is most commonly attributed to calcium debris within the posterior semi-circular canal, known as canalithiasis. This debris likely represents loose otoconia (calcium carbonate crystals) within the auricular sac. These are normal structures that are displaced from the utricle. There are three variants:

1. Posterior canal (prototype/classical)
2. Anterior canal (superior canal)
3. Horizontal canal.

Posterior Canal Benign Paroxysmal Positional Vertigo (Prototype/Classical)

Recurrent episodes of vertigo lasting 1 minute or less. Although individual episodes are brief, these typically recur periodically for weeks-to-months without therapy.

Episodes are provoked by specific types of head movements, such as looking up while standing or sitting, lying down or getting up from bed, and rolling over in bed. The spells may wax and wane over the time.

The vertigo may be associated with nausea and vomiting.

Examination

Nystagmus is optimally provoked by the Dix–Hallpike (sensitivity 50–88%) or Barany maneuvers.

Nystagmus is an involuntary movement of the eye characterized by a smooth pursuit eye movement followed by a rapid saccade in the opposite direction of the smooth pursuit eye movement.

Dix–Hallpike Maneuver

- With the patient sitting, the neck is extended and turned to one side.
- The patient is then placed supine rapidly, so that the head hangs over the edge of the bed.
- The patient is kept in this position until 30 seconds have passed if no nystagmus occurs.
- The patient is then returned to upright, observed for another 30 seconds for nystagmus, and the maneuver is repeated with the head turned to the other side.

Diagnostic Criteria

Diagnostic criteria employing the Dix–Hallpike maneuver have been proposed for posterior canal BPPV.

- Nystagmus and vertigo usually appear with a latency of a few seconds and last less than 30 seconds.
- It has a typical trajectory, beating upward and torsionally, with the upper poles of the eyes beating toward the ground.
- After it stops and the patient sits up, the nystagmus will recur but in the opposite direction.
- The patient should then have the maneuver repeated to the same side; with each repetition, the intensity and duration of nystagmus will diminish.

Management of Peripheral Vertigo

Epley's maneuver (**Fig. 1** and **Table 3**) should be performed for all patients with confirmed BPPV. This procedure alone provides significant symptom relief in many patients. Oral medications may then be added for symptomatic management.

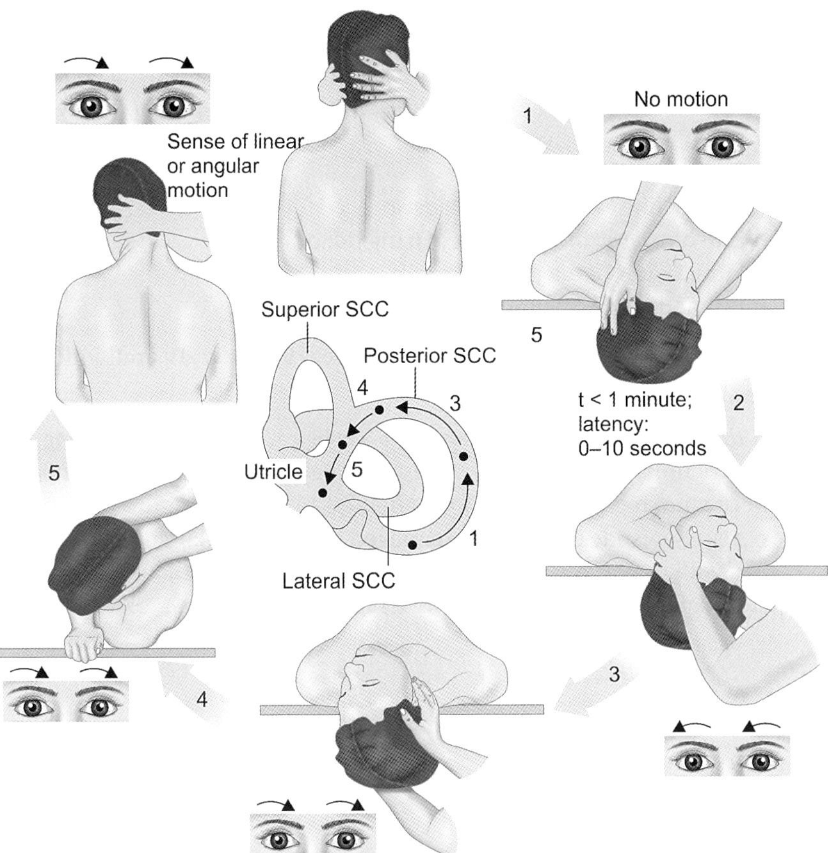

FIG. 1: Epley's maneuver for right-sided benign paroxysmal positional vertigo.

TABLE 3: Particle repositioning maneuver (Epley's maneuver).

The Epley's Maneuver for Right Side BPPV	
Step 1	Patient is made to sit facing forward
Step 2	Turn the head 45° to the right and then rapidly bring the patient into supine position with the head extending just beyond the examining table with the right ear down
Step 3	Examiner should move to the head end of the table
Step 4	Turn the head quickly to the left side with the right ear upward and hold this position for 30 seconds
Step 5	Roll the patient to the left lateral position and rotate the head until the nose faces the floor. Hold this position for 30 seconds
Step 6	Rapidly lift the patient into sitting position
Entire sequence is repeated until no nystagmus can be elicited	

Medications for Vertigo

The neurons involved in the vestibular system are mediated by acetylcholine. Anticholinergic drugs or antihistamines with anticholinergic activity are extremely useful in treating vertigo.

- Tablet Cinnarizine 25 mg tid; or
- Tablet Betahistine (Vertin) 16 mg tid; or
- Tablet Prochlorperazine (Stemetil) 10 mg tid; or
- Tablet Flunarizine 10 mg tid; or
- Tablet Promethazine (Avomine/Phenergan) 25 mg bd.

Acute bacterial labyrinthitis: Patients may require admission , IV antibiotics and if severe, surgical drainage and debridement.

Meniere's disease (classic triad of episodic vertigo, tinnitus and hearing loss): Dietary restrictions (low sodium and caffeine) and lifestyle modifications (cessation of smoking and alcohol) are helpful in decreasing the frequency of episodes. Acute episodes should be managed with vestibular suppressants and antiemetics with or without additional diuretics. Glucocorticoid therapy may be required for patients with refractory and disabling symptoms.

CHAPTER 89

Deep Neck Space Infections

RETROPHARYNGEAL ABSCESS

Once almost exclusively a disease of children, retropharyngeal abscess (RPA) is observed with increasing frequency in adults. Patients who present at an early are often misdiagnosed as pharyngitis and are treated inadequately.

Clinical Features

Clinical features include fever, sore throat, dysphagia, odynophagia, neck pain, and stridor. Patients may present with signs of airway obstruction. Physical signs prior to this stage include posterior pharyngeal edema, cervical adenopathy, drooling, and neck stiffness.

Causes

Retropharyngeal abscess usually occurs through contiguous spread from upper respiratory or oral infections. Pharyngeal trauma from endotracheal intubation, nasogastric tube insertion, endoscopy, foreign body ingestion, and foreign body removal may cause a subsequent RPA. Common organisms include *Streptococcus* species, *Staphylococcus aureus*, *Klebsiella*, *Bacteroides,* and *Escherichia coli.*

Investigations

If a RPA is suspected, ask for X-ray soft tissue neck lateral view. Widening of the retropharyngeal soft tissues is seen in most cases. This is defined as soft tissue swelling.
- >7 mm at C2, or
- >22 mm at C6, or
- More than two-thirds of the width of the vertebral body.

Management

- *Initiate antibiotics*: Amoxicillin-Clavulanate
- Refer urgently to ENT
- Urgent incision and drainage may be required, if airway is compromised.

PERITONSILLAR ABSCESS (QUINSY)

- Peritonsillar abscess is usually a complication of acute tonsillitis and is the most common deep space infection of the neck.
- It is a collection of pus in the peritonsillar space (between the tonsillar capsule and the superior constrictor and palatopharyngeus muscles). The infection begins as a cellulitis and progresses to abscess formation, most commonly near the superior pole of the tonsil.
- Symptoms and signs include fever, odynophagia, foul breath, 'hot potato voice,' earache, and trismus.
- Microbial etiology includes *S. pyogenes* (group A *Streptococcus*) and oral anaerobes like *Fusobacterium*.
- Start antibiotics (Amoxicillin-Clavulanate) and refer to ENT for needle aspiration or incision and drainage of the abscess.
- Complications include airway obstruction, cavernous sinus thrombosis, rupture and aspiration of the contents, epiglottitis, septicemia.

LUDWIG'S ANGINA

- Ludwig's angina is a bilateral infection of the submandibular space. Infection usually begins in the 2nd or 3rd mandibular molar teeth.
- It is typically a polymicrobial infection involving the flora of the oral cavity (alpha-hemolytic streptococci, staphylococci, and *Bacteroides*).
- Clinical features include odynophagia, fever, and brawny cellulitis without lymphadenopathy.
- Airway compromise due to rapid posterior displacement of the tongue is a potential complication.
- Treatment includes urgent surgical drainage and antibiotic therapy. Injection clindamycin 600 mg IV q6–8h × 2 weeks or injection Amoxicillin/Clavulanate 1.2 mg IV q12h × 2 weeks.
- Difficulty in managing secretions and stridor may necessitate emergency airway management.

Urological Emergencies

INTRODUCTION

Epididymitis refers to inflammation of the epididymis. If the infection extends to the scrotum, it is called "epididymo-orchitis". It causes significant morbidity among men in the age group 18–60 years. The clinical presentation of epididymitis is similar to torsion testes, but it is critical to identify torsion testes since torsion is a true urologic emergency and requires immediate intervention.

ETIOLOGY

- *Bacterial*:
  - *Sexually active age group*: *Chlamydia trachomatis* and *Neisseria gonorrhoeae.*
  - *Older men*: *E. coli*, other coliforms, and *Pseudomonas* species.
- *Viral*: Mumps (may cause isolated orchitis) and cytomegalovirus.
- *Others:* Epididymitis may also be caused by noninfectious causes such as trauma and autoimmune diseases, but these usually present as subacute or chronic epididymitis.

CLINICAL FEATURES

Epididymo-orchitis may be acute (lesser than 6 weeks) or chronic (≥6 weeks):
- The clinical features are fever, testicular pain and swelling, and tenderness.
- Epididymitis is characterized by local testicular pain tenderness on the posterior part of the scrotum where the epididymis is located.
- In contrast to torsion testes, manual elevation of the scrotum relieves pain (positive Prehn's sign) due to epididymo-orchitis.
- In epididymo-orchitis, the cremasteric reflex is positive, in contrast to torsion testes where it is typically absent.
- The above two clinical findings help in differentiating torsion testes from epididymo-orchitis.

LABORATORY INVESTIGATIONS

The following examinations should be done:
- Complete blood count (CBC) and renal function tests
- Urinalysis and urine culture to confirm the infective etiology
- Doppler ultrasonography to rule out testicular torsion.

MANAGEMENT

- *Most patients can be managed on an outpatient basis with oral antibiotics, local application of ice,* nonsteroidal anti-inflammatory drugs (NSAIDs), and opioids if necessary.
- *Antibiotics*: Empiric antimicrobial therapy should be started in the ED pending culture sensitivity results and depends on the risk of acquiring sexually transmittable diseases (STD)
- *Patients at high risk of acquiring STDs*: Empiric antibiotics should cover *N. gonorrhoeae* and *C. trachomatis*
  Injection Ceftriaxone 500 mg IV stat plus Tab. doxycycline 100 mg bd × 10 days
  (Tab Azithromycin 1g stat single dose is an alternate to doxycycline)
- *Patients at low risk of acquiring STDs*: Empiric antibiotics should cover enteric gram negative bacteria
  Tablet levofloxaxin 500 mg od × 10 days
  or
  Tablet trimethoprim-sulfamethoxazole double strength bd × 10 days
- Scrotal elevation is a very useful adjunct and must be advised to all patients till symptomatic relief. Ambulatory patients must be advised to wear scrotal supporter and be careful not to do maneuvers that increase intra-abdominal pressure like lifting heavy objects or straining while passing stools.
- Complications include scrotal abscess, testicular infarction, testicular atrophy, and infertility.

93

PHIMOSIS

Phimosis is a condition seen in uncircumcised males in which the foreskin (prepuce) cannot be retracted over the glans penis (**Fig. 1**). The foreskin may normally be nonretractile up to 5 years of age.

Pathologic phimosis may present with painful erections, painful prepuce, recurrent urinary tract infections, hematuria, or a weakened urinary stream.

Management

- Patients with phimosis rarely requires any emergency intervention and can be managed by conservative therapy by application of dexamethasone cream thrice daily for 1 week and referring to Urology.
- If the patient has severe symptoms, refer to Urology. A dorsal slit can be performed for immediate relief.

PARAPHIMOSIS

Paraphimosis is a urologic emergency in which the retracted foreskin cannot be reduced back to is normal position. It is seen in uncircumcised males.

It is often caused by medical professionals (during examination and procedures like catheterization) and parents who retract the foreskin improperly for a long period. This may result in painful swelling of the glans penis. Decreased blood supply eventually results in gangrene and amputation of the glans penis (**Fig. 1**).

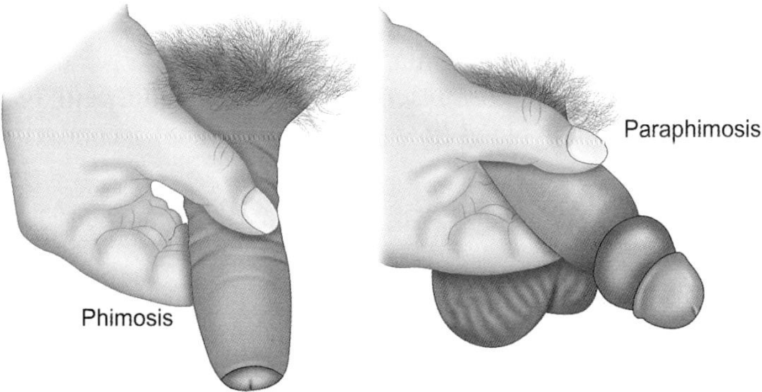

FIG. 1: Phimosis and paraphimosis.

Management

- Administer a penile ring block, which is similar to a digital ring block.
- Apply gentle and constant pressure for 5 minutes to reduce the edema and then attempt manual reduction to reduce the glans back into the preputial fold.
- Before attempting manual reduction, soak the penis in a glove full of ice. This helps to reduce the edema around the glans.
- If manual reduction fails, an emergency dorsal slit may have to be performed. Refer urgently to Urology.

PENILE FRACTURE

- A penile fracture refers to an acute tear or rupture of the tunica albuginea of one or both corpus cavernosa. It occurs in young adults from trauma during sexual intercourse or other sexual activities.
- A typical snapping sound occurs followed by loss of erection, rapid swelling, bruising and deviation of the penis. The penis appears acutely swollen, discolored, flaccid, and tender.
- Ultrasonography is useful to delineate the exact location and extent of the tear.
- *Management:* Surgical intervention is required in most cases and may require hematoma evacuation and suture opposition of the ruptured tunica albuginea.

PRIAPISM

Priapism is a urological emergency characterized by a persistent, pathological, painful erection of the penis. Both the corpora cavernosa are engorged with stagnant blood. It is classified as follows:

- *Low flow (ischemic) priapism:* The most common type is very painful and results from impaired venous drainage, thus increasing cavernosal pressures. If prolonged, it can result in irreversible ischemic changes and permanent erectile dysfunction. It is commonly caused by intracavernosal injection of vasoactive substances (papaverine, prostaglandin E) for impotence, prothrombotic disorders (sickle cell anemia) or some oral medications (hydralazine, prazosin, chlorpromazine, trazodone).
- *High flow (nonischemic) priapism:* Usually, nonpainful and results from dysregulation of penile blood flow (traumatic fistulae) secondary to trauma or surgery.

Management

Low flow priapism is a urological emergency.

- Administer adequate analgesia. Systemic analgesia like morphine/tramadol can be given but may not be adequate. Consider a dorsal penile nerve block by landmark technique or under ultrasound guidance (**Fig. 2**).

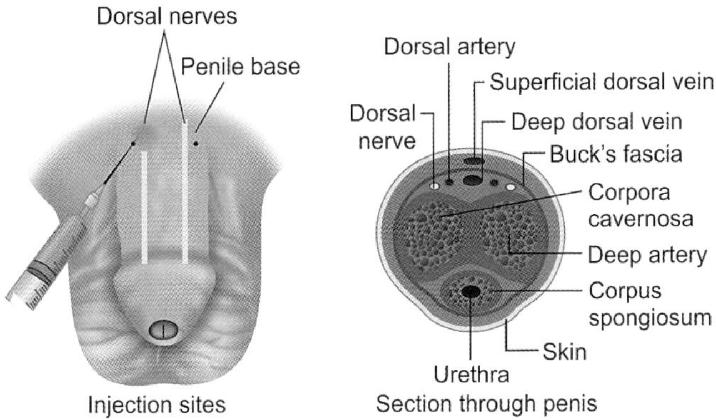

FIG. 2: Dorsal-Penile-Nerve-Block.

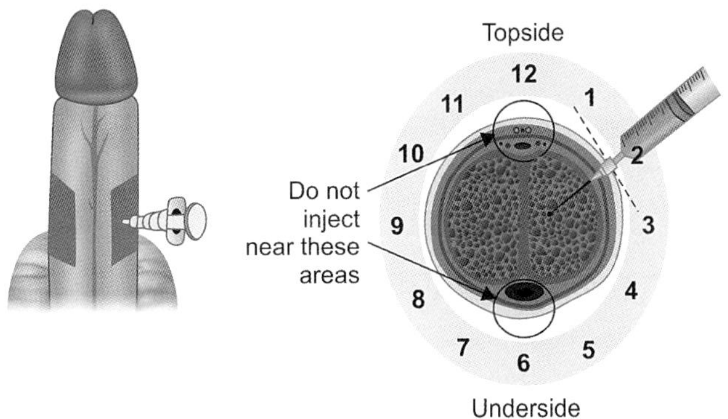

FIG. 3: Intracorporal-Injection.

- Apply warm compress for vasodilation that would improve blood flow and relieve pain
- Priapism due to sickle cell disease can be reversed by adequate hydration and if required, a simple exchange transfusion.

Invasive management: Intracorporal injection of an alpha-adrenergic agonist (phenylephrine) can cause cavernous smooth muscle contraction, thus allowing venous outflow. Phenylephrine (250–500 µg diluted in 1 mL NS) or Adrenaline (0.1 mg diluted in 1 mL NS) can be injected at either '2 o'clock' or at '10 o'clock' position at the base of the penis using a 25 or 26 guage needle. Advance needle at 45 degrees angle to the skin till blood is aspirated (**Fig. 3**). A repeat injection can be given after 30 minutes. Bilateral injection is not necessary as the corpora cavernosa communicate.

Definitive management incudes aspiration and irrigation with a vasoactive substance such as phenylephrine or adrenaline using a 19 guage butterfly needle at the same site described above. Irrigation is done if inadequate blood returns on aspiration or detumescence is not achieved.

Surgical Emergencies

Skin and Soft Tissue Infections

CELLULITIS

Cellulitis and erysipelas are superficial infections of the skin and soft tissue that are caused by bacteria (*Staphylococcus* and group A streptococci) breaching the skin barrier through open wounds.

Erysipelas: Infection of the upper dermis and superficial lymphatics, with an area of erythema and well-demarcated, raised borders, usually involving the lower extremities or the face.

Cellulitis: Infection of the deeper dermis and subcutaneous fat, with ill-defined borders, most commonly involving the extremities.

Necrotizing fasciitis (NF): NF is characterized by infection of the deep fascia and necrosis of the subcutaneous tissues. This represents the other end of the spectrum of skin and soft tissue infections and results from untreated cellulitis or erysipelas.

Investigations

Investigations include complete blood count (CBC), electrolytes, creatinine, and blood culture and sensitivity (c/s).

Management

- $MgSO_4$ dressing twice daily to reduce edema. Treat skin dryness with topical agents like moisturizers.
- Limb elevation for drainage of edema.
- *Antibiotics*:
    - Cefazolin 1 g IV q8h × 7–10 days; or
    - Cloxacillin 500–1,000 mg PO q6h × 7–10 days; or
    - Cephalexin 500 mg PO q6h × 7–10 days.
- Refer to general surgery.

It is important to differentiate cellulitis and necrotizing fasciitis (NF) clinically

- Cellulitis is a superficial infection of the skin and requires only conservative management.
- Necrotizing fasciitis is a deeper infection of the subcutaneous tissues, has skin discoloration/blebs/necrosis. Urgent surgical debridement is essential.
- Do not send preoperative tests [prothrombin time (PT), activated partial thromboplastin time (aPTT), and blood borne virus screen (BBVS)] for clinical diagnosis of cellulitis.

NECROTIZING FASCIITIS

Necrotizing fasciitis is an acute bacterial infection involving the skin and deeper layers of the fascia, resulting in necrosis of the skin and subcutaneous tissue. It is a rapidly progressive condition characterized by skin color changes, blisters, and gangrene and requires urgent surgical intervention.

Fournier gangrene: Necrotizing fasciitis involving the scrotum, penis and perineum is called Fournier gangrene. It typically presents abruptly with severe pain and may rapidly spread to the anterior abdominal wall or the gluteal muscles.

Microbiology

- *Type I infection*: It is the most common type and is a polymicrobial infection caused by obligate and facultative anaerobes like *Bacteroides, Clostridium*, or *Peptostreptococcus*. It usually involves the trunk and perineum with diabetes mellitus being the risk factor.
- *Type II infection*: It is monomicrobial, most common organism being Group A beta-hemolytic *Streptococcus*. It usually affects the extremities.
- *Type III infection*: It is also monomicrobial caused by *Clostridium* species, gram-negative bacteria, *Vibrio vulnificus*, or *Aeromonas hydrophila*.
- *Type IV infection*: It is usually caused by fungi (*Candida* species and Zygomycetes) in the immunocompromised host.

Investigations

The investigations include CBC, electrolytes, creatinine, blood c/s, chest X-ray, ECG, PT, aPTT, and BBVs rapid.

Management

- Limb elevation for drainage of edema
- *Antibiotics*: Piperacillin-Tazobactam 4.5 g IV stat and q6–8h, or
  Crystalline penicillin 20 L Units IV q4h + Clindamycin 600 mg IV q6h
- Refer to general surgery for urgent surgical debridement.
  In large tertiary care hospitals with high rates of antibiotic resistance, the following protocol may be followed:
  - Moderate infection (local infection with erythema >2 cm or involving structures) involving skin and subcutaneous tissues (e.g., abscess, osteomyelitis, septic arthritis, fasciitis): Piperacillin tazobactam 4.5 g IV q8h plus Vancomycin 15 mg/kg IV q12h.
  - Severe infection (life-threatening/gangrene/septic shock): Meropenem 1 g IV q8h plus Vancomycin 15 mg/kg IV q12h.
- Surgical debridement is a limb and life-saving intervention and must be performed as soon as possible. Debridement, necrosectomy, or fasciotomy may have to be repeated till fresh viable tissue starts appearing. Any delay in surgical intervention may lead to irreversible necrosis and gangrene resulting in amputation of the limb or death due to septic shock.

Duodenal Ulcer Perforation

INTRODUCTION

Peptic ulcer disease is a common condition that may be complicated by bleeding, perforation, or gastric outlet obstruction.

Duodenal ulcer perforation should be suspected in patients who suddenly develop severe, diffuse abdominal pain. It is important to take history of chronic antiplatelets, nonsteroidal anti-inflammatory drugs (NSAIDs) and steroid use in patients suspected to have duodenal perforation.

Consider the differentials shown in **Table 1** while evaluating a patient with acute abdominal pain.

CLINICAL MANIFESTATIONS

- *Initial phase (within 2 h of onset)*: Abdominal pain is usually sudden, sometimes producing collapse or syncope. Usually, localized to the epigastrium.
- *Second phase (usually 2–12 h after onset)*: Abdominal pain may lessen, usually generalized, often markedly worse upon movement. Abdomen shows marked board-like rigidity.
- *Third phase (usually >12 h after onset)*: Abdominal distension increases but abdominal pain, tenderness, and rigidity may be less evident. Hypovolemia and shock may result due to third spacing into the peritoneal cavity.

TABLE 1: Causes of acute abdominal pain in adults.

Surgical	Gynecological	Medical
• Acute appendicitis	• Ectopic pregnancy	• Acute pancreatitis
• Acute cholecystitis	• Pelvic inflammatory disease	• Inferior wall myocardial infarction
• Biliary colic	• Rupture/torsion of ovarian cyst	• Peptic ulcer disease
• Duodenal ulcer perforation	• Endometriosis	• Acute hepatitis
• Intestinal obstruction	• Mittelschmerz	• Diabetic ketoacidosis
• Ureteric colic		• Urinary tract infection
• Testicular torsion		• Gastroenteritis
• Aortic dissection		• Irritable bowel syndrome
• Diverticulitis		
• Mesenteric ischemia		
• Large bowel perforation		
• Nonspecific abdominal pain		

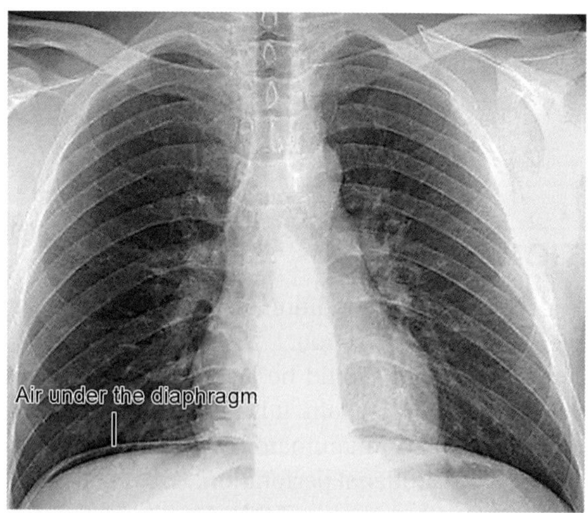

FIG. 1: Air under the diaphragm.

INVESTIGATIONS

The investigations include complete blood count (CBC), electrolytes, creatinine, urea, blood culture and sensitivity, rapid blood borne virus screen (BBVS), prothrombin time, activated partial thromboplastin time (aPTT), ECG, chest X-ray erect, and X-ray abdomen supine. Look for air under the diaphragm (**Fig. 1**).

If clinical diagnosis is doubtful, amylase, lipase, or cardiac enzymes may have to be sent depending on the history and examination findings.

MANAGEMENT

- Obtain IV access and start fluid resuscitation.
- Insert a nasogastric (NG) tube and keep the patient nil per oral (NPO)
- Prove adequate analgesia (Morphine/Tramadol).
- Give proton pump inhibitor and antiemetics (Injection Pantoprazole 40 mg + Injection Metoclopramide 10 mg IV stat.)
- *Administer empiric antibiotics:*
  - In hemodynamically stable patients: Cefazolin 1 g IV + Gentamicin 1.5–2 mg/kg IV + Metronidazole 500 mg IV stat.
  - In patients with systemic inflammatory response syndrome/shock: Piperacillin-Tazobactam 4.5 g IV or Injection Ertapenem 1 g IV stat.
- Refer to general surgery for further management.

Acute Appendicitis

INTRODUCTION

Appendicitis is one of the most common causes of acute abdomen presenting to the emergency department. It refers to an inflammation of the vestigial vermiform appendix.

CLINICAL MANIFESTATIONS

The clinical presentation is characterized by the following symptoms:
- *Abdominal pain*: Classically, pain starts in the periumbilical region and migrates to the right lower quadrant (right anterior iliac fossa) with increasing inflammation.
- Anorexia
- Nausea and vomiting

PHYSICAL EXAMINATION

Palpate gently for areas of tenderness. It is unnecessary and unkind to attempt to repeatedly elicit rebound tenderness. Tenderness on percussion or palpation is ample evidence of peritonitis.

Common physical signs include:
- *McBurney's sign* is described as maximal tenderness at the McBurney's point (**Fig. 1**), which lies at one-third of the distance from the anterior superior iliac spine (ASIS) to the umbilicus (sensitivity 50–94%; specificity 75–86%).
- *Rovsing's sign*: Palpation of the left lower quadrant elicits pain in the right lower quadrant. This sign is also called "indirect tenderness" and is indicative of right-sided local peritoneal irritation.
- The *psoas sign* is associated with a retrocecal appendix, which may manifest by right lower quadrant pain with passive extension of the right hip.
- The obturator sign is associated with a pelvic appendix. In this sign, right lower quadrant pain is elicited on flexing the patient's right hip and knee followed by internal rotation of the right hip.

  Rectal examination, although often advocated, has not been shown to provide additional diagnostic information in cases of appendicitis.

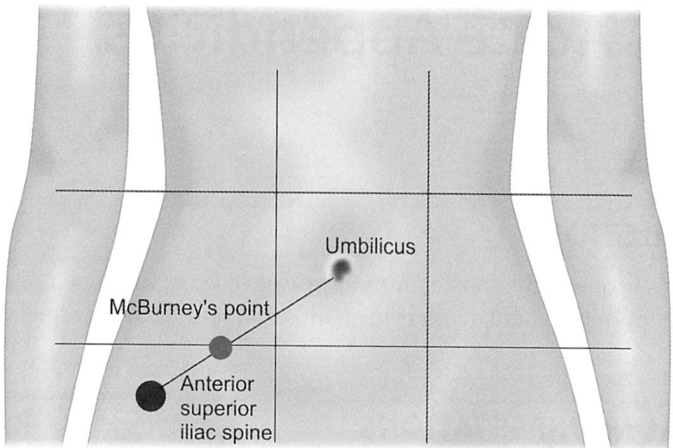

FIG. 1: McBurney's point.

INVESTIGATIONS

- The investigations include complete blood count (CBC), electrolytes, creatinine, liver function test (LFT), chest X-ray (CXR) (to rule out hollow viscus perforation), and urinalysis (to look for RBC in urine s/o renal calculi).
- Acute appendicitis is a clinical diagnosis. Ultrasonography (USG) of abdomen is only indicated in female patients with nonspecific abdominal pain to rule out a gynecological cause. An inflamed appendix may be seen as a noncompressible tubular structure of 7–9 mm in diameter on a USG.
- In women of reproductive age group, perform a pelvic examination and do a pregnancy test (urine precolor) to rule out obstetric causes.
- Send rapid blood borne virus screen (BBVS) and prothrombin time (PT), and activated partial thromboplastin time (aPTT), if surgical intervention is likely. Calculate the probability of acute appendicitis by using the modified Alvarado score (**Table 1**)

MANAGEMENT

- Commence IV fluids if there is evidence of dehydration.
- Give IV opioid and antiemetic (Tramadol 50 mg IV/Morphine 0.1 mg/kg IV stat plus Metoclopramide 10 mg IV stat. Repeat if necessary).
- If appendicectomy is planned, start antibiotics: Piperacillin-Tazobactam 4.5 g IV stat. Preoperative administration of antibiotics decrease postoperative wound infections.
- Insert a nasogastric (NG) tube and keep the patient nil per oral (NPO)
- Management depends on whether the appendix is perforated or nonperforated at the time of presentation.

TABLE 1: Modified Alvarado score for acute appendicitis.

	Conditions	Score	Interpretation
M	Migratory right iliac fossa pain	1	0–3: Low risk
A	Anorexia	1	
N	Nausea or vomiting	1	4–6: Probable
T	Tenderness in the right iliac fossa	2	
R	Rebound tenderness in the right iliac fossa	1	7–9: Very probable
E	Fever >37.5°C	1	
L	Leukocytosis	2	
S	Shift to the left	1	

- *Nonperforated:* This refers to simple/uncomplicated appendicitis without clinical or radiological signs of perforation. Appendectomy is the standard of care for most patients, either by laparoscopic or by open approach.
  - *Perforated appendix:* About 10-20% of patients with acute appendicitis may have a perforation and would require emergency appendectomy.
- Refer to General surgery for further management

Acute Cholecystitis

INTRODUCTION

The term cholecystitis refers to inflammation of the gallbladder.

- *Acute cholecystitis*: Acute cholecystitis refers to inflammation of the gallbladder, usually caused by a gallstone obstructing the biliary drainage (**Fig. 1**). It is characterized by right upper quadrant abdominal pain, fever, and leukocytosis.
- *Acalculous cholecystitis*: This is clinically similar to acute cholecystitis but is not associated with gallstones. It usually occurs in critically ill patients or severe trauma.

HISTORY

Right upper quadrant or epigastric pain that is steady and severe is the typical presentation. The pain may radiate to the right shoulder or back. Episodes of biliary pain keep recurring in most patients. Approximately, 60–70% of patients report a previous episode of biliary pain that resolved spontaneously.

PHYSICAL EXAMINATION

Patients with acute cholecystitis are usually ill appearing, febrile, and tachycardic.

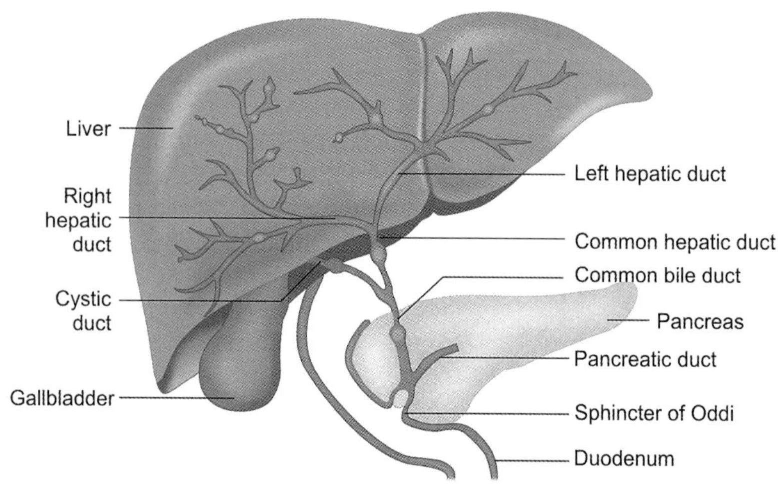

FIG. 1: Anatomy of the pancreaticobiliary drainage.

Murphy's sign: Right hypochondrial tenderness on deep inspiration in sitting position.

INVESTIGATIONS

- Complete blood count (CBC), electrolytes, creatinine, and liver function test.
- *Ultrasonography abdomen*: To look for gallstones, CBC dilatation. Ultrasonic Murphy's sign may be elicited to confirm the diagnosis.
- Rapid blood borne virus screen (BBVS) and prothrombin time (PT), and activated partial thromboplastin time (aPTT), if surgical intervention likely.

DIAGNOSIS

Diagnosis of acute cholecystitis is generally made on the basis of typical history and examination findings. The classical triad of sudden onset right upper quadrant (hypochondrial) pain, fever and leukocytosis (WBC count: 10–15,000/mm^3) is highly suggestive of acute cholecystitis.

MANAGEMENT

- Intravenous (IV) fluid resuscitation
- Provide analgesia (Tramadol 50 mg IV/Morphine 0.1 mg/kg IV stat plus Metoclopramide 10 mg IV stat). Repeat if necessary.
- Start broad-spectrum IV antibiotics after taking a blood culture
- Refer urgently to general surgery
- Percutaneous cholecystostomy tube placement (for surgically high risk or critically ill patients) or cholecystectomy (definitive treatment) may be required if there is no clinical improvement with antibiotics and supportive care.

What Causes Elevation of Alkaline Phosphatase Levels?

Alkaline phosphatase level (ALP) is produced from only four sites in the body. It is usually elevated due to cholestasis. If ALP is elevated, think of the following sources.

- *Liver*:
  - *Mild elevation*: Hepatitis, heavy alcohol consumption, and sepsis.
  - *High levels*: Biliary obstruction, infiltrative process (malignancy, tuberculosis, amyloidosis, and sarcoidosis), and primary biliary cirrhosis.
- *Gastrointestinal (GI) tract*: GI malignancies and GI tuberculosis.
- *Bone*: Fractures, Paget's disease, and osteomalacia.
- *Placenta*: Pregnancy.

  Gamma-glutamyl transpeptidase (GGT) also reflects cholestasis and is rarely elevated in conditions other than liver disease. If ALP and GGT are both elevated, the source of ALP is the liver. If ALP is elevated and GGT is normal, the source of ALP is the GI tract/bone/placenta.

Intestinal Obstruction

INTRODUCTION

Intestinal obstruction may be mechanical or paralytic in nature. The causes of intestinal obstruction are shown in **Table 1**.

HISTORY

- Classic symptoms are abdominal pain, distension, vomiting, and constipation.
- Ask for history of previous surgery.
- Severe pain suggests strangulation and developing ischemia in a closed loop.

EXAMINATION

- Look for evidence of dehydration and shock.
- Carefully examine the hernial orifices and inspect for scars of previous surgery.
- Look for distension and areas of tenderness.
- Perform a per rectal examination. Impacted stools may be the cause for obstruction especially in the elderly.

INVESTIGATIONS

The investigations include:
- Complete blood count (CBC), electrolytes, creatinine, and liver function test (LFT)

TABLE 1: Causes of intestinal obstruction.	
Mechanical causes	*Paralytic causes*
• Adhesions after previous surgery	• Postoperative ileus
• Obstructed hernia	• Electrolyte disturbance: Hypokalemia
• Tumors (gastric, pancreatic, and large bowel)	• Pseudo-obstruction
• Volvulus (sigmoid, gastric, and cecal)	
• Inflammatory mass (diverticular and Crohn's)	
• Peptic ulcer disease	
• Gallstone ileus	
• Intussusception	

- Chest X-ray (CXR) erect and X-ray abdomen supine
- Rapid blood borne virus screen (BBVS), prothrombin time (PT), and activated partial thromboplastin time (aPTT), if surgical intervention is likely.
- The site and nature of the bowel loops may suggest the site of obstruction.

MANAGEMENT

- Insert an intravenous (IV) cannula and start IV fluid resuscitation.
- Insert a nasogastric tube and keep the patient nil per oral.
- Prove adequate analgesia (Morphine/Tramadol).
- Give an antiemetic (Metoclopramide/Ondansetron).
- Refer to surgical team for further management.

INTESTINAL PSEUDO-OBSTRUCTION

This is due to chronic impairment in gastrointestinal (GI) motility, especially seen in the elderly taking tricyclic antidepressants or other anticholinergic drugs. Any part of the GI tract may be involved, but colonic distention is the most common. Treatment of acute colonic pseudo-obstruction is decompression using a colonoscopy.

When to do a CT Abdomen?

In patients with intestinal obstruction and signs of peritonitis who require immediate intervention and in postoperative patients where the etiology is known, computed tomography (CT) abdomen is not needed.

CT scan of the abdomen is useful to identify:
- Specific sites of obstruction (transition points)
- Severity of obstruction (partial vs. complete)
- Determining the etiology like hernias, masses, or inflammatory changes
- Identifying complications like ischemia, necrosis, or perforation.

Do not ask for CT abdomen with oral contrast in a patient with signs of perforation.

Mesenteric Ischemia

CHAPTER 99

INTRODUCTION

Acute mesenteric ischemia refers to the sudden onset of small intestinal hypoperfusion, which is usually due to acute embolic occlusion of the intestinal blood supply, most commonly the superior mesenteric artery (SMA).

Mesenteric ischemia can be divided into arterial and venous. Arterial disease can be further sub divided into non occlusive (low flow state) and occlusive (embolic or thrombotic).

OCCLUSIVE MESENTERIC ARTERIAL DISEASE

1. *Mesenteric arterial embolism*: The source of emboli is the heart (left atrium, left ventricle, and valves) or a dislodged thrombus from the proximal aorta. Increased risk among patients with cardiac arrhythmias, valvular heart disease, infective endocarditis, recent myocardial infarction, ventricular aneurysm and aortic aneurysm.
2. *Mesenteric arterial thrombosis*: Acute thrombosis of the mesenteric circulation usually occurs in patients with chronic mesenteric ischemia due to progressively worsening atherosclerotic plaque in the mesenteric arteries. It may also occur in patients with vascular injuries due to abdominal trauma, infection, or mesenteric dissection.

CLINICAL FEATURES

Usually presents with sudden onset severe diffuse abdominal pain. Typically, the severity of the pain initially far exceeds the associated physical signs. Pain due to embolism to the proximal superior mesenteric artery is typically sudden, severe, peri-umbilical and associated with nausea or vomiting. Pain due to thrombotic etiology is usually insidious in onset with post-prandial worsening.

PHYSICAL EXAMINATION

- Initially there may only be mild diffuse abdominal tenderness. Shock, absent bowel sounds, abdominal distension, and tenderness are late signs.
- Carefully examine the cardiovascular system for any embolic source (atrial fibrillation and valvular heart disease).
- Perform a per rectal examination to look for altered blood in stools that suggests progression of the ischemia.

DIAGNOSIS

Diagnosis may be difficult as the clinical presentation mimics other acute intra-abdominal emergencies. A high index of suspicion is required for diagnosis, especially in the elderly (>60 years) and those with atrial fibrillation, myocardial infarction or congestive heart failure.

- Arterial blood gas typically reveals a severe metabolic acidosis and elevated lactate. These findings in a patient with severe abdominal pain should arouse a strong suspicion of mesenteric ischemia.
- A computed tomography (CT) angiography confirms the diagnosis. It can differentiate between embolic and thrombotic etiologies and provide information for operative planning, such as distal arterial reconstitution and choice of inflow vessel for surgical bypass.

MANAGEMENT

- Resuscitate with intravenous fluids and oxygen, if required
- Nasogastric tube and keep the patient nil per oral
- Prove adequate analgesia. Administer Morphine 5 mg IV/SC or Tramadol 50 mg IV and repeat doses as required.
- Administer proton pump inhibitors (Pantoprazole 40 mg IV stat) and an antiemetic (Metoclopramide 10 mg IV stat)
- Consider broad-spectrum antibiotics (Meropenem/Piperacillin-Tazobactam)
- Administer anticoagulants (unfractionated heparin or low molecular heparin) to limit thrombus propagation
- Refer to general surgery for urgent surgical intervention. Immediate surgery is indicated for patients with acute mesenteric ischemia with clinical symptoms or signs of bowel gangrene (e.g., peritonitis, septic shock, pneumatosis intestinalis). Surgery consists of abdominal exploration/damage control and revascularization (embolectomy/mesenteric bypass). Despite best efforts, prognosis remains poor with a high mortality rate.

INTRODUCTION

Gas gangrene or clostridial myonecrosis is a rapidly progressive infection of the muscles caused by *Clostridium* species and can be fatal.

It may develop at the site of trauma or may get seeded in the muscle by hematogenous spread from the gastrointestinal (GI) tract. Clostridial gas gangrene may therefore present in two ways: Traumatic and spontaneous.

1. *Traumatic gas gangrene*: Most common etiology is *C. perfringens*. Some conditions that predispose to traumatic gas gangrene include crush injuries, gun shot wounds, knife wounds, bowel and biliary tract surgery, abortion, and retained placenta.
2. *Spontaneous gangrene*: Most common etiology is *C. septicum*.

CLINICAL FEATURES

- Sudden onset of severe pain at the site of surgery or trauma.
- The mean incubation period is <24 hours (range 6 h to several days).
- Characteristic yellowish-brown or bronze appearance of the skin, followed by blebs or hemorrhagic bullae. The skin becomes tense and exquisitely tender.
- Serosanguinous exudate with a characteristic foul odor.
- Signs of systemic toxicity develop rapidly including tachycardia and fever, followed by shock and multiorgan failure.

DIAGNOSIS

- Pain at a site of traumatic injury together with signs of systemic toxicity and gas in the soft tissue support the diagnosis of gas gangrene. The most specific finding to confirm gas gangrene is demonstration of crepitus in the soft tissue.
- Gas within the soft tissue can be detected by X-ray, CT scan, or MRI scan.
- Definitive diagnosis of gas gangrene requires demonstration of large, gram-variable rods at the site of injury. Tissue culture and blood culture (aerobic and anaerobic) should be obtained.

MANAGEMENT

- Resuscitate with intravenous (IV) fluids and oxygen if required
- Isolate the patient in side observation area after resuscitation
- *Antibiotic therapy*: Injection crystalline penicillin 40 L units q4h plus injection clindamycin 600 mg IV q8h. Carbapenems are an alternative.
- *Surgical debridement*: Extensive debridement of devitalized tissue is life-saving. The affected limb may have to be amputated.

INTRODUCTION

The most common nail bed emergencies are injuries (crush injury or subungual hematoma) and infections (paronychia).

NAIL BED INJURIES

Fingertip and nail bed injuries are common components of hand injuries. Nail bed is the soft tissue below the nail and helps in nail growth. Crush injuries of the nail bed and fractures of the distal phalanx result in stunted, deformed, or absent nail growth.

Subungual hematomas are frequently associated with nail bed injuries and can be excruciatingly painful. The nail bed has a rich vascular supply and bleeding results in increased pressure under the nail and can cause significant discomfort.

Management

- Administer digital ring block (with 2% lignocaine without adrenaline) for immediate pain relief. Assess the neurological status of the finger before administering anesthesia.
- If the nail plate is mobile, remove it and inspect the matrix for nail bed lacerations.
- Irrigate the nail bed with sterile normal saline (NS) using a 26-G needle.
- Clean and remove debris.
- Reinsert the nail plate and reappose the nail folds.
- Apply sterile nonadherent dressing and splint.
- Small subungual hematomas resolve spontaneously and hence require no treatment. However, painful and large hematomas should be evacuated via nail trephination (i.e., making a hole in the nail for drainage of blood).

Nail Trephination (Fig. 1)

- Paint the nail with 10% povidone-iodine (Betadine) solution.
- Puncture the nail with a hot metal wire (e.g., an electrocautery device or a carbon dioxide laser). The hole should be large enough (3–4 mm) for continued drainage, which may occur for 24–36 hours after the injury.
- Alternatively, insert an insulin syringe needle (29-G) underneath the nail at the distal hyponychium and advance it proximally and parallel to the nail

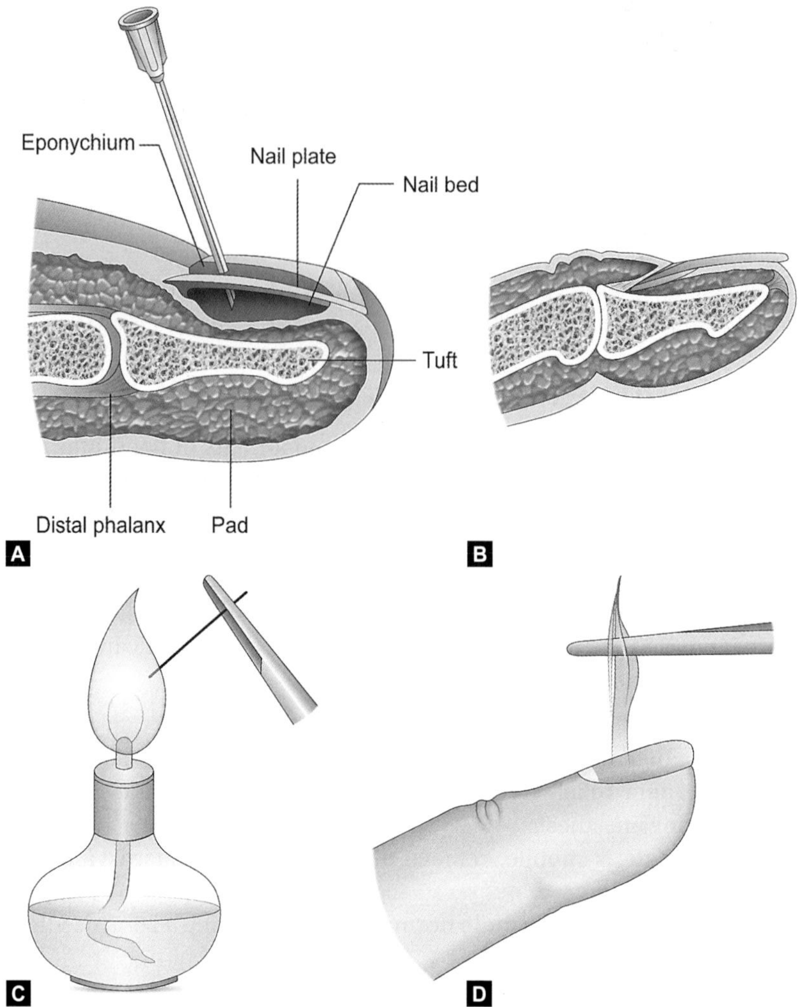

FIGS. 1A TO D: Nail trephination.

plate with gentle suction on the syringe until the hematoma begins to drain. Apply light pressure to the nail to complete evacuation.

- Cover the puncture site with sterile gauze dressing while the wound continues to drain.

PARONYCHIA

Paronychia is the most common infection of the hand, occurring along the edge of the finger nail or toe nail. The infection is most often caused by *Staphylococcus aureus* or *Streptococcus* species. Mixed bacterial and gram-negative etiology is common in diabetic patients.

Management

- Early acute paronychia without abscess formation can be treated with warm water soaks, oral antibiotics (Cloxacillin) and analgesics.
- Incision and drainage is required, if an abscess develops.

Paronychia Drainage (Fig. 2)

- Prepare the skin with 10% povidone-iodine (Betadine) solution.
- Administer mid-dorsal digital block with 2% lignocaine without adrenaline.
- Using a small blunt instrument like the back of a sterile blade or a metal probe, gently elevate the lateral eponychial fold and allow the pus to drain.
- If required, make a longitudinal incision using a No. 11 or No. 15 blade away from the nail fold. This drains the pus without disturbing the eponychial folds.
- Irrigate the cavity with NS using a 24-G syringe.
- Excise the lateral nail if pus has tracked under the nail, such as in ingrown toe nail.
- Removal of the entire nail is usually not indicated.
- Oral antibiotics (Cloxacillin 500 mg q6h or Cefazolin 500 mg q6h for 1 week).
- Administer adequate analgesia (nonsteroidal anti-inflammatory drugs or Tramadol).
- Review and change dressing after 48 hours.

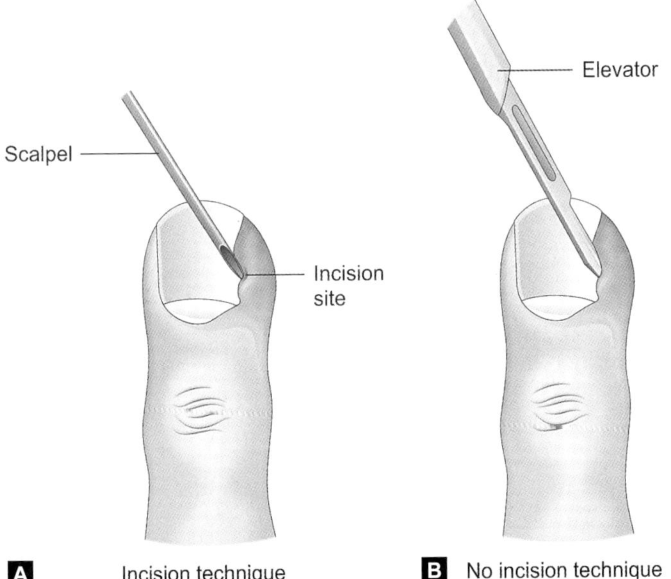

FIGS. 2A AND B: Paronychia drainage.

FELON

- A felon is a subcutaneous pyogenic infection or abscess of the pulp space of the distal finger or thumb that may cause increased pressure and ischemic necrosis of the surrounding tissue, osteomyelitis, flexor tenosynovitis or septic arthritis of the distal interphalangeal joint.
- Infection begins with minor trauma and patients present with severe throbbing pain and a tense, red pulp space.
- The infection may spread between septae of the pulp space, forming compartmental abscesses.
- Management:
  - In the early stages, patients may respond to warm soaks, elevation, rest and oral antibiotics (Cloxacillin 500 mg PO q6h or Cephalexin 500 mg PO q6H × 5–7 days)
  - Severe cases require incision and drainage or even debridement of the abscess cavity (**Fig. 3**).

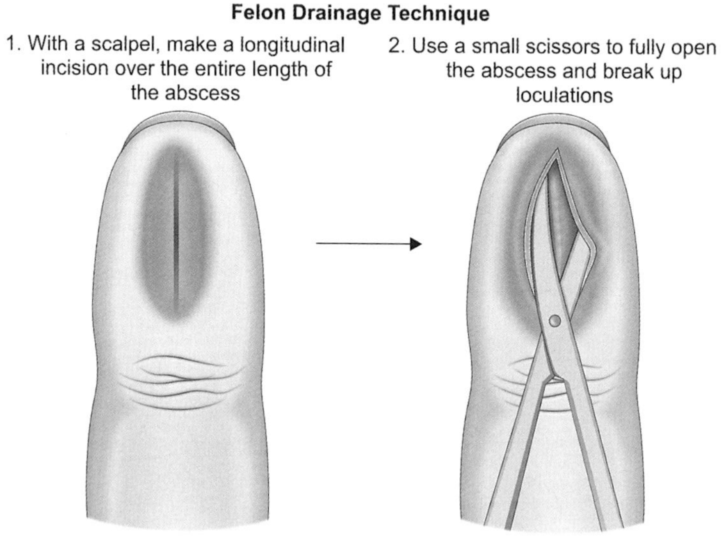

FIG. 3: Incision and drainage of a felon.

HEMORRHOIDS

Hemorrhoids or piles refer to enlarged or swollen veins in the anal canal and rectum and increase in incidence with age. They are of two types: External and internal.

1. *External hemorrhoids* form at the anus and protrude out. They may be complicated by thrombosis, hygiene-related problems, infection, or bleeding per rectum. They are usually associated with significant pain, itching, and incomplete bowel movements. A skin tag is usually a sign of a healed external hemorrhoid.
2. *Internal hemorrhoids* arise in the lower rectum and may not protrude out though the anus. As they do not have any cutaneous innervations, they typically cause painless, bright red bleeding associated with defecation, but blood is not mixed in stools.

A thrombosed hemorrhoid may present as an acute emergency and is usually quite painful. It may necessitate immediate surgical intervention to remove the thrombosed vessel.

Management

- Advice high-fiber diet.
- Prescribe stool softeners (naturolax powder 2 teaspoon od/bd) and analgesics.
- *Warm sitz baths*: Advice the patient to sit in a shallow tub filled with warm water and soak the rectal area for 10–15 minutes, 2–3 times daily.
- Refer to general surgery for surgical intervention or conservative management.

ANAL FISSURE

Anal fissures may cause severe pain on defecation and for a few hours afterward. Most fissures are located posteriorly in the midline just inside the anal orifice.

Management

- Advice high-fiber diet.
- Prescribe stool softeners and analgesics.
- Topical analgesic jelly or creams (e.g., 2% lidocaine jelly) may be prescribed.
- Topical vasodilators like nifedipine (0.2–0.3% ointment, 2–4 times daily) or topical nitroglycerine (0.4% rectal ointment twice daily) increase the local blood flow and reduce the anal sphincter pressure.

- *Warm sitz baths*: Advice the patient to sit in a shallow tub filled with warm water and soak the rectal area for 10–15 minutes, 2–3 times daily.
- Most heal spontaneously but the presence of significant ulceration, hypertrophied tissue, skin tags suggests chronicity and needs surgical follow up.

PILONIDAL ABSCESS

- Pilonidal cysts usually form in young individuals (15–35 years), probably due to impacted hair follicles in the natal cleft. They may be itchy and painful and cause discomfort while sitting.
- A pilonidal sinus is formed when a pilonidal cyst ruptures through the skin forming a tract that discharges material or pus from the cyst. This may become chronic.
- A pilonidal abscess is formed when a pilonidal cyst or a sinus becomes infected. This requires immediate surgical intervention as patients pre- sent with a fluctuant swelling in the natal cleft, which is extremely painful and tender.

Etiology of a Pilonidal Abscess

Most common pathogens are anaerobic bacteria such as *Bacteroides*, but *Enterococci, Staphylococci,* and hemolytic *Streptococci* have also been implicated. Anaerobes are usually associated with postoperative wound reinfections.

Management

Broad-spectrum antibiotics (Metronidazole/Piperacillin-Tazobactam) and immediate surgical drainage of the abscess.

ANORECTAL ABSCESS

An anorectal abscess (perineal abscess) is formed if an anal crypt and gland gets infected. The infection can easily spread through the loose intersphincteric space, ischiorectal space, or the supralevator space. These are more common in young and middle-aged males.

*The types of anorectal abscess shown in **Figure 1** are:*
- Perianal (60%)
- Ischiorectal (20%)
- Intersphincteric (5%)
- Supralevator (4%)
- Submucosal (1%)

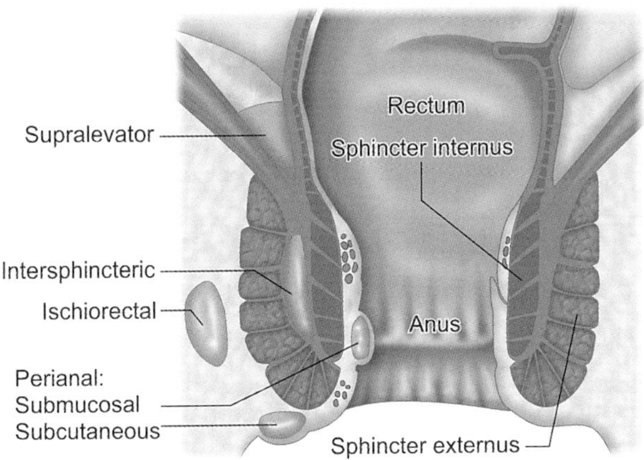

FIG. 1: Location of anorectal abscesses.

Symptoms

Persistent dull, throbbing pain made worse by walking or sitting and prior to defecation. Pain is a prominent symptom followed by signs of local inflammation. Examination shows a localized fluctuant red tender swelling close to the anus.

Management

Administer analgesics (NSAIDs or opiates). Definitive treatment is incision and drainage. Isolated, simple, superficial, fluctuant perianal abscesses may be drained in the ED under local analgesia or procedural sedation.

FISTULA IN ANO

- *Fistula in ano* refers to an abnormal tract lined with epithelium and granulation tissue, connecting the anal canal with the skin.
- These tracts usually result from perianal or ischiorectal abscesses and may also be associated with Crohn's disease, colonic malignancies, anal fissures or sexually transmitted diseases.
- *Goodsall's rule:* Anterior opening fistulas follow a simple direct course to the anal canal while posterior opening fistulas often follow a devious, curving path including horseshoe-shaped tracks.
- Patients present with persistent, blood-stained, foul smelling discharge. Recurrent abscesses may form due to blockade of the tracts due to inflammation.
- Analgesics, antipyretics, antibiotics (metronidazole) may be started for patients with significant symptoms awaiting surgical consultation.
- The only definite treatment is surgical excision of the fistula.

RUPTURED ABDOMINAL AORTIC ANEURYSM

Rupture of an abdominal aortic aneurysm (AAA) carries significant mortality. Early diagnosis, prompt resuscitation, and early surgical intervention are of paramount importance.

Most AAA is saccular and found in the infrarenal part of the aorta.

Clinical Presentation

- The presentation is highly variable ranging from severe pain to syncope or cardiac arrest. The pain is usually sudden onset, severe, and located to the central abdomen or low back.
- Examination may show tachycardia, hypotension, one or both absent femoral pulse or a tender pulsatile abdominal mass.

Diagnosis

- Diagnosis of a ruptured AAA is confirmed by CT angiogram. In patients with a known AAA, an emergency USG may be sufficient and safer rather than shifting the unstable patient for a CT scan.
- Close differentials are ureteric colic and acute pancreatitis.

Management

- Obtain intravenous (IV) access and start fluid resuscitation.
- Send cross match for blood products.
- Provide adequate analgesia (Morphine if BP is normal, else Tramadol).
- Give Pantoprazole and an antiemetic (Ondansetron 8 mg IV stat).
- Refer to vascular surgery immediately if clinical suspicion is high.

AORTIC DISSECTION

Aortic dissection is caused by a circumferential or transverse tear of the intima of the ascending aorta or the descending thoracic aorta. According to the Stanford classification, they can be of two types:
- Type A/Proximal dissection involving the ascending aorta
- Type B/Distal dissection involving the descending aorta only

Clinical Features

- Abrupt onset of severe pain in the chest or between the scapulae is the most common presentation
- Examination findings may include hypertension or hypotension, loss of distal (lower limb) pulses, or pulmonary edema
- Dissection into the carotid artery may result in syncope or hemiplegia
- Paraplegia may result if arterial supply to the spinal cord is interrupted
- Aortic regurgitation, hemopericardium, and cardiac tamponade may complicate a proximal dissection

Diagnosis

- *Chest X-ray*: CXR findings of a thoracic dissection usually are, a widening of the mediastinum, pleural effusion, deviation of the trachea, mainstem bronchi or esophagus.
- *Echocardiography*: Transesophageal ECHO is quite sensitive at identifying dissections involving ascending and descending thoracic aorta. Aortic regurgitation and pericardial effusion can also be visualized.
- *CT/MRI angiography*: These are the diagnostic tests of choice for identifying intimal flap and extent of the dissection.

Management

- *Medical management*: In the ED, initiate medical management as soon as diagnosis is suspected
- Treat like a hypertensive emergency and rapidly lower the blood pressure. Administer a beta blocker (injection labetolol 20 mg IV stat or injection esmolol 250–500 µg loading dose over 1 min) refer Chapter 37.
- Add a vasodilator like nitroprusside (0.5 µg/kg/min IV) for further antihypertensive effect
- If the patient presents with hypotension, administer fluids and blood products if required
- *Surgical management*: Urgent open or endovascular surgical intervention is the definite treatment of an aortic dissection. Refer to cardiothoracic surgery and vascular surgery.

ACUTE LIMBISCHEMIA

Acute limb ischemia secondary to a thrombus or embolism requires immediate intervention for limb salvage. The term 'critical limb ischemia' is used when chronic progressive peripheral arterial disease results in ischemic pain at rest, ulceration or gangrene. The following are common causes of arterial occlusion:

- *Thrombus (most common)*: Atherosclerosis or thrombus of native vessels and bypass grafts

- *Embolic*: Cardiac source (atrial fibrillation, RHD, mechanical valves, infective endocarditis)
- *Others*: Vasculitis (rheumatoid arthritis, lupus, polyarteritis nodosa), Raynaud disease, thromboangiitis obliterans (Buergers disease), Takayasu arteritis

Clinical Features

The cardinal features of acute limb ischemia are summarized by the six **Ps**.

1. **P**ain
2. **P**aresthesia
3. **P**allor
4. **P**ulselessness
5. **P**aralysis (due to muscle damage)
6. **P**oikilothermia

Pain may be either constant or elicited by passive movement of the involved extremity.

The history should include a history of intermittent claudication, previous leg bypass or other vascular procedures, and history suggestive of embolic sources, such as cardiac arrhythmias and aortic aneurysms.

Examination

- Look for skin changes. A clear demarcation between normal and ischemic skin suggests an embolic cause.
- Palpate all pulses carefully. The presence of normal pulses in the contralateral limb suggests an embolic source, whereas absent or weak contralateral pulse makes thrombosis more likely.
- Look for potential sources of emboli (irregular pulse, murmurs, clicks, or bruits).

Investigations

Investigations include complete blood count (CBC), creatinine, urea, electrolytes, prothrombin time (PT), activated partial thromboplastin time (aPTT), ECG, chest X-ray (CXR), rapid blood borne virus screen (BBVS), and hand Doppler screening.

Administer unfractionated heparin (80 U/kg bolus followed by 18 U/kg/h infusion) immediately, if acute limb ischemia is suspected clinically (unless there is a contraindication for heparin).

Administer heparin before sending any blood investigation or referring to vascular surgery.

Management

- Obtain IV access and start fluid resuscitation.
- Unfractionated heparin 80 U/kg bolus followed by 18 U/kg/h infusion.
- Prove adequate analgesia (Morphine/Tramadol).

- Refer to vascular surgery immediately. Revascularization is required within 6 hours to prevent muscle necrosis and complications like renal failure.
- If the etiology is embolus, embolectomy is required.
- If the etiology is thrombosis, angiography is needed to define the site and extent of the lesion. Thrombolysis with or without reconstructive surgery would then be required.

ACUTE DEEP VEIN THROMBOSIS

Deep vein thrombosis (DVT) results due to abnormal clotting in the deep venous system of the legs (popliteal) or pelvis (femoral or iliac). Acute mortality is due to pulmonary embolism. About 50% of those with DVT will develop post-thrombotic syndrome with lifelong pain and swelling of the leg.

Risk Factors for DVT

- Recent surgery (especially orthopedic, abdominal, spinal, or obstetric done under general anesthesia)
- Pregnancy
- Obesity
- Smoking
- Malignancy
- *Prothrombotic states*: Antithrombin III deficiency, protein C or protein S deficiency, factor V Leiden mutation, and prothrombin gene mutation.

Clinical Features

Classical symptoms of DVT include leg pain, swelling, warmth, tenderness, and dilated superficial veins in the affected leg. However, clinical signs depend on the size and extent of the thrombus and are highly variable.

Investigations

Investigations include CBC, creatinine, electrolytes, D-dimer, PT, aPTT, ECG, CXR, and venous Doppler.

Administer unfractionated heparin (80 U/kg bolus followed by 18 U/kg/h infusion) immediately, if acute DVT is suspected clinically (unless there is a contraindication for heparin).

Administer heparin before sending any blood investigation or referring to vascular surgery.

Management

- Obtain IV access and start fluid resuscitation.
- Unfractionated heparin (80 U/kg bolus followed by 18 U/kg/h infusion)
- Prove adequate analgesia (Morphine/Tramadol)
- Refer to vascular surgery.

ACUTE MASTITIS AND BREAST ABSCESS

Acute inflammation of the breast tissue (mastitis) may or may not be accompanied by infection and presents with erythema, edema, and tenderness with or without fever.

- *Lactational mastitis*:
  - This condition is most common in the first 3 months of breastfeeding. Most episodes are caused by *Staphylococcus aureus*.
  - Initial management of mild lactational mastitis consists of symptomatic treatment to reduce pain and swelling (nonsteroidal inflammatory agents, cold compresses). The mother should be encouraged to completely empty the breast of milk via ongoing breastfeeding, pumping, or hand expression.
  - Moderately severe cases with fever require a course of antibiotics (Cloxacillin 500 mg PO q6h or Cephalexin 500 mg PO q6H × 5–7 days)
  - Patients with an organized breast abscess will require incision and drainage or surgical debridement.
- *Nonlactational mastitis*:
  - Periductal mastitis (mammary duct ectasia) is an inflammatory condition of the subareolar ducts resulting in periareolar inflammation. Secondary infection of inflamed ducts may result in duct rupture or abscess formation.
  - This condition is seen in women over 40 years of age and presents with constant mastalgia associated with nipple retraction and discharge.
  - Management includes pain relief and a course of antibiotics. Refer to general surgery for definitive management.

MASTALGIA

- Mastalgia (mastodynia) is a common cause of breast pain among menstruating women and must be differentiated from acute mastitis.
- Cyclical mastalgia usually presents in the immediate premenstrual phase and resolves completely after menstruation.
- The pain is usually bilateral, but may be more severe in the upper outer quadrants of the breasts
- Symptoms are relieved by occasional use of nonsteroidal anti-inflammatory drugs (NSAIDs).

Section **16**

Trauma

Early Management of Trauma

CHAPTER 105

PRIORITIES IN EARLY MANAGEMENT OF TRAUMA

Certain caveats in the early management of a trauma victim are:
- Treat it as the greatest threat to life first.
- Lack of a definitive diagnosis should never impede the application of an indicated treatment.
- A detailed history is not a prerequisite to begin the evaluation of an acutely injured patient.

The main steps in the early management of trauma are:
1. Primary assessment
2. *Resuscitation*: Perform primary assessment and resuscitation together
3. Reassessment of airway, breathing, and circulation (ABC)
4. Secondary assessment

PRIMARY ASSESSMENT

The purpose of a primary assessment is to identify life and limb-threatening injuries. It should be conducted in a sequential manner as follows:
A—Airway with in-line cervical spine immobilization
B—Breathing with oxygen supplementation
C—Circulation with hemorrhage control
D—*Disability*: Neurological status, as expressed by the patient
E—Exposure of the entire body, looking for occult injuries

RESUSCITATION

Resuscitation should follow the ABC pattern of the primary assessment, and should be performed simultaneously.
- If the airway is compromised, the primary assessment should be suspended till the airway is secured.
- If breathing is compromised, then that should be dealt with. This may require decompression of a tension pneumothorax or a massive hemothorax. It may also involve endotracheal intubation and mechanical ventilation in a patient, who is not breathing adequately.
- Resuscitation of circulation includes insertion of two large bore cannulae and infusing 2 L of normal saline/Ringer's lactate solution. At the same time, take a blood sample for crossmatch, electrolytes, and hemoglobin (Hb).

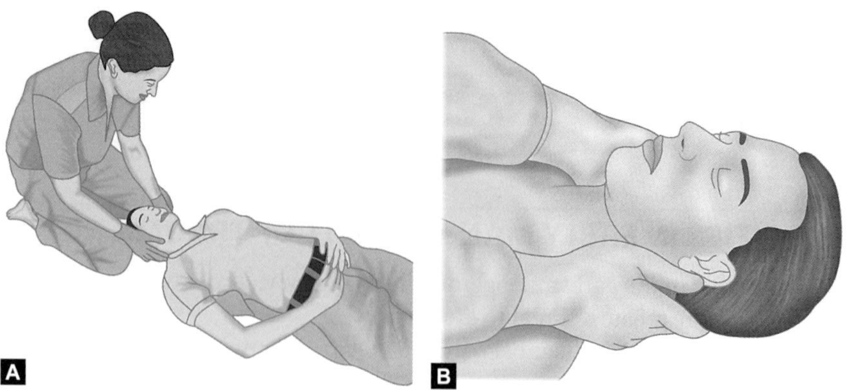

FIGS. 1A AND B: Manual in-line stabilization of the spine.

- While examining or intubating a trauma victim, ask an assistant to perform a manual in line stabilization of the neck in order to minimize un-intentional movement of the cervical spine.

  This maneuver is performed by an assistant standing at the head end or side of the trolley and using the fingers and palms of both hands stabilizes the patient's occiput and mastoid processes. This should be done while moving a trauma victim, performing a logroll and during intubation (**Figs. 1A** and **B**).

REASSESSMENT OF THE ABC

Reassessment of the ABC is an integral component to ensure that there has been no decompensation after initial resuscitation. This should be done as each step of the primary assessment is completed or if there is a time lag between components.

By the end of the primary assessment and resuscitation, the following should be achieved.

- Airway established and maintained
- Supplemental oxygen initiated
- Cervical spine immobilized
- Two large bore intravenous lines started
- Blood drawn for baseline investigations and crossmatch
- External hemorrhage control achieved
- ECG, BP, and saturation of oxygen (arterial blood) (SpO_2) monitoring
- Brief neurological examination completed
- Full exposure and environmental control done.

SECONDARY ASSESSMENT

The secondary assessment should be performed after the completion of primary assessment. It is a head-to-toe systematic and comprehensive evaluation of all organ systems. It is during this phase of management that the patient's detailed history should be elicited. A useful system for history elicitation is the AMPLE:

A—Allergies

M—Medications (especially anticoagulants, insulin, and cardiovascular medications)

P—Previous medical or surgical history

L—Last meal (time)

E—*Event*: Details regarding the biomechanism of injury

Examination of the Head and Face

Immobilize the neck with a hard cervical collar until cervical spine X-ray is done and cleared. With an assistant immobilizing the head, remove the cervical collar and examine the neck for any lacerations, tenderness, bogginess, or step deformities indicating the possibility of a cervical spine injury.

- Scalp lacerations tend to bleed profusely because of abundant vascular supply. Apply direct pressure to control any bleeding. Check the continuity of the cranium with a gloved hand, palpating gently with the fingertips. Beware of small puncture wounds of the scalp, which may indicate penetrating injury of the brain.
- Assess the Glasgow Coma Scale.
- Examine the nose and ears for bleeding and leakage of cerebrospinal fluid.
- Inspect the mouth for lacerations, broken teeth, or vomitus, since they could jeopardize the airway.

Examination of the Thorax

Although assessed during primary assessment, the thorax should again be reviewed for injuries. Check SpO_2 to assess peripheral oxygen saturation.

Examination of the Abdomen

- Abdominal assessment includes inspection for contusions, abrasions, and distension. Discoloration of the flanks may indicate retroperitoneal bleeding. Any wound above the umbilicus may have penetrated the thorax.
- Femoral pulse should be simultaneously palpated bilaterally and assessed for equality.
- The integrity of the pelvis should be evaluated by pushing on the wings of the iliac bone to determine, if this action elicits pain.
- Examine the urinary meatus for the presence of blood, which may indicate ruptured urethra.
- Perform a digital pelvic examination in females to look for the presence of vaginal bleeding.
- The patient should be logrolled with the head aligned to the body and the spine evaluated for asymmetry and the presence of tenderness (**Fig. 2**).

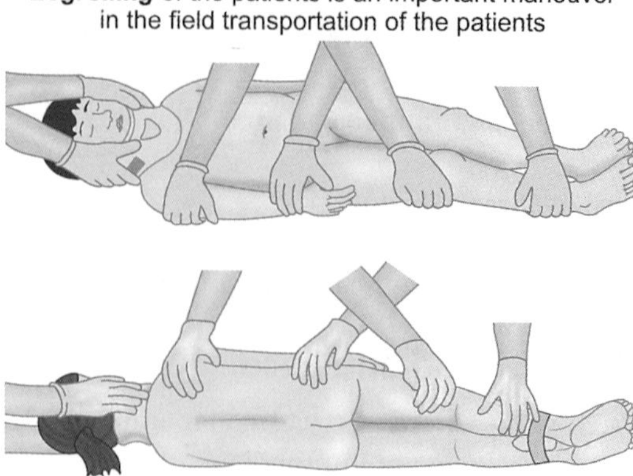

FIG. 2: Logrolling of the patient.

- During the logroll, perform a rectal examination to evaluate sphincter tone and presence of blood.

Examination of the Extremities

- Palpate the extremities for tenderness, crepitus, and deformities.
- Evaluate for quality and integrity of pulses. Diminished pulses suggest disrupted blood vessels. Traction generally restores blood flow.
- If the patient is conscious, assess sensory and motor functions.
- Suspected fractures and dislocations should be splinted for further radiographic and diagnostic evaluation.

Adjuncts to Secondary Assessment

- *Urinary catheter* is a vital adjunct for polytrauma management. The urine output is an excellent way of assessing perfusion in patients with an intact renal function. Moreover, blood in the urine may indicate renal trauma. Urinary catheter should be inserted only after ensuring that there are no pelvic fractures that could have injured the urethra. Blood in the meatus, perianal hematoma or a high riding prostate on rectal examination should raise suspicion of a urethral injury. Under these circumstances, urinary catheterization should only be attempted after an ascending urethrogram.
- *Nasogastric tube* needs to be inserted, to avoid stomach distension and to reduce the risk of aspiration. When a base of skull fracture is suspected, the gastric tube should be inserted orally to prevent intracranial passage.
- If available, obtain an arterial blood gas test to assess the hematocrit, partial pressure of arterial oxygen and the degree of acidosis.

Mandatory X-rays in trauma evaluation for all high velocity accidents includes chest, lateral cervical spine, and pelvis. Focused assessment with sonography for trauma (FAST) is indicated, if intra-abdominal injury is suspected.

Hemorrhagic Shock

INTRODUCTION

The blood volume is 7% of an adult body weight. It is slightly higher in children at 80–90 mL/kg body weight. Clinically, it is possible to estimate the volume of blood lost in a patient. Four classes of hemorrhagic shock are recognized as tabulated in **Table 1**.

From **Table 1**, it is evident that fall in blood pressure occurs only when more than 30% of blood loss has occurred.

MANAGEMENT OF HEMORRHAGIC SHOCK

Hemorrhagic shock in trauma is one of the potentially preventable causes of death. The first step in treatment is recognition of shock, as bleeding may often be covert. The average amount of blood lost with some common fractures is as follows: Humerus (750 mL), tibia (750 mL), femur (1,500 mL) and pelvis (>3 L). Tachycardia is often the first abnormal vital sign of hemorrhagic shock. BP may be normal till 30% of the blood volume is lost (750–1,500 mL). Hence, prolonged capillary refill time (normally <3 s) is a very useful test to identify early decrease in peripheral perfusion due to hemorrhagic shock.

TABLE 1: Blood loss and hemodynamic compensation due to hemorrhagic shock.

Parameter	Class I	Class II	Class III	Class IV
Blood loss	<750 mL	750–1,500 mL	1,500–2,000 mL	>2,000 mL
Blood volume lost	<15%	15–30%	30–40%	>40%
Heart rate	<100/min	100–120/min	120–140/min	>140/min
Capillary refill time	Normal	Delayed	Delayed	Delayed
Systolic BP	Normal	Normal	Low	Low
Diastolic BP	Normal	Raised	Low	Often unrecordable
Respiratory rate	Normal	20–30/min	30–40/min	>35/min
Urine output	>30 mL/h	20–30 mL/h	<20 mL/h	<20 mL/h
Mental state	Mildly anxious	Anxious	Confused	Confused/ drowsy
Resuscitation	Crystalloid	Crystalloid	Crystalloid and blood	Crystalloid and blood

- In the acute phase, the therapeutic priority is control of hemorrhage by pressure bandage or ligation of bleeders.
- Start 2 large bore IV cannulae (14/16G) in the antecubital fossa and start fluid resuscitation with ringer lactate. In severe trauma, do not give >1 L of crystalloids due to the risk of dilutional coagulopathy.
- For significant hemorrhage, transfuse O negative blood followed by type specific blood.

Tranexamic Acid: Early administration in trauma victims with significant hemorrhage has been of proven benefit and should be administered to patients who present within 3 hours of the incident.

Dose: 1 g intravenous (IV) over 10 minutes, followed by IV infusion of 1 g over 8 hours.

Evaluating the type of response to initial resuscitation is important to determine further management of the patient. The response to the initial resuscitation may be of three types.

1. **Rapid responders:** These are patients in whom bleeding has either been contained or controlled and the initial resuscitation fluid restores the lost volume.
2. **Transient responders:** These patients show a good response to the initial resuscitation but deteriorate when fluids are slowed. They require group specific blood in addition to crystalloids. A search for the source of bleeding should be made and a surgical opinion sought.
3. **Non-responders:** These are patients who continue to deteriorate despite resuscitation and indicate an ongoing hemorrhage. These patients require immediate blood transfusion and surgical intervention.

MASSIVE TRANSFUSION PROTOCOL

Severe bleeding results in dilutional anemia and dilutional coagulopathy and hence, plasma substitutes are required in addition to packed red cells. The "lethal triad" of trauma is acidosis, hypothermia, and coagulopathy. In patients with trauma presenting with severe bleeding and expected to require large amount of blood product transfusion, massive transfusion protocol (MTP) should be initiated (**Flowchart 1**).

Massive blood transfusion is most practically defined as:

- Transfusion of >4 units of packed red blood cells (PRCs) in 1 hour when ongoing need is foreseeable
- Replacement of 50% of total blood volume within 3 hours.

When to Activate?

- Polytrauma or severe crush injuries or multiple long bone injuries with hemorrhagic shock despite fluid resuscitation.
- Thoracic or abdominal trauma with persistent hypotension due to blood loss.

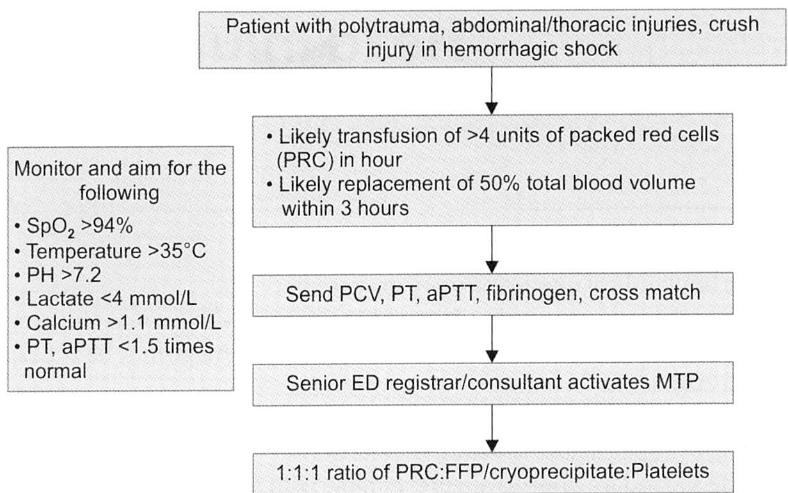

(aPTT: activated partial thromboplastine time; FFP: fresh frozen plasma; MTP: massive transfusion protocol; PCV: packed cell volume; PT: prothrombin time)

FLOWCHART 1: Massive transfusion protocol.

Massive transfusion protocol should be activated by the senior emergency department physician when the need for massive transfusion is perceived and usually after 2–3 units of PRCs are transfused. The most acceptable recommendation for MTP is a predefined ration of 1:1:1 of PRCs:Fresh frozen plasma (FFP)/cryoprecipitate:Platelets. Once activated, the blood bank should ensure rapid supply of these blood products for transfusion.

- *Packed red cells*: 4 mL/kg body weight
- *FFP*: 10–15 mL/kg body weight
- *Cryoprecipitate*: 1 unit for every 5–10 kg body weight
- *Platelets*: 1 unit

Complications of Massive Transfusion

- Volume overload
- Hypothermia (monitor temperature)
- Excessive citrate may cause metabolic acidosis and hypocalcemia (monitor pH and calcium)
- Hyperkalemia

INTRODUCTION

Traumatic brain injury may be primary or secondary:
- Primary injury occurs at the time of head injury with axonal shearing and disruption and areas of hemorrhage. The primary damage may be widespread (diffuse axonal) or localized.
- Secondary injury occurs later and may be due to hypoxia, hypovolemia and cerebral hypoperfusion, seizures, or infection.

Many of the secondary injuries are preventable with aggressive resuscitation.

GLASGOW COMA SCALE

This scale is now almost universally used to assess the severity of brain injury, and also to guide management and prognosticate. It has three components with a total of 15 points. The minimum score of 3 points indicates maximal severity, and a score of 15 is considered normal. In children, the Glasgow Coma Scale (GCS) is slightly modified. The total GCS is used to classify the severity of head injury (**Table 1**).
- *Severe*: 8 or less
- *Moderate*: 9–13
- *Mild*: 14–15

A cervical spine X-ray before a CT brain is mandatory for all patients with suspected head injury.

MANAGEMENT

- Initial assessment of a patient with head injury includes airway, breathing, and circulation management. Airway and breathing may be compromised due to low sensorium and/or bleeding. Patients with GCS of <8 with airway compromise will require urgent intubation and those with normal oxygenation and stable airway will need elective intubation.
- Examine the scalp for lacerations. Scalp wounds can result in significant blood loss and should be managed by full thickness interrupted suturing at the earliest.
- Palpate the skull for deformities or tenderness. Signs of base of skull fracture such as Battle's sign (Mastoid hematoma), bilateral racoon eyes, and CSF otorrhea or rhinorrhea should be noted.

TABLE 1: Glasgow Coma Scale (GCS).

Eye opening	Score	Verbal response	Score	Motor response	Score
GCS: Adult					
Spontaneous eye opening	4	Oriented	5	Obeys commands	6
Opens eyes to call	3	Confused	4	Localizes painful stimuli	5
Opens eyes to painful stimuli	2	Inappropriate words	3	Withdraws to pain	4
No eye opening	1	Incomprehensible sounds	2	Abnormal flexion to pain	3
		No verbal response	1	Abnormal extension to pain	2
				No motor response to pain	1
GCS: Infant (<1 year)					
Spontaneous	4	Coos and babbles	5	Moves spontaneously	6
To verbal stimuli	3	Irritable cries	4	Withdraws to touch	5
To pain only	2	Cries to pain	3	Withdraws to pain	4
No response	1	Moans to pain	2	Abnormal flexion	3
		No response	1	Abnormal extension	2
				No response	1

- Observe for bleeding or cerebrospinal fluid leak from the ear or nose.
- Start fluid resuscitation and oxygen therapy if saturation is low.
- Decrease intracranial pressure if there is evidence of intracranial herniation or a dropping GCS. Start 20% mannitol 100 mL stat and q8h.
- Start antiepileptics (phenytoin) if there is any parenchymal injury or a depressed skull fracture.
- Administer tetanus-diphtheria (Td) vaccine for open injuries if not adequately vaccinated. At discharge, advice the patient to complete the vaccination schedule (2 more doses 4 weeks apart).

INTRODUCTION

Significant spinal cord injuries are caused by road traffic accidents, heavy weights falling on a person, fall from a height, etc.

Injudicious movement after trauma and inadequate immobilization during transportation can cause "secondary spinal cord injury". In fact, about 10–25% of neurological deficits occur because of improper prehospital handling.

Principles of Assessment and Management of Suspected Cervical Spine Injuries

- Assume that all trauma victims have spinal cord injury until proven otherwise, especially in unconscious patients.
- During transportation of a trauma victim, total spinal immobilization along with the head, neck, chest, pelvis, and lower extremities should take utmost priority.
- In spinal cord injuries, there is a high probability of cord edema, which may cause respiratory arrest. Hence, airway and ventilation must be adequately addressed during transportation of a trauma victim.
- *C-spine immobilization*: This can be achieved by using a rigid cervical orthosis, sandbags, strapping, or a spine board.
- Immobilize spine in the same position the victim presents to you. *Do not attempt to straighten or manipulate the neck.*
- General examination of any suspected case of spinal injury must be carried out with patient in a neutral position and without any movement of the spine. No spinal segment should be mobilized until it has been specifically cleared by appropriate radiography.
- A conscious patient with paralysis is usually able to localize the site of an injury because of tenderness or loss of sensation below that level.
- Paralysis and loss of sensation mask severity of intra-abdominal and lower extremity injuries.

Classification of Spinal Injuries

- *Unstable*: Subluxation, bilateral facet dislocation, atlanto-occipital dislocation, odontoid fracture with lateral displacement, posterior neural arch fracture (C1), Jefferson's fracture (C1), and Hangman's fracture (C2).
- *Stable*: Unilateral facet dislocation, wedge fracture, Clay Shoveler's fracture (C7), and transverse process fracture.

HOW TO CLEAR A C-SPINE CLINICALLY

History and physical examination can be sufficient in clearing the cervical spine. Notable clinical prediction rules to determine the need for radiological imaging are:

1. National Emergency X-Radiography Utilization Study (NEXUS) criteria
2. Canadian C-Spine rules (more sensitive and specific)

However, we recommend the following SMART-D assessment of patients with suspected cervical spine injuries. (**Table 1**).

Follow **Flowchart 1** to determine indications for C-spine imaging and for clinical clearance of cervical spine.

RADIOLOGICAL EVALUATION OF CERVICAL SPINE

- Plain radiography is the basic investigation (Lateral/Swimmers cervical spine X-ray). If the lateral view is inadequate and does not show C7 lower end plate, then traction can be given to the hand or a swimmers view (the arm closer to the cassette over the head and the other arm depressed) can be performed.
- This is a crucial investigation as early cord injury, which requires surgery for good prognosis can be picked up on basis of fractures.
- Delayed recognition may lead to irreversible injury
- All radiographs must be taken with the cervical collar in situ.

TABLE 1: SMART-D assessment of C-spine in the emergency department (ED).		
S	SENSORIUM	• Alertness—whether fully awake and conscious • Alcohol intoxication
M	MECHANISM OF INJURY	• Painful distracting injury: Refers to any injury to the body producing pain sufficient enough to distract the patient from neck injury. (long bone fractures, visceral injuries, crush and degloving injuries, burns) • Dangerous mechanism of injury (Fall from height >3 feet/5 stairs, axial load to the head, high velocity motor vehicle accidents, rollover, or ejection motor vehicle injuries)
A	AGE	• Age >65 years
R	ROTATION OF NECK	• Ability to rotate the neck 45 degree left and right (This step must be performed ONLY if all the other factors of SMART-D assessment are negative)
T	TENDERNESS OVER NECK	Assess posterior midline cervical tenderness (from occiput to T1)
D	DEFICITS	• Paresthesia in extremities • Focal neurological deficits

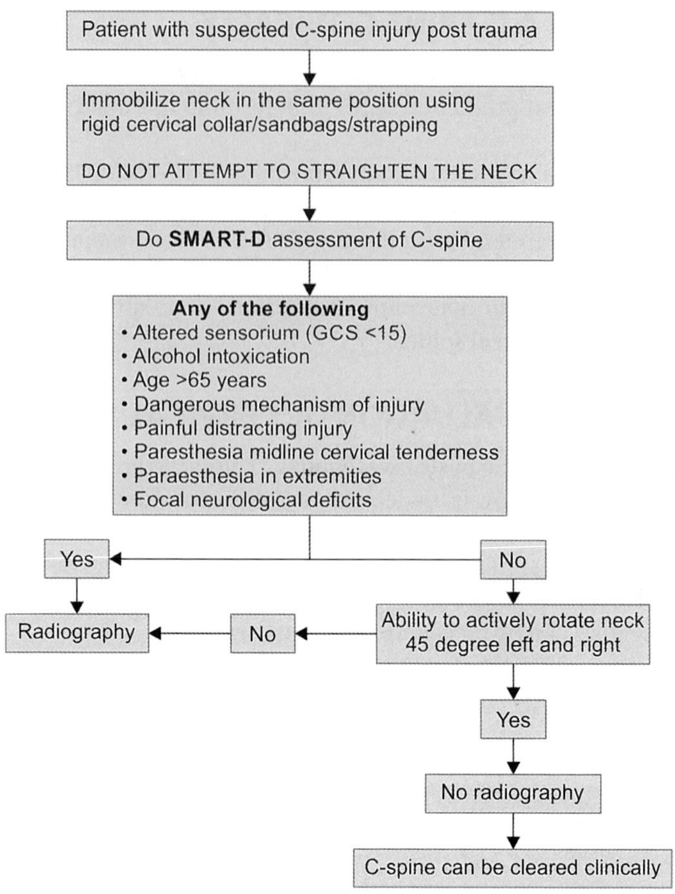

(GCS: Glasgow Coma Scale)

FLOWCHART 1: C-spine assessment.

INTERPRETATION OF THE CERVICAL SPINE X-RAY

Carefully look for the following components while interpreting a cervical spine X-ray.

- **A: Adequacy and Alignment:**
  - Adequacy of a spine X-ray is determined by the clear visibility of C7/T1 junction. If this is not visible on a lateral X-ray, a simmers view may be performed.
  - In a normal C-spine X-ray, all four longitudinal lines shown in **Fig. 1B** would be aligned. The four longitudinal lines are
    a. Anterior contour line
    b. Posterior contour line
    c. Spinolaminal line
    d. Spinous process line

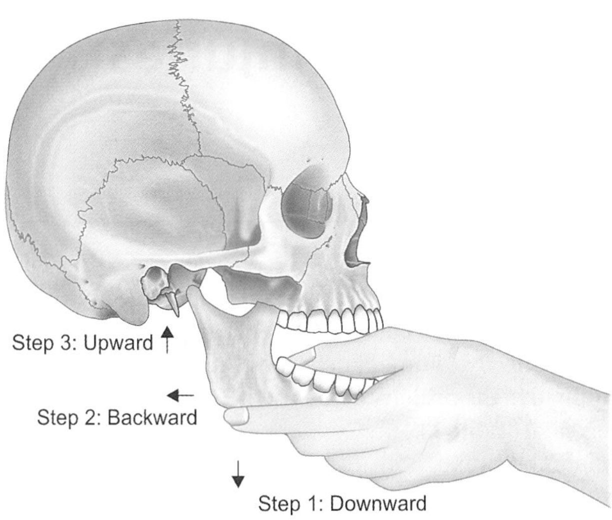

FIG. 2: Reduction of anterior dislocation of temporomandibular joint.

6. Refer to maxillofacial surgeon (dental surgery) for further follow up.

Downward → Backward → Upward

After successful reduction of a TMJ dislocation, do an orthopantomogram (X-ray mandible lateral view) to ensure adequate reduction and to exclude an avulsion fracture.

Following reduction, the patient should receive the following instructions:
- Avoid extreme opening of the jaw for 3 weeks
- Support the lower jaw when yawning
- Apply warm compresses to the TMJ area for 24 hours
- Take nonsteroidal anti-inflammatory drugs as needed for pain and swelling.

The following patients should be urgently referred to an oral and maxillofacial surgeon:
- Patients with an anterior TMJ dislocation in association with a fracture
- Patients who fail reduction of an anterior TMJ dislocation despite multiple attempts
- Patients who have had more than two prior TMJ dislocations
- Patients with superior or posterior dislocations.

INTRODUCTION

- About 25% of deaths due to trauma are a result of thoracic injuries.
- Majority of deaths (60–70%) occur after patient reaches a hospital.
- The following are the five immediately life-threatening chest injuries that should be identified in the primary assessment. Failure to identify these could be immediately fatal (**Table 1**).
    - Tension pneumothorax
    - Open pneumothorax

TABLE 1: Clinical features and management of common thoracic injuries.

	Tracheal position	Chest wall movement	Breath sounds	Percussion	Treatment
Tension pneumothorax	Away	Decreased	Decreased or absent	Hyper-resonant	• Immediate: Needle thoracostomy • Definitive: Tube thoracotomy
Open pneumothorax	Midline	Decreased	May be decreased	May be hyper-resonant Usually normal	• Immediate: Occlusive dressing over the wound, which is taped on three sides • Definitive: Tube thoracotomy
• Massive hemo- thorax • Defined as accumulation of >1,500 mL of blood in the thoracic cavity	Midline	Decreased	Dimini-shed, if large Normal, if small	Dull, especially posteriorly	• Fluid replacement • Tube thoracotomy • Surgical thoracotomy, if initial blood loss via chest tube >1,500 mL or a persistent need for blood transfusion

Continued

Continued

	Tracheal position	Chest wall movement	Breath sounds	Percussion	Treatment
Flail chest + pulmonary contusion	Midline	Paradoxical movement of the flail segment	Normal may have crackles	Normal	• Adequate ventilation, humidified O_2, analgesics and fluid resuscitation • Endotracheal intubation in case of impending respiratory failure

- ○ Flail chest
- ○ Massive hemothorax
- ○ Cardiac tamponade

TENSION PNEUMOTHORAX

If the air leak occurs through "one-way valve" from the lung or through the chest wall, the air is forced into the thoracic cavity completely collapsing the affected lung. This condition, known as tension pneumothorax causes cardio-respiratory collapse by shifting the mediastinum to the contralateral side and compression of the great vessels of the thorax. Immediate decompression by needle thoracostomy is warranted. Common causes of tension pneumothorax are mechanical ventilation with positive end-expiratory pressure, ruptured emphysematous bullae, blunt trauma, in which parenchymal leak which has not sealed.

OPEN PNEUMOTHORAX

Open pneumothorax is caused by a large wound in the chest wall, that remain open. Equilibrium between intrathoracic and atmospheric pressure occurs almost immediately. If the opening is greater than two-thirds the diameter of the trachea, air passes through the defect from the atmosphere thus impairing ventilation.

Emergency management: If a patient has an open wound in the thorax causing tension pneumothorax, apply a sterile occlusive dressing over the wound and tape it on 3 sides (**Fig. 1**). The 3 way occlusive dressing provides a flutter type valve and prevents air from entering from outside.

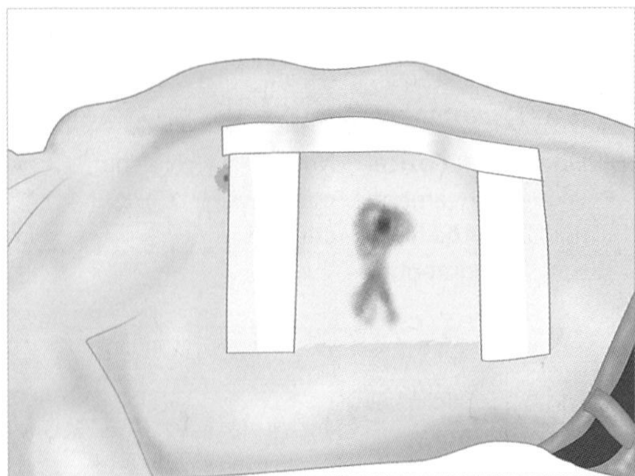

FIG. 1: 3 way occlusive dressing.

FLAIL CHEST + PULMONARY CONTUSION

These occur when there are fractures of two or more ribs at two or more sites. A bony segment moves independent of the rest of the thoracic cavities. The pathophysiology arises from underlying lung injury, along with impaired pulmonary mechanics. The flail segment does not move with the rest of the lung during respiration. Although chest wall instability leads to paradoxical motion of the chest wall with inspiration and expiration, this defect alone does not cause hypoxia. Associated pain with restricted chest wall movement and underlying lung injury contribute to the patient's hypoxia. The injured lung in flail segment is sensitive to both under and over hydration and hence adequate care must be taken during fluid resuscitation.

Tension pneumothorax is a clinical diagnosis. Do not wait for radiological confirmation to intervene.

CARDIAC TAMPONADE

Relatively small amount of blood (150 mL) in the pericardial sac can increase the pressure around the heart leading to impaired cardiac filling and decreased cardiac output. The classic Becks triad of cardiac tamponade includes distended neck veins, muffled heart sounds, and hypotension. Most patients will have at least one of these signs; all three rarely appear simultaneously. Urgent pericardiocentesis is warranted and the removal of as little as 10–15 mL of blood from the pericardial cavity results in remarkable improvement.

CHAPTER 111

Abdominal Injuries

INTRODUCTION

- Abdominal trauma is a cause of preventable deaths, which can easily go unnoticed if one does not search for it.
- When assessing the "C" in trauma, the abdomen and pelvis are important areas to rule out bleeding.
- Any mechanism of injury involving the torso, such as blunt or penetrating injuries or deceleration injuries can cause abdominal injuries.
  - Blunt trauma occurs in 85% while penetrating trauma accounts for only 15% of all abdominal traumas.
  - Large amounts of blood can accumulate in the peritoneal and pelvic cavities without any significant or early changes in the physical examination findings.
- In the case of blunt injuries, the following is the incidence:
  - *Spleen*: 40–55%
  - *Liver*: 35–45%
  - *Bowel*: 5–10%
- In the case of stab injuries, the following is the incidence:
  - *Liver*: 40%
  - *Small bowel*: 30%
  - *Diaphragm*: 20%
  - *Colon*: 15%
- In the case of gunshot injuries, the following is the incidence:
  - *Small bowel*: 50%
  - *Colon*: 40%
  - *Liver*: 30%

EVALUATION

- Assessment of hemodynamic stability is the most important initial concern in the evaluation of a patient with abdominal trauma.
- Chest X-ray to look for diaphragmatic hernia, hemothorax, or air under the diaphragm.
- Extended focused assessment with sonography in trauma (eFAST) (**Fig. 1**) is the dominant imaging modality used in the early assessment of abdomino-thoracic trauma. In a hemodynamically unstable patient with a negative eFAST, it may be prudent to repeat it after 10 minutes. If a hemodynamically stable patient has a positive eFAST, a CT thorax and abdomen needs to be performed.

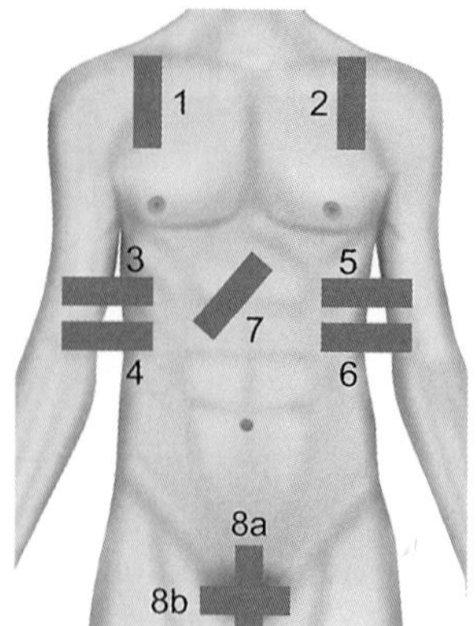

(eFAST: extended focused assessment with sonography in trauma)

FIG. 1: The sequence of 8 views that make up the eFAST examination.

- A CT scan though has the highest positive yield rate, should be reserved only for persistently stable patients.

Do not shift a hemodynamically unstable patient for a CT scan.

MANAGEMENT

Emergency Department Management

- Secure airway and breathing
- Start 2 wide bore IV lines above the diaphragm and start fluid resuscitation
- Avoid femoral central line
- Tranexamic acid 10 mg/kg IV (1 g in adults) over 10 minutes, if the patient presents within 3 hours of trauma
- If the penetrating object is still in place, DO NOT ATTEMPT TO REMOVE IT
- Avoid palpating the prostate by digital rectal examination (DRE). It must be done only to assess bleeding PR, or anal tone

Surgical management may involve either operative intervention (laparotomy) or conservative management.

Indications for Emergency Laparotomy

- Bowel or bladder rupture
- Peritonitis
- Uncontrolled shock despite adequate resuscitation
- *Penetrating injuries*: Relative indication
- Air under the diaphragm
- Massive intra-abdominal bleed.

Nonoperative Management

This involves frequent monitoring of hemodynamic status and bleeding manifestations.

- Hemodynamically stable patients with positive eFAST findings require a CT scan to define the nature and extent of their injuries and thus augment the decision to manage by nonsurgical intervention.
- Operative treatment is not indicated in every patient with positive eFAST results, since this could result in an unacceptably high laparotomy rate. Most pediatric patients can be resuscitated and treated nonoperatively. Hemodynamically stable adults with solid organ injuries, primarily those to the liver and spleen, may be candidates for nonoperative management.

FRACTURES

Definition

A fracture is any break in the continuity of the bone.

- *Open versus Closed*: Open fractures occur when either the fractured bone communicates with the exterior by breaching the muscle planes and skin or as a result of an external injury exposing the bone at the fractured site. Open injuries need to be prioritized over closed fractures to limit infection.
- *Based on pattern*: Fractures can be radiologically described as transverse, oblique, segmental, comminuted, or with bone loss.

Signs and Symptoms

Signs and symptoms can be as overt as gross deformity of the limb, restriction of movements of joints with pain or as subtle as tenderness with limb shortening.

Gustilo and Anderson Classification

This is a useful tool for assessing open fracture severity (**Table 1**).

TABLE 1: Gustilo open fracture classification.

Gustilo grade	Definition
I	Open fracture, clean wound, and wound <1 cm in length
II	Open fracture, wound >1 cm but <10 cm in length without extensive soft-tissue damage, flaps, and avulsions
III	Open fracture with extensive soft-tissue laceration (>10 cm), damage, or loss or an open segmental fracture. This type also includes open fractures caused by farm injuries, fractures requiring vascular repair, or fractures that have been open for 8 h prior to treatment
III A	Type III fracture with adequate periosteal coverage of the fracture bone despite the extensive soft-tissue laceration or damage
III B	Type III fracture with extensive soft-tissue loss, periosteal stripping, and bone damage. Usually associated with massive contamination. Will often need further soft-tissue coverage procedure (i.e., free or rotational flap)
III C	Type III fracture associated with an arterial injury requiring repair, irrespective of degree of soft-tissue injury

Source: Gustilo RB, Mendoza RM, Williams DN. Problems in the management of type III (severe) open fractures: A new classification of type III open fractures. J Trauma. 1984;24:742-6.

Compound or open fractures occur when a fracture is open through a skin wound. These may be associated with gross soft tissue damage, hemorrhage, or vascular injuries.

Basic Principles of Management of Fractures

- Obtain proper history of the mechanism of injury.
- Administer analgesia prior to handling the wound.
- Administer tetanus-diphtheria (Td) vaccine as prophylaxis, if not adequately immunized.
- Start antibiotics only in open injuries.
- Realign limb to minimize deformity and pain.
- Document any neurovascular deficit.
- Using sterile techniques, wash the wound with normal saline and apply sterile padding.
- Immobilize the affected limb one joint above and below the fracture site with appropriate splint or traction.
- Keep the limb elevated to minimize swelling.

X-rays

- Order only minimal, relevant imaging to clinch a diagnosis.
- X-rays of a fractured limb should involve one joint above and below the fractured site.
- Always order two views of a limb [anteroposterior (AP) and lateral].
- In children, order X-rays of the normal limb too, for comparison and to avoid confusion over growth plates.

Investigations

The investigations include packed cell volume (PCV), creatinine, electrolytes, and rapid blood borne virus screen (BBVS) (if surgery is required).

Preservation of Amputated Part

Remember only clean cut amputations can be salvaged; crushed, or ragged body parts are nonsalvageable.

- Wash part in isotonic solution
- Wrap in sterile gauze soaked in penicillin (100,00 units in 50 mL of Ringer's lactate)
- Wrap this in a sterile moist towel
- Place in a plastic bag
- Keep in crushed ice and avoid freezing
- *Call* the hand surgery team on arrival of patient itself, as time to surgery is the key to a good prognosis.

COMMON FRACTURES SEEN IN THE EMERGENCY DEPARTMENT

Hand Fractures

Hand fractures are commonly seen but commonly missed.
- *Initial treatment*: Follow basic principles of management.
- Fingers can be buddy-splinted by strapping the injured finger to a neighboring unaffected finger (**Fig. 1**).
- *X-rays*: Anteroposterior and oblique views for full hand.
- *For isolated finger injuries*: AP and lateral views focusing on the specific finger.

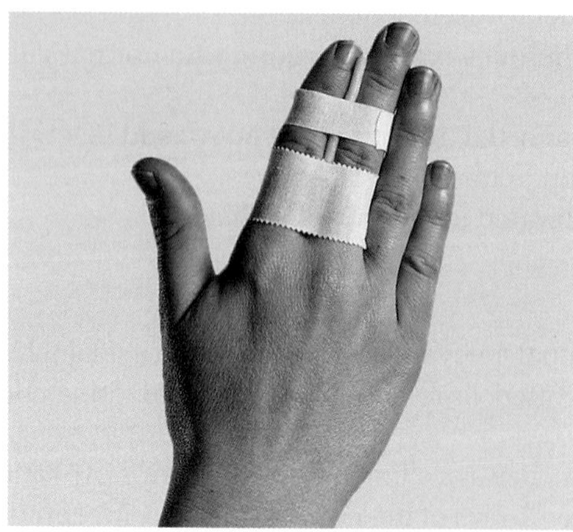

FIG. 1: Buddy taping of fingers.

Colles Fracture

It is the most common distal radius injury (fracture at the base of the ulnar styloid process). This results from a fall on the out stretched hand with the wrist in dorsiflexion. Carefully examine the median nerve and motor function of the finger flexors.
- Intra-articular fractures require an orthopedic intervention.
- Extra-articular fractures can be close reduced and sent to outpatient department in a cast or splint.

Reduction Technique (Figs. 2A to C)

- Administer a hematoma block; allow it to take effect.
- Then reduce the fracture by giving a sustained linear traction, with one assistant pulling on the proximal part at the elbow while another assistant holds the thumb separately with one hand and the rest four fingers with the other giving a counter traction distally in 30 degree of ulnar deviation and 10 degree of palmar flexion.

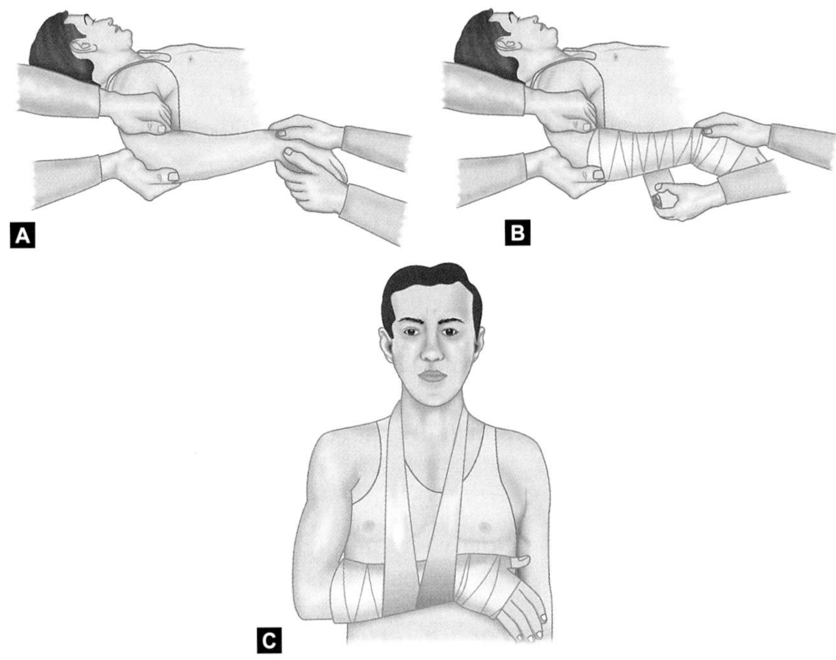

FIGS. 2A TO C: Reduction of Colles fracture.

- Placing your hands on the fracture site, manually realign the fracture by reversing the position of the displaced fragments.
- Then maintaining the traction-countertraction, now apply a padded Colles cast to maintain the reduction.

X-rays

Anteroposterior and lateral of the wrist with forearm; repeat check X-rays after reduction.

Pelvic Fractures

This is a potentially life-threatening condition which should be recognized immediately. An "open book" fracture with diastasis of more than 2 cm is considered unstable.

When to Suspect?

- High-velocity trauma
- Falls from height
- All trauma patients presenting with unexplained hypotensive shock.

Pelvic Compression Test

This test is done to confirm a pelvic fracture. This is done by giving downward and inward compression to both iliac crests simultaneously. If one feels a "give" it is considered to be positive for an unstable pelvis. Perform this test only once.

X-rays

Pelvis anteroposterior view.

Treatment

- Avoid moving the patient unnecessarily
- Apply a pelvic binder (any broad sheet or cloth can be used for this purpose)
- Fluid resuscitation as required and maintain the blood pressure
- Avoid catheterization till urethral injury has been ruled out.

Hip Fractures

These are very common in the elderly and mostly result from fall on the level ground. This can be associated with acetabular fractures.

Neck of Femur versus Intertrochanteric Fractures

These can be easily diagnosed clinically by observing the attitude of the lower limb.
- *Neck of femur fracture*: Being an intracapsular fracture, patients present with slight shortening and mild external rotation of the lower limb.
- *Intertrochanteric fractures*: Being an extracapsular fracture, patients present with ecchymosis of the overlying skin, shortening and gross external rotation of the lower limb.

X-rays

Pelvis with both hips (in 10 degree of internal rotation)—anteroposterior and lateral view of affected hip. Follow the Shenton's line for finding obscure fractures (**Fig. 3**).

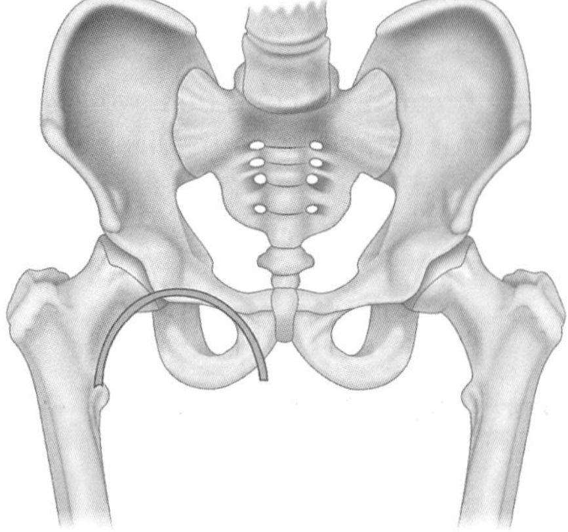

FIG. 3: Shenton's line.

Treatment

Initial treatment consists of immobilizing the lower limb with skin traction. There is no role for splints.

Shaft of Femur and Tibia Fractures

Both these injuries are common in road traffic accidents. Always assess the neurovascular status in these limbs, as the incidence of neurovascular injuries is quite high. Monitor for compartment syndrome.

X-rays

Anteroposterior/lateral views visualizing both the joint above and below the shaft.

Always request for an additional X-ray of the pelvis with both hips, as fracture dislocation is often associated with these injuries.

Treatment

Immobilize with a Below Knee (B/K) splint for a tibia fractures and Above Knee (A/K) splint for a femur fracture.

Alternately, a Thomas splint may be used for these fractures, which is also the best way to transfer a patient.

DISLOCATIONS

- *Dislocation* is a complete loss of articular contact between two opposing joint surfaces.
- *Subluxation* is a partial loss of articular contact between two opposing joint surfaces.

Signs and Symptoms

A dislocation is more painful than sustaining a fracture and therefore needs immediate attention. However, they are often associated with a fracture.

Based on the joint involved, the presentation is usually classical for that joint.

Always check the neurovascular status of the limb.

Investigations

No routine blood investigations are required for dislocations.

Role of X-ray

X-ray is not needed in habitual or recurrent dislocations. In first time dislocations, an X-ray may be warranted to rule out other injuries as well. However, *do not* delay getting it done as one needs to reduce the dislocation soon after.

The following are some of the more common dislocations one would encounter in the emergency department (ED).

SHOULDER DISLOCATIONS

Anterior glenohumeral (AGH) (**Fig. 4**) dislocations are the most common, while posterior (PGH) accounts less than 1%. Luxatio erecta (inferior dislocation) and superior are extremely rare (**Table 2**).

Clinical Examination (Focused)

- *Anterior glenohumeral dislocation*: Arm is usually held in abduction and slight external rotation with shoulder appearing "squared off", i.e., loss of normal rounded contour. Humeral head (HH) is palpable and anterior to shoulder joint.
- *Posterior glenohumeral dislocation*: Arm is usually adducted and internally rotated making the anterior shoulder appear flat. Prominence of the coracoid and HH is palpable posterior to the shoulder joint.
- *Inferior dislocation*: HH is palpable in the lateral chest wall with the arm fully abducted, elbow flexed, and forearm lying behind or on the head.
- Look for axillary nerve injury by checking sensation over the deltoid region.
- Check for brachial and radial artery pulsation.

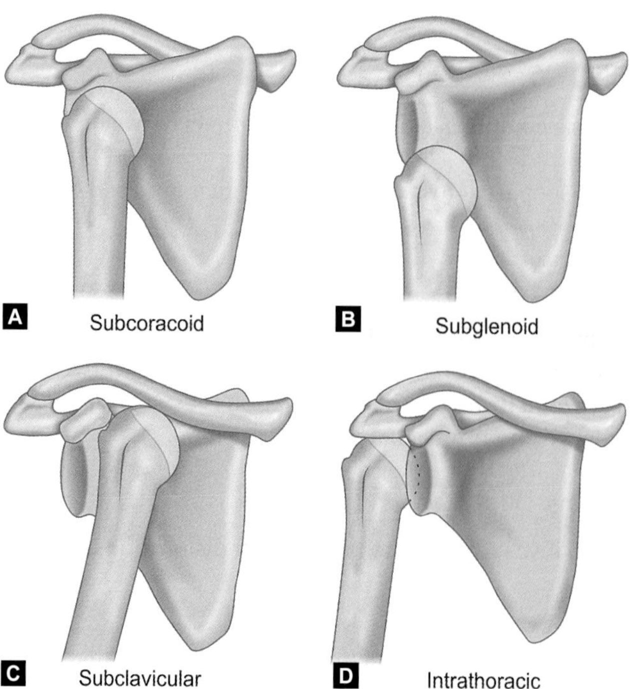

FIGS. 4A TO D: Types of anterior glenohumeral dislocation.

TABLE 2: Types of shoulder dislocation.

Types	Subtypes	Description of injury	Associated injuries
Anterior (MOI: Indirect blow with arm in abduction, extension, and external rotation)	Subcoracoid (most common)	HH displaced anterior to glenoid and inferior to coracoid	Fracture greater tuberosity, humeral neck, anterior glenoid rim (Bankart fracture), and axillary artery injury
	Subglenoid	HH lies inferior and anterior to the glenoid	
	Subclavicular	HH displaced medial to coracoid below the clavicle	
	Intrathoracic	HH lies between the ribs and thoracic cavity	
Posterior (MOI: Indirect forced internal rotation and adduction)	Subacromial (most common)	HH posterior to glenoid and inferior to acromion	Fracture of posterior glenoid rim, humeral head, and shaft and lesser tuberosity
	Subglenoid	HH lies inferior and posterior to glenoid	
	Subspinous	HH lies inferior to spine of scapula	
Inferior (MOI: Continuous hyperabduction force at shoulder)		Neck of humerus is levered against the acromion and inferior capsular tear	Severe soft tissue injury, rotator cuff tear, neurovascular injury, and fracture proximal humerus

(HH: humeral head; MOI: mechanism of injury)

X-rays

- X-ray of anteroposterior view of the shoulder.
- X-ray of scapular Y view—to classify the dislocation further.

Treatment

- Posterior and inferior glenohumeral dislocations need expertise and should be reduced and managed only by orthopedicians.
- Anterior dislocations are commoner and may be reduced in the ED. Under sedation, all attempts to reduce the dislocation should be done by one of the following techniques available. Most techniques use either leverage or traction-countertraction mechanisms.

Stimson's Technique

This is very useful in a busy ED where one cannot attend to the patient immediately or in a situation where an anticipated difficult reduction (as in a dislocation which occurred many hours earlier) is expected (**Fig. 5**).

- Administer a good dose of analgesic before the procedure.
- Place the patient in prone position with the affected arm hanging down by the side of the table.
- Place a folded sheet under the clavicle of the affected side and attach a weight of approximately 3–5 kg to the wrist of the affected hand.
- The muscles will slowly relax and gravity helps to reduce the dislocation in 20–30 minutes.
- In addition to above steps, a manual rotation of tip of the dislocated scapula medially with one hand and stabilizing upper scapula with the other hand help in much easier reduction with a success rate close to 96% (Scapular manipulation).
- Monitor the neurovascular status periodically.

Kocher's Technique

This technique was first described in 1870 as a painless procedure and since then many modifications have been proposed. This method uses leverage alone and does not involve traction (**Figs. 6A to D**).

- Place the patient supine and stand by the side of the affected arm.
- Bend the arm at 90 degree at the elbow and adduct it against the body.
- Grasp the wrist and the point of the elbow.
- Externally rotate the arm by 70–85 degree until a resistance is felt.
- Lift the externally rotated arm in the sagittal plane as far forward as possible.

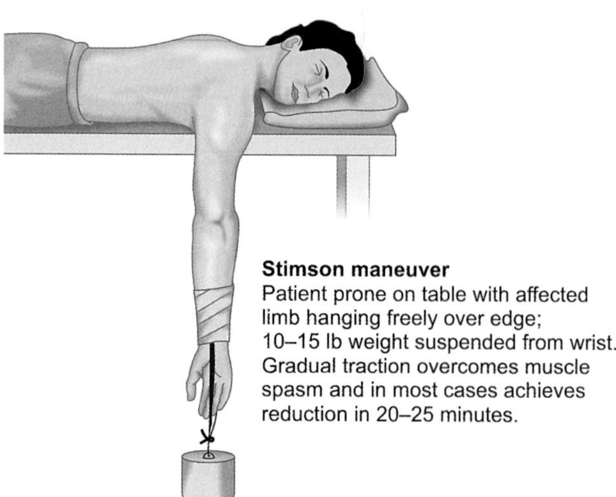

FIG. 5: Stimson's technique for shoulder.

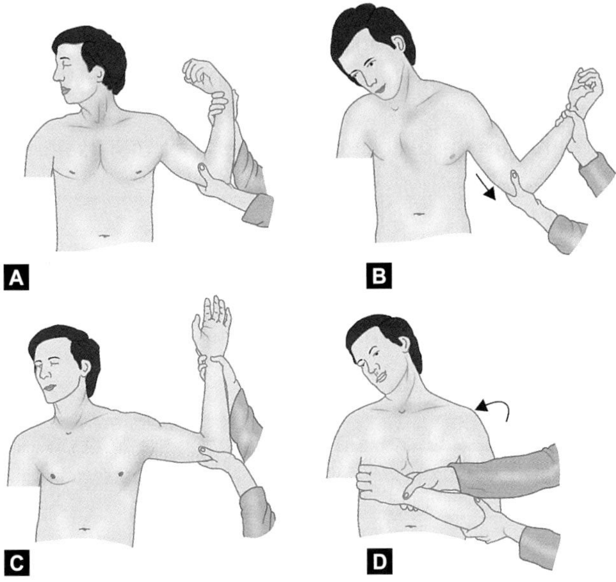

FIGS. 6A TO D: Kocher's technique for shoulder reduction.

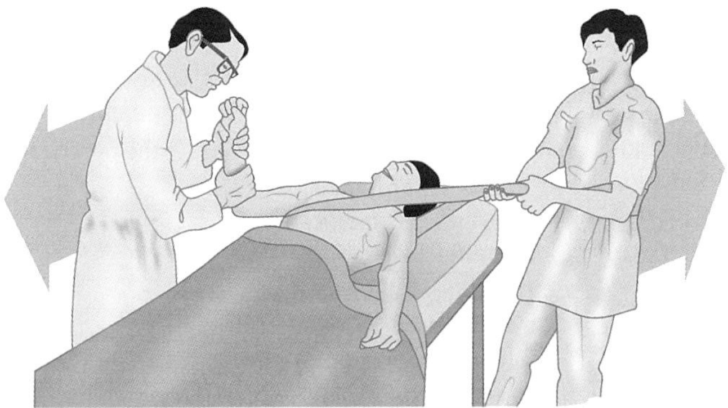

FIG. 7: Matsen's traction—countertraction method.

- Now internally rotate the shoulder to bring the patient's hand toward the opposite shoulder.
- This should result in the femoral head slipping into the glenoid fossa.
- Patient can be discharged after a check X-ray, on an arm pouch.

Matsen's Traction—Countertraction Method

This technique employs the traction-countertraction principle and requires an assistant (**Fig. 7**).

- Place the patient in the supine position.
- Wrap a sheet around the patient's thorax under the axilla that is held by the assistant standing on the other side to provide countertraction.

- With the elbow of the affected arm flexed at 90 degree, grasp the forearm, lean back, and apply traction at 30–40 degree abduction.
- The assistant should pull on the sheet toward the opposite shoulder to provide countertraction.
- This usually unhinges the dislocated shoulder back into its normal position.

HIP DISLOCATIONS

Hip dislocations are classified into anterior hip dislocation (AHD), posterior hip dislocation (PHD), central, and inferior (luxatio erecta) (**Table 3**) and are usually associated with motor vehicle accidents without seat belt usage.

TABLE 3: Types of hip dislocation.

Types	Subtypes and description of dislocation	Associated injuries
Anterior (10%) (MOI—forceful extension, abduction and external rotation of the leg. Femoral head levers out of the acetabular cup)	Epstein classification of anterior hip dislocation (**Fig. 8**) • Superior dislocation (pelvis) • Inferior dislocation (obturator)	• Fracture and impaction of femoral head • Fracture of acetabulum • Femoral artery and nerve injury
Posterior (90%) [MOI—axial force over the femur with knee and hip flexed, adducted, and internally rotated (dash board injury)]	Thompson and Epstein classification of posterior hip dislocation (**Fig. 9**) • Simple dislocation with or without an insignificant posterior wall fragment • Dislocation associated with a single large posterior wall fragment • Dislocation associated with a comminuted posterior wall fragment • Dislocation associated with fracture of the acetabular floor • Dislocation associated with fracture of the femoral head	10% incidence of sciatic nerve injury especially the peroneal branch
Central (rare)	Entire femoral head is forced centrally through comminuted acetabular fracture	Acetabular fracture
Inferior (very rare)	Exclusively in children <7 years	

(MOI: mechanism of injury)

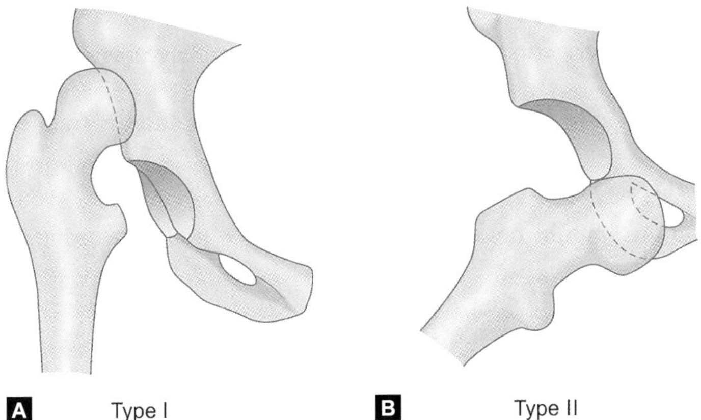

A   Type I   **B**   Type II

FIGS. 8A AND B: Epstein classification of anterior hip dislocations.

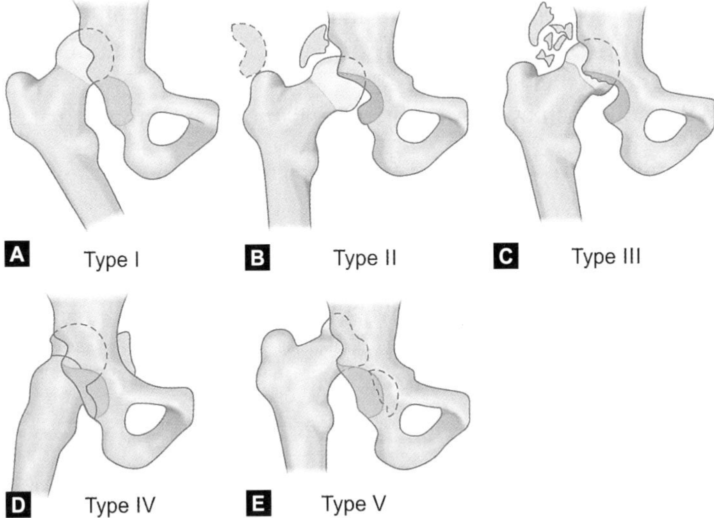

A   Type I   **B**   Type II   **C**   Type III

D   Type IV   **E**   Type V

FIGS. 9A TO E: Thompson and Epstein classification of posterior hip dislocations.

Examination (Focused)

- Anterior hip dislocation—the dislocated limb lies in abduction, external rotation, and in slight flexion.
- *Posterior hip dislocation*: The dislocated limb lies flexed, adducted, and internally rotated such that the knee rests on the unaffected limb. There is shortening of the dislocated limb, prominence of greater trochanter, and buttock.
- Do not forget to examine for distal pulsation, especially in AHD.
- Check peroneal nerve injury by dorsiflexion of the ankle and extension of extensor hallucis longus against resistance (PHD).

X-rays

- X-ray of the pelvis with both the hip joints' AP and lateral view (if the patient cooperates).
- X-ray of Judet view of the pelvis—look for acetabular and rim fractures.

Treatment

Hip dislocations should be reduced in less than 6 hours in order to prevent avascular necrosis.

Reduction of a Posterior Hip Dislocations

Allis Technique

- After adequate procedural sedation, place the patient on the floor from the trolley or bed.
- Ask the assistant to stabilize the pelvis by applying pressure over both the anterior and superior iliac spine and the physician should flex patient's dislocated hip and knee to 90 degree with inline continuous traction as demonstrated in the **Figure 10**.
- The reduction is achieved by slight internal and external rotation at the hip.

Anterior hip dislocation is relatively rare and earlier referral to orthopedic team for reduction is ideal.

Complications

- Osteonecrosis, the incidence of which is directly proportional to the time taken for reduction.
- Post-traumatic osteoarthritis on long term

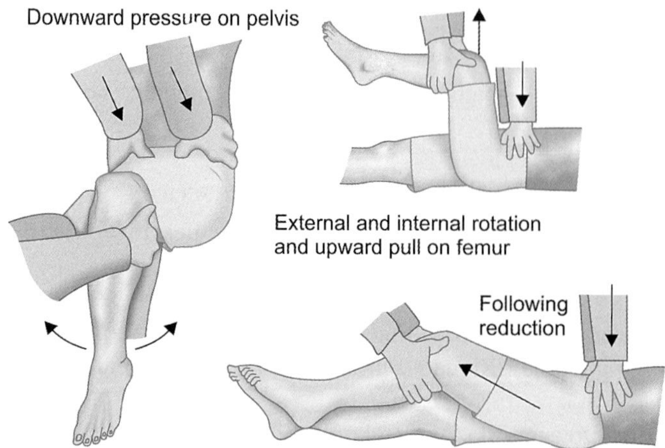

FIG. 10: Allis technique for reduction of posterior dislocation.

- Recurrent dislocation (2%)
- Neurovascular injury.

PATELLAR DISLOCATIONS

Patellar dislocations occur due to twisting injury on an extended knee resulting in severe pain and deformity of the knee. Without exception, patellar dislocations are lateral due to the pull of the stronger lateral ligaments. Habitual or recurrent dislocations can also occur.

Attitude

Knee is semiflexed with a bony prominence seen or felt usually lateral to the knee joint.

Treatment

Under sedation all attempts to reduce the dislocation should be attempted by the technique described (**Fig. 11**).
- Flex the hip, hyperextend the knee and slide the patella medially back into place.
- This maneuver results in immediate relief of pain.

Perform an X-ray to rule out a fracture or an intra-articular loose body. Apply a knee brace for primary dislocations after the relocation procedure to allow healing.

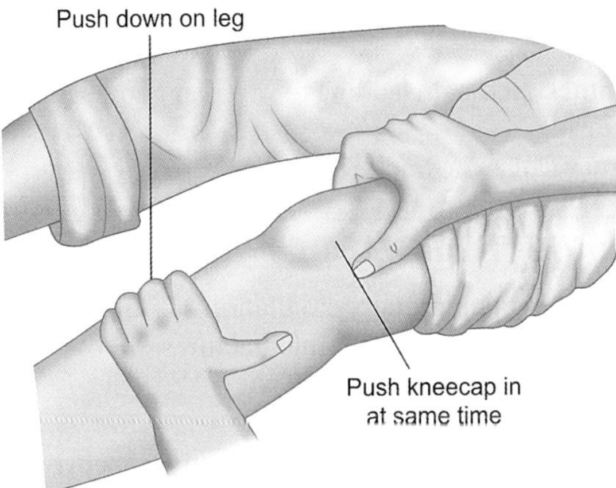

FIG. 11: Reduction of patellar dislocation.

CASTS AND SPLINTS

- *Plaster of Paris (POP)*: POP is cheap and easily available. Disadvantages are susceptibility to damage or disintegration and longer time (<48 h) for large casts to dry fully after the application of cast.
- *Resin casts*: These are costlier, but lighter and stronger than POP. They are also more resistant to water. They set in 5–10 minutes and gain maximum strength after 30 minutes. However, they are more rigid and harder to mold and hence more difficult to apply and remove.

Steps in Applying a POP Slab

- *Prepare the cotton base*: Apply a 6-inch bandage roll to the desired length and apply to a thin layer of nonabsorbable cotton over the bandage.
- *Prepare the POP roll*: Spread the POP roll to the exact length of the limb. Layer the POP roll over itself 9–10 times for the upper limb and 10–11 times for the lower limb.
- *Prepare the slab*: Soak the plaster roll in a pail containing water for 5 seconds. Squeeze gently without twisting or wrinkling to remove excess water and stretch out the roll. Place the POP layer over the cotton base and fold the edges of the base over it.
- *Apply the slab*: Place the slab over the posterior aspect of the limb with the cotton base in contact with the skin and the limb in the desired position. Apply 2–3 layers over the slab and await setting and to hold the slab in position. It sets firmly in position in about 30 minutes.

Complications

- Local irritation
- Excessive tightness and pain leading to vascular compromise
- Pressure necrosis
- A loose slab may cause the fracture to worsen.

FAT EMBOLISM SYNDROME

Presence of fat globules in pulmonary circulation 24–72 hours following an initial insult like long bone fractures and multiple fractures.

Triad of Fat Embolism

- Early pulmonary symptoms (Hypoxemia, dyspnea, tachypnea, and ARDS)
- Neurological symptoms (Minor global dysfunction, seizures, and focal deficits)
- Cutaneous manifestations (Petechial rash on conjunctiva, neck and axilla)

Management

- Early immobilization of fracture reduces incidence of fat embolism syndrome
- Early fixation (External fixation/Open reduction and Internal fixation)
- Administer oxygen if the patient is hypoxic (SpO_2 <94%). There is no role for prophylactic oxygen administration

CHAPTER 113

Wound Management

INTRODUCTION

Instructions to be followed as part of wound management are:

Wound Wash

- All open wounds should be thoroughly washed before and after wound debridement as it clears the debris and hematoma whilst providing optimal exposure, reducing contamination, and bacterial load.
- Wound irrigation should be done before and after wound debridement as it clears the debris, hematoma and provides optimal exposure, reduces contamination and bacterial load. It should be a part of routine wound management.
- Low pressure irrigation can be performed in the emergency department (ED) using a syringe/bulb and is usually adequate to remove material from the surface of most wounds.
- Warm, isotonic, normal saline is typically used for wound irrigation. There is no advantage of adding soap/antiseptics/antibiotics to lavage fluid.
- Use of hydrogen peroxide, alcohol solution, povidone iodine, and other chemical agents may impair osteoblast function, inhibit wound healing and cause cartilage damage and hence *should not be used.*
- Adequate quantity of lavage fluid must be used for cleaning the wound based on the principle *"the solution for pollution is dilution".* Typically, >9 L of fluid is required for Gustillo type IIIb injuries.

Tetanus Prophylaxis

- Diphtheria-tetanus (dT) vaccine and human tetanus immunoglobulin (TIG) should be administered to all patients with open wounds.
- At discharge, advice the patient to complete the full course of tetanus vaccination with 2 more doses of dT given at 4 weekly intervals.

Analgesia

Be generous in administering analgesics like opioids as soon as the patient presents to the ED.

SUTURE MATERIALS

Suture materials are classified as absorbable or nonabsorbable, natural or synthetic, and braided or monofilament.

- *Absorbable suture materials*: Defined by the loss of most of their tensile strength within 60 days after placement. These are best suited for closure of deep structures such as dermis and fascia.
  - *Natural absorbable sutures*: Catgut (made from sheep or cattle intestines)
  - *Synthetic braided sutures*: Polyglycolic acid (Dexon) and polyglactin 910 (Vicryl)
  - *Synthetic monofilament sutures*: Polydioxanone (PDS), polytrimethy lene carbonate (Maxon), poliglecaprone (Monocryl), glycomer 631 (Biosyn), and polyglytone 6211 (Caprosyn).
- *Nonabsorbable suture materials*: Defined by their resistance to degradation by living tissues. These are most often used to close the outermost layers of the skin or for repair of tendons.
  - *Natural absorbable sutures*: Silk, cotton, and linen
  - *Synthetic braided sutures*: Composed of nylon and polyester (infrequently used)
  - *Synthetic monofilament sutures*: Nylon (Ethilon), polypropylene (Prolene), and polybutester (Novafil).
- Monofilament synthetic sutures (nylon or polypropylene) have the lowest rates of infection.
- Braided sutures are usually easier to handle and tie, but can harbor bacteria between strands and cause higher infection rates.

The higher the number of zeros (1-0 to 10-0), the smaller the size and the lower the strength:

- *Hand and finger lacerations*: 5-0 sutures
- *Facial laceration*: 5-0 or 6-0 sutures
- *Scalp lacerations*: 3-0 or 4-0 sutures
- *Other lacerations*: 4-0 sutures

SUTURE NEEDLES

- *Cutting*: Have opposing cutting edges.
- *Conventional cutting*: Have a third cutting edge on the inside concave curvature of the needle.
- *Reverse cutting*: Have a third cutting edge located on the outer convex curvature of the needle. It is used for thick skin like the palm and soles.

Scalp Laceration

INTRODUCTION

Scalp laceration is a common injury presenting to the emergency department (ED).

The scalp consists of five layers, best remembered by the mnemonic SCALP:
- *S*: Skin
- *C*: Subcutaneous tissue
- *A*: Aponeurosis and muscle (contains the middle meningeal artery)
- *L*: Loose areolar tissue and subgaleal fascia
- *P*: Periosteum

  In lacerations, separation usually occurs at the layer of loose areolar tissue. Clinical evaluation should identify associated serious head injury, laceration of the galea, or bony defect of the skull. Removal of all foreign debris and blood will allow for proper assessment.

MANAGEMENT

Hemostasis

Bleeding may be profuse and substantial blood loss can occur with scalp lacerations. Hemostasis should be achieved by applying direct pressure for 5–15 minutes with or without local injection of lidocaine and adrenaline. If this fails, the edges of the laceration should be everted and rapidly closed with simple interrupted sutures.

Wound Debridement and Cleansing

After hemostasis is achieved and the wound should be irrigated using a syringe with 26-G needle, administer local or regional anesthesia prior to initiating irrigation and wound cleansing to improve patient comfort.
- Small and clean wounds can be irrigated with isotonic 0.9% normal saline (NS).
- Larger, more extensive laceration (animal or human bites and contaminated wounds) should be irrigated with a mixture of 10% povidone iodine solution (Betadine® solution) and 0.9% NS.

Wound Closure

It is not necessary to shave or cut scalp hair prior to wound closure; shaving increases the likelihood of a wound infection.
- Small scalp lacerations may be closed with 3-0 or 4-0 nonabsorbable or absorbable (Vicryl) simple, interrupted sutures.

- Deep scalp lacerations may also benefit from the placement of a pressure dressing for the first 24 hours to prevent hematoma formation.
- Scalp wounds should be left open to air unless they require a pressure dressing to prevent hematoma formation.
- After 24–48 hours, wounds closed with staples or nonabsorbable sutures can be cleansed gently with soap and water.
- Staples or nonabsorbable sutures should be removed after 7–14 days.
- Administer tetanus-diphtheria (Td) vaccine for open injuries, if not adequately vaccinated. At discharge, advice the patient to complete the vaccination schedule (2 more doses 4 weeks apart).

Compartment Syndrome

DEFINITION

In general, compartment syndrome is a condition in which the circulation within a closed compartment of one of the extremities is compromised by an increase in pressure within the compartment, causing necrosis of muscles and nerves and eventually of the skin because of excessive swelling.

Any injury or insult that causes a decrease in compartment size or increase in compartment pressure can initiate compartment syndrome. Compartment syndrome may be acute or chronic.

CAUSES OF COMPARTMENT SYNDROME

- *Acute*:
  - Closed fractures
  - Crush or compression injuries
  - Burns
  - Tight or constricting casts
  - Intra-arterial injections
  - Infections
  - Snakebites
- *Chronic*:
  - Excessive exercise
  - Anomalous insertions of the foot muscles

CLINICAL FEATURES

Severe pain (out of proportion to findings) on passive extension is the most important sign. In addition, look for paresis, pallor, tense swelling, and pulselessness (late sign).

COMMON SITES

The common sites are forearm and leg; and the less common sites are foot, hand, thigh, and abdomen.

DIAGNOSIS

- It is essentially based on clinical judgment of signs and symptoms.
- Bedside invasive measurement of compartment pressures (>30 mm Hg of the diastolic pressure of the patient) is an adjunct. This in invasive and not performed in the ED. Unilateral swelling with severe pain and/or pulselessness should alert the physician of the possibility of compartment syndrome.
- In unconscious patients, it may be useful to assess with serial girth measurements of the limb.
- Bedside doppler and/or USG can also be done to look for subcutaneous edema and/or reduced pulsatility of arteries.

Other investigations include routine blood tests, serum creatine phosphokinase (CPK), and X-ray of affected limb.

MANAGEMENT

Refer to the treating department immediately without any delay:
- *Medical*: Keep limb slightly elevated up to heart level:
  - Administer adequate analgesia (Morphine/Tramadol)
  - Remove any constricting padding
  - Serial measurements of limb circumference
  - *Start mannitol*: 100 mL intravenous stat and q8h till improvement in limb swelling.
- *Surgical*: The definitive treatment of compartment syndrome is urgent fasciotomy, preferably done within 12 hours of onset of symptoms. Make a surgical incision along the length of the compartment to relieve the pressure and leave the wound open. After a few days, once the edema resolves, the patient may be take to the operating room for wound closure.

INTRODUCTION

Trauma is a leading cause of non-obstetric morbidity and mortality in pregnant women where two lives are at stake instead of one. Pregnancy causes major anatomical and physiological changes in almost every system of the body. The initial treatment and stabilization are the same as for non-pregnant patients. The best initial resuscitation of the fetus is the optimal resuscitation to the mother.

ANATOMICAL CONSIDERATIONS FOR NORMAL PREGNANCY

- The major anatomical considerations are due to the enlarged gravid uterus. The enlarging uterus reaches the umbilicus by 20 weeks and the costal margin by 34–36 weeks. As the bowel gets pushed cephalad, the risk of intestinal injuries decreases. But complex intestinal injuries can occur, in the case of penetrating upper abdominal trauma. The gravid uterus can also cause compression of major vessels, thereby decreasing cardiac return.
- The placenta, which is not as flexible as the uterine myometrium, is highly susceptible to abruption when shearing forces are involved. Pelvic injuries and fractures can cause direct fetal injuries in late gestation.

PHYSIOLOGICAL CONSIDERATIONS FOR NORMAL PREGNANCY

- *Cardiovascular changes:*
  - Blood volumes increase in pregnancy till the 34th week with a smaller increase in RBC volume, resulting in physiological anemia of pregnancy.
  - Due to increased intravascular volume, healthy pregnant patients can lose up to 1.5 L of blood volume before developing tachycardia or hypotension, resulting in delayed recognition of shock. However, due to decreased perfusion of the placenta, the fetus may show signs of distress early.
  - Hypotension can be precipitated by the compression of the inferior vena cava (IVC) by the gravid uterus, whereas hypertension may represent preeclampsia.
  - When supine, compression of the vena cava by the gravid uterus results in decreased venous return to the heart, and can decrease the cardiac output by up to 30%.

- ○ Heart rate increases by 10–15/min in pregnancy. Consider this factor while assessing a tachycardic response to hypovolemia.
- *Pulmonary changes*:
  - ○ Due to increase in tidal volume, minute ventilation increases in pregnancy, hence hypocapnia is relatively common in late pregnancy. Therefore, a $PaCO_2$ of 35–40 mm Hg may indicate impending respiratory failure.
  - ○ Due to elevation of the diaphragm, chest tubes must be placed in the midaxillary line, but 2 cm higher than usual, to avoid damage to the liver or spleen.
- *Other systems*:
  - ○ Due to delayed gastric emptying during pregnancy, early gastric decompression by a nasogastric tube is recommended to prevent aspiration.
  - ○ By the 7th month, the symphysis pubis widens to 4–8 mm and the sacroiliac joint spaces widen. Consider these factors while interpreting X-rays of the pelvis.
  - ○ Blunt trauma to the abdomen may result in massive retroperitoneal hemorrhage due to the large, engorged pelvic vessels surrounding the uterus.

RESUSCITATION AND MANAGEMENT

- Standard trauma algorithm (primary survey and secondary survey) must be followed for evaluation of a pregnant patient with trauma. Obstetric team should be called along with the trauma team.
- Secure the airway early to prevent aspiration, provide adequate ventilation and effective circulation to the mother.
- In an unconscious patient, gently palpate the abdomen and measure fundal height to estimate the gestational age.
- Displace the uterus manually to the left side to relieve compression on the IVC.
- IV access should be above the diaphragm, avoiding femoral lines. At least 2 wide bore IV lines should be placed. Initiate crystalloid fluid resuscitation and early type specific blood administration. Vasopressors should be the last resort as they reduce uterine blood flow and cause fetal hypoxia.
- Fibrinogen and other clotting factors level are higher than normal in pregnancy. A normal level in cases of trauma could be suggestive of early disseminated intravascular coagulation (DIC).
- Perineal examination and per vaginal examination by an obstetrician are indicated in all cases of trauma to rule out abruption or early onset of labor.
- The main causes of fetal death are maternal shock, maternal death, abruption, and uterine rupture. Identify if present and address these immediately
  - ○ *Abruptio placenta*: This should be suspected even in minor trauma especially in late pregnancy. Presence of vaginal bleeding, uterine tenderness, uterine contractions or uterine tetany suggests an abruption.

- ○ *Uterine rupture*: Abdominal tenderness, guarding, rebound tenderness may suggest a uterine rupture if associated with shock. Other signs of rupture include inability to palpate the fundus (due to fundal rupture), easy palpation of fetal parts (due to extrauterine location).
- Monitor the fetal heart continuously by tocodynamometer. The normal range for fetal heart rate is 120–160 beats/min. The following are signs of impending fetal distress and warrants urgent obstetric consultation
  - ○ Abnormal fetal heart rate
  - ○ Repetitive decelerations
  - ○ Absence of beat-to-beat variability or accelerations
  - ○ Frequent uterine activity
- Fetomaternal hemorrhage results in isoimmunization if the mother is Rh negative. Administer Rh immunoglobulin (300 microgram) to all pregnant Rh negative trauma patients with suspected abdominal trauma (within 72 h of injury).
- If a pregnant mother has a cardiac arrest, perimortem cesarean section can be a lifesaving intervention for both mother and fetus. In case of maternal death, perform perimortem caesarian section within 5 minutes of the arrest.

CHAPTER 117

Pediatric Trauma

INTRODUCTION

Evaluation and management of injuries in children have the same principles as for adults. Due to unique anatomical and physiological characteristics, children sustain a distinct pattern of trauma.

- Smaller body mass, lesser fat, lesser subcutaneous tissue, and close proximity of vital organs often result in multiple injuries.
- Due to a proportionately larger head in smaller children, head injuries are more common. Blunt injuries to the head often result in apnea, hypoventilation and hypoxia with hypovolemia and hypotension being much less common. Hence, the need for more aggressive management of airway and breathing.

AIRWAY MANAGEMENT

- If the airway is partially obstructed, use jaw-thrust maneuver with bimanual inline stabilization of the spine to open the airway. Clear the mouth and oropharynx of secretions or debris and administer supplemental oxygen.
- *Oral airway:* If the child is unconscious, insert an oral airway directly into the oropharynx. Do not perform the maneuver of inserting the airway backward and rotating 180 degrees as in adults, as this could result in trauma to the soft tissue structures of the oropharynx in children.
- *Preoxygenation:* Before attempting to mechanically establish an airway, all children must be adequately preoxygenated.
- *Infants:* Infants (<1 year) have a profound vagal response to laryngeal stimulation during endotracheal intubation, resulting in bradycardia. Consider pretreatment with atropine (0.01–0.03 mg/kg) for infants 1–2 minutes before intubation. Atropine also dries oral secretions, enabling visualization of landmarks for intubation
- *Endotracheal (ET) tube:* A simple way to determine the size of the ET tube is to approximate the diameter of the tube to the child's nares or the tip of the small finger. A cuffed ET tube can be used even in infants as the currently available ET tubes are safe and do not cause tracheal necrosis. However, check the cuff pressure after intubation and <30 mm Hg is considered safe.
- *Intubation:* Orotracheal intubation with manual in line stabilization of the spine is the preferred method of securing the airway. Do not perform a nasotracheal intubation due to the relatively acute angle in the nasopharynx in children, making the procedure very difficult. Position the ET tube 3–4 cm

below the level of the vocal cords. For correct ET tube placement, it should be fixed at the gums/teeth at the number 3 times the size of the ET tube.

Breathing and Ventilation

- Use a pediatric bag mask for children <30 kg as an adult bag mask can cause significant barotrauma in children.
- Hypoxia due to hypoventilation is the most common cause of cardiac arrest in children and hence must be addressed by providing optimum oxygenation and ventilation.
- Tension pneumothorax must be decompressed at the 2nd intercostal space in the midclavicular line as in adults.
- Chest tubes, when required are proportionately smaller and should be inserted in the 4th to 5th intercostal space, just anterior to the midaxillary line as in adults.

Circulation

- *Normal parameters in children:* The mean normal systolic blood pressure (SBP) in children is 90 mm Hg plus twice the age in years. The lower limit of normal SBP is 70 mm Hg plus twice the age in years. The diastolic blood pressure (DBP) should be two-thirds the SBP. A child's blood volume is 70 mL/kg while an infant's blood volume is 80 mL/kg.
- Children have increased physiological reserve and hence can maintain BP even in the presence of shock. Hypotension manifests only after a 30% decrease in circulating blood volume. Tachycardia and decrease skin perfusion may be the only early markers of hypovolemia in children, and must be recognized to initiate appropriate fluid resuscitation.
- Other subtle signs of blood loss in children include weakening of the pulse, narrow pulse pressure (<20 mm Hg), cold extremities, decreased sensorium, and dulled response to pain.
- If two attempts at peripheral percutaneous venous access fail, obtain an intraosseous line at the anteromedial tibia or distal femur (refer Chapter 149).
- *Fluid resuscitation:* Crystalloid administration is based on the weight of the child. Administer three boluses of 20 mL/kg (total of 60 mL/kg) to replace the estimated 25% blood loss. Consider the use of packed red blood cells (pRBC) while administering the third fluid bolus. Administer pRBC at boluses of 10 mL/kg and consider additional products like plasma and platelets.
- *Response to fluid resuscitation:* The following are indicators of adequate fluid response.
  ○ Slowing of heart rate (age dependent)
  ○ Improving sensorium
  ○ Increased strength of the pulse
  ○ Increased warmth of extremities
  ○ Return of normal skin color

- ○ Increased blood pressure and pulse pressure
- ○ Improving urinary output
- *Urine output:* If the child requires substantial fluid resuscitation, insert a urinary catheter to accurately measure urine output. The target urine output for infants (<1 year) is 2 mL/kg/h, for younger children is 1.5 mL/kg/h and for older children is 1 mL/kg/h.
- *Hypothermia:* Significant blood loss results in hypothermia which in turn worsens trauma associated coagulopathy and makes resuscitation ineffective. Initiate warming measures like thermal blankets, warming the intravenous fluids, and room heaters.

DISABILITY AND EXPOSURE

Chest Trauma

In children, mobility of the mediastinal structures often results in tension pneumothorax, which is the most common immediately life-threatening injury.

Abdominal Trauma

- Most children swallow large amounts of air due to the stress and pain of trauma. If the upper abdomen is distended, insert a nasogastric tube to decompress the stomach.
- Avoid deep, painful forceful palpation of the abdomen that may induce voluntary guarding from the child, hence confusing the findings.
- Isolated intraparenchymal bleed which account for one third of solid organ injuries in children can not be identified by an E FAST. Hence, bedside ultrasonography alone cannot be relied upon as the sole diagnostic test for intra-abdominal injuries in children.

Head Trauma

- Hypotension from hypovolemia and hypoxia can have a devastating combination on an injured child's brain and hence must be addressed as priority.
- Vomiting and amnesia are common in children, post-head trauma and do not necessarily indicate raised intra cranial pressure (ICP). However, persistent or more frequent vomiting is an alarming sign and warrants a CT imaging of the head.
- Infants with open fontanelles and uncalcified cranial sutures have more tolerance for a large intracranial hematoma and may not show signs of raised ICP early on. They may present with a bulging fontanelle or suture diastases, which must be treated as signs of raised ICP due to an intracranial bleed.

- The following drugs can be used to decrease cerebral edema and ICP: Hypertonic saline 3% (3–5 mL/kg) or Mannitol (0.5–1 g/kg). However, diuresis with mannitol may worsen hypovolemia and hence should not be given in the early stages of resuscitation of head trauma.

Spinal Cord Injury

- Pseudosubluxation (anterior displacement of C2 on C3) may be seen on a lateral X-ray in 20–40% of children. This radiographic abnormality can be corrected by placing the child's head in a neutral position (place a 2.5 cm thick padding under the body from shoulders to the hips, but not the head). True subluxation will persist on the X-ray with this maneuver.
- Spinal cord injury without radiographic abnormalities (SCIWORA) is more commonly seen in children than in adults. Therefore, if history and neurological examination suggest spinal cord injury, and if X-ray imaging of the spine is normal, continue spinal immobilization till further imaging with CT/MRI can be done and obtain neurosurgical consultation.

Musculoskeletal Trauma

- In children, crush injuries to the physis (growth plates) have the worst prognosis with significant long-term disability.
- Long bone and pelvic fractures result in proportionately less blood loss in children than in adults.
- *Green stick fractures*: Fractures of long bones often result in incomplete fracture with angulated bones, due to immature, pliable nature of bones in children.
- Simple splinting of fractured extremities in children usually is sufficient until definitive orthopedic evaluation can be performed.

Geriatric Trauma

INTRODUCTION

The geriatric age group (>65 years) is vulnerable to trauma and has a higher mortality rate due to physical impairment, degenerative diseases, cognitive decline, and the presence of comorbidities. Hence, the above factors must be considered during assessment and management of geriatric trauma.

Remember that minimal trauma may result in fractures and significant disability. The common locations of fractures among the elderly are the ribs, hip, proximal femur, wrist, and the humerus.

The following are important points to note during early management of geriatric trauma.

AIRWAY

- Factors that affect management of the airway in the elderly include dentition, nasopharyngeal fragility, microstomia, macroglossia, and cervical spine arthritis.
  - Remove any broken dentures. If the dentures are intact and well-fitted, it is best to leave them in place till airway is secured.
  - Be careful while placing a NG tube as nasopharyngeal friability, especially around the turbinate, may result in profuse bleeding.
  - Arthritis of the temporomandibular joints and the cervical spine may make endotracheal intubation difficult and even dangerous with a risk of spinal injury during manipulation of the arthritic spine.

BREATHING AND VENTILATION

- Ageing and chronic inhalation of pollutants and smoking results in decreased compliance of the lungs and chest wall and increased work of breathing. This alteration places elderly trauma patients at high risk for respiratory failure.
- Chest wall injuries, rib fractures, and even simple pneumothorax are not well-tolerated by the elderly and need close monitoring.
- Aging causes a suppressed heart rate response to hypoxia; respiratory failure may present insidiously in older adults.
- Adequate pain control with analgesics and opioids is crucial for pain relief, but must be balanced with the increased risk of respiratory depression.

CIRCULATION

- Ageing heart and coronary artery stenosis results in progressive loss of function. The maximum tachycardia response decreases with age. The maximal heart rate can be calculated by the formula: 220 minus current age.
- With aging, total blood volume decreases and circulation time increases. In a hypertensive elderly, a systolic blood pressure (SBP) of about 110–120 mm Hg post-trauma may actually represent hypotension.
- Early stages of shock may be masked by the absence of tachycardia and hypotension. Hence, in the elderly, "normal BP" and "normal heart rate" DO NOT necessarily indicate normovolemia.
- Elderly on chronic medications like diuretics may be volume contracted and more prone for serious electrolyte imbalances and to volume overload during resuscitation.
- As the kidneys lose mass after the age of 50 years, creatinine clearance decreases in the elderly, and the aged kidney is more susceptible to damage from hypovolemia, nephrotoxins, and medications.
- Consider the early use of advanced monitoring [e.g., central venous pressure (CVP), echocardiography and ultrasonography] to guide optimal resuscitation, given the risks of preexisting cardiovascular disease.

DISABILITY

- In the elderly, brain mass shrinks causing the dura to become more adherent to the skull, thereby increasing the risk of subdural and intraparenchymal hematomas with injury. Hence, liberal use of imaging of the brain is advised in the elderly.
- Take a detailed history of antiplatelet and anticoagulant use as these increases the risk and severity of intracranial hemorrhage.
- Age related changes that predispose the elderly to injuries include reduced cerebral blood flow due to atherosclerosis, auditory and visual decline, demyelination, memory loss, and other preexisting medical conditions.
- In the spine, age related degeneration of the intervertebral discs, osteoporosis and osteoarthritis increases the likelihood of injuries.

EXPOSURE AND ENVIRONMENT

- Age related decrease in skin integrity, results in decreased thermal regulation, decreased barrier function, and impaired wound healing.
- Hypothermia significantly worsens outcome and care must be taken to prevent this complication.

INTRODUCTION

Prompt and focused imaging of trauma victims must be planned in the ED based on a thorough clinical examination through primary and secondary surveys. The standard trauma series is composed of X-rays of the chest, pelvis, and cervical spine. Following is a comprehensive list of X-rays required to assess the extent of injury in trauma victims.

TABLE 1: X-rays in trauma.

Region	X-rays	Comments
Clavicle and rib	Chest AP	In case of suspected clavicular fracture, include the acromioclavicular and sternoclavicular joints
Cervical spine	Lateral	• Look for alignment—integrity of the anterior and posterior spinal lines, the spinolaminar line and the spinous process line • Look for cortical breaks in the outline of cervical vertebrae
	Swimmers view	If C7-T1 intervertebral disk space is not visualized on lateral view
	AP	If one of the spinous processes is misaligned, a facet dislocation may be seen
	Open-mouth odontoid view	If predentate space is >3 mm in adults and 5 mm in children on lateral X-ray
Shoulder	AP and lateral (Y-view)	In case of shoulder dislocation
Elbow	AP and lateral	Supracondylar fracture, radial head fracture or elbow dislocation
Wrist	AP and lateral	Include forearm if fracture of radius or ulna is suspected
	Scaphoid series	In case of suspected scaphoid bone fracture (oblique and PA with ulnar deviation)
Hand	AP and oblique	For entire hand
	Lateral	Isolated finger injury in addition to AP view

Continued

Continued

Region	X-rays	Comments
Pelvis with hip	AP with both hip joints	Neck of femur fracture or intertrochanteric fracture
	Lateral hip joint view	
Femur	AP and lateral	Proximal and distal joints to be included
Knee	AP and lateral	Include distal femur and proximal tibia
	Skyline	For suspected patellar dislocation or fracture
Ankle	AP and true lateral	For suspected ankle fracture
	Mortise view	To visualize the lateral malleolar joint space
Foot	AP	To visualize 1st and 2nd metatarsal, medial, and intermediate cuneiforms, tarsometatarsal joint and metatarsophalangeal joints
	Oblique	To visualize 3rd, 4th, and 5th metatarsals, lateral cuneiform, navicular, cuboid, phalanges, and interphalangeal joints

(AP: anteroposterior; PA: posteroanterior)

The following are the common eponyms of fractures/dislocations in trauma (**Table 1**).

TABLE 1: Eponyms in trauma.

Eponym	Description	Bones/Joints involved	Comment
ARM			
Bankart fracture	Avulsion fracture of the anteroinferior glenoid rim	Scapula (glenoid rim)	Associated with recurrent anterior shoulder dislocation
Hill–Sachs fracture	Compression fracture of posterolateral humeral head	Humeral head	Associated with recurrent anterior shoulder dislocation when glenoid rim hits the posterior part of humeral head
Holstein–Lewis fracture	Spiral fracture of the distal third of shaft of humerus	Shaft of humerus	Radial nerve entrapment
FOREARM			
Barton fracture	Fracture-dislocation of radiocarpal joint involving the volar or dorsal lip (volar/reverse Barton or dorsal Barton fracture)	Radiocarpal joint	Distal radius intra articular fracture. Fall on outstretched hand
Hume fracture	Fracture of the olecranon with an associated anterior dislocation of radial head	Elbow joint	Usually seen in children. Hyperextension of elbow with pronation of forearm
Colles fracture/ Pouteau fracture	Fracture of the distal radial metaphyseal region with dorsal angulation and impaction	Distal radius	Extra articular distal radius fracture. Fall on outstretched hand
Smith fracture	Fracture of the distal radial metaphyseal region with volar angulation	Distal radius	Extra articular distal radius fracture. Fall on flexed wrist

Continued

Continued

Eponym	Description	Bones/Joints involved	Comment
Essex-Lopresti fracture-dislocation	Fracture of the radial head, dislocation of the distal radioulnar joint (DRUJ) and rupture of the antebrachial interosseous membrane	Radial head, DRUJ	Longitudinal force on the outstretched hand with the elbow in extension
Galeazzi fracture-dislocation/ Piedmont fracture	Distal third radial shaft fracture with associated DRUJ injury	Distal Radius, DRUJ	Surgical fixation
Monteggia fracture	Proximal third ulna fracture with dislocation of radial head	Proximal ulna and radial head	Common in children. Posterior interosseous nerve (PIN) neuropathy
Chauffeur fracture/ Hutchinson fracture/backfire fracture	Intra-articular fracture of the radial styloid process	Radial styloid	Forced ulnar deviation of the wrist causing avulsion of the radial styloid
Nightstick fracture	Isolated fracture of the ulnar shaft, typically transverse and located in the mid-diaphysis	Ulna	Direct blow to the medial forearm
Golfer's elbow	Medial epicondylitis	Medial epicondyle of humerus	An overuse syndrome of the flexor-pronator mass origin
Tennis elbow	Lateral epicondylitis	Lateral epicondyle of humerus	Overuse injury involving at the origin of common extensor tendon
HAND			
Bennett fracture	An intra-articular, simple, oblique fracture at the base of the first metacarpal. Usually, a 2-part fracture	Base of first metacarpal bone	Axial force applied to the thumb in flexion
Rolando fracture	Three-part or comminuted intra-articular fracture-dislocation of the base of the 1st MCP	Base of first metacarpal bone	Axial force applied to the thumb in flexion

Continued

Continued

Eponym	Description	Bones/Joints involved	Comment
Boxer's fracture	Minimally comminuted, transverse fractures of the 5th metacarpal neck	Neck of fifth metacarpal bone	Direct trauma to a clenched fist
Gamekeeper's thumb/Skier's thumb/Break-dancer's thumb	Avulsion or rupture of the ulnar collateral ligament (UCL) of the first MCP joint	First MCP	Valgus force on the abducted MCP joint, leading to a ruptured UCL
Mallet finger/Baseball finger	Finger deformity caused by disruption of the terminal extensor tendon distal to DIP joint	Extensor tendon injury of DIP joint	Traumatic impaction blow (sudden forced flexion) to the tip of the finger in the extended position. Lack of active DIP extension
Jersey finger/Rugby finger	Avulsion injury of flexor digitorum profundus (FDP) from insertion at base of distal phalanx	Flexor tendon injury of DIP joint	Hyperextension of finger at DIP joint while proximal portion of finger is flexed. Inability to flex at DIP joint
PELVIS			
Duverney fracture	Isolated iliac wing fracture. Stable injury	Ilium	Direct blow to the ilium
Malgaigne's fracture	Unstable pelvic ring fracture. Vertical shear injury causing vertical orientation of pubic rami fracture, disruption of SI joints, vertical displacement of hemipelvis	Pelvic bone	Due to high energy impact to pelvis (front to back)
KNEE			
Stieda fracture	Bony avulsion injury of the medial collateral ligament (MCL) at the medial femoral condyle	MCL	Valgus knee loading and forceful shifts of direction (e.g., skiing, football, ice hockey)
Segond fracture	Lateral tibial plateau avulsion fracture with ACL tear	ACL	Due to internal rotation and varus stress of the knee

Continued

Continued

Eponym	Description	Bones/Joints involved	Comment
LEG			
Gosselin fracture	V-shaped fracture of distal tibia with extension into the tibial plafond dividing it into anterior and posterior segments	Tibia	Axial loading of weight bearing surface of tibia
Pilon fracture	Articular fracture of distal tibia involving the tibial plafond	Tibia	Axial loading of weight bearing surface of tibia
Toddler's fracture	Undisplaced spiral fracture of distal tibia in children	Tibia	Common in children in early years of walking (9 months to 3 years)
Bumper fracture	Compression fracture of lateral tibial plateau	Tibia	Forced valgus of knee when struck from side by car bumper
Runner's fracture	Stress fracture of distal fibula 3–8 cm above the lateral malleolus	Fibula	Due to repeated axial stress on fibula
ANKLE			
Bosworth fracture	Bimalleolar fracture dislocation of the ankle with entrapment of fibula behind the posterior tubercle of distal tibia	Ankle joint	Extreme external rotation
Chopart fracture-dislocation	Fracture dislocation of mid-tarsal joints (Talonavicular and Calcaneocuboid joints)	Midtarsal joint	Fall from height/MVA/ twisting injuries
Cotton fracture	Fracture of the ankle involving both malleoli and posterior process of the tibia	Ankle joint	Trimalleolar ankle fracture
Dupuytren fracture	Fracture of the distal portion of the fibula above the lateral malleolus, with rupture of distal tibiofibular and deltoid ligaments	Ankle joint	Type of bimalleolar ankle fracture causing ankle instability

Continued

Continued

Eponym	Description	Bones/Joints involved	Comment
Lisfranc fracture-dislocations	Dislocation of the articulation of the tarsus with the metatarsal bases	TMT joint	Direct crush injury or indirect load onto a plantar flexed foot
Maisonneuve fracture	Spiral fracture of the proximal third of fibula with distal tibiofibular syndesmotic disruption	Fibula	Pronation-external rotation injury
Pott's fracture	Fracture affecting one or both of the malleoli	Tibia/fibula	Twisting injury while walking/running
Shepherd fracture	Fracture of the lateral tubercle of the posterior process of the talus	Posterior process of Talus	Inversion or extreme equinus
Stieda process fracture	Fracture of elongated lateral tubercle of the posterior process of the talus	Posterior process of Talus	Inversion or extreme equinus
Cedell fracture	Fracture of the medial tubercle of the posterior process of the talus	Posterior process of Talus	Forced dorsiflexion and pronation
Tillaux fracture	Fracture through the anterolateral aspect of the distal tibial epiphysis	Tibia	Abduction-external rotation force on foot causes ATFL to avulse the anterolateral corner of distal tibial epiphysis
Aviator fracture	Coronal fracture of the neck of the talus	Talus	Forced dorsiflexion of the ankle. Proximal avascular necrosis is a potential complication of neck fractures
Paratrooper's fracture	Fracture of posterior malleolus or posterior lip of distal tibia	Distal tibia	Injuries sustained due to improper landing techniques from height
FOOT			
Jones fracture	Extra-articular fracture at the base of the fifth metatarsal	5th metatarsal	Significant adduction force to the foot with heel raised and foot in plantar flexion

Continued

Continued

Eponym	Description	Bones/Joints involved	Comment
Pseudo jones fracture	Tuberosity avulsion fractures	5th metatarsal	Inversion and plantar flexion of foot
Dancer's fracture	Long spiral fracture extending into the distal metaphyseal area	5th Metatarsal	Dancer rolling over their foot/while landing a jump
March fracture	Metatarsal fracture caused by repetitive stress	Most commonly 2nd, 3rd metatarsals	Repetitive stress/fatigue
Nutcracker fracture	Cuboid impaction fracture, associated with navicular avulsion fracture	Cuboid	Forced plantar flexion and abduction, crushing the cuboid between calcaneus and 4th, 5th metatarsals
SPINE			
Jefferson fracture	Burst fracture of the ring of C1 with lateral displacement of both articular masses	C1 vertebrae	Axial compression injury
Hangman's fracture	Traumatic anterior spondylolisthesis of the axis (C2) due to bilateral fracture of pars interarticularis	C2 vertebrae	Hyperextension injury
Clay-shoveler fracture	Avulsion-type spinous process fracture in the lower cervical or upper thoracic spine	Most commonly C7, but can affect C6 to T3	Direct trauma to posterior spinous process or sudden muscular/ligamentous pull in flexion or extension
Chance/seatbelt fracture	Flexion-distraction type injuries of the spine that extend to involve all three spinal columns	Most commonly lower thoracic and upper lumbar spine	Flexion distraction injury. Associated with intra-abdominal injuries. Unstable fracture: All 3 columns involved

Continued

Continued

Eponym	Description	Bones/Joints involved	Comment
Holdsworth fracture	Unstable fracture dislocation of the thoraco-lumbar junction of the spine	Thoraco-lumbar junction	Flexion-rotation injury
FACE			
Le Fort fractures	Fractures of the midface. Separation of all or a portion of the midface from the skull base	Mid face	Divided into Le Fort I, II and III

Pediatric Emergencies

- *M*: Medications (regular medications for comorbid conditions)
- *P*: Past medical history (comorbidities, previous surgery)
- *L*: Last meal (time of last meal for administration of anesthesia if needed)
- *E*: Events preceding the injury/illness.

Focused Physical Examination

Infants and toddlers are always most comfortable and cooperative when examined in the parent's lap.

TERTIARY ASSESSMENT

Tertiary assessment is mainly done by "doing diagnostic tests" to identify the problems. The following diagnostic tests can be done in pediatric emergency.

- Random blood sugar
- Urine analysis
- Hemoglobin, complete blood count (CBC)
- Chest X-ray (CXR), ultrasonography (USG)
- ECG, ECHO
- Arterial/Venous blood gas.

The formulas for estimating the weight for age is shown in the **Table 4**. The emergency department should have an adequate supply of the resuscitative equipment as shown in the **Table 5**.

TABLE 4: Formula for estimating weight for age for normal children.	
Age	*Weight (kg)*
3–12 months	$\dfrac{\text{Age in months} + 9}{2}$
1–6 years	(Age in years × 2) + 8
7–12 years	$\dfrac{(\text{Age in years} \times 7) + 5}{2}$

TABLE 5: Pediatric resuscitative equipment.

Equipment	Newborn/Small infant (3–5 kg)	Infant (6–9 kg)	Toddler (10–11 kg)	Small Child (12–14 kg)	Child (15–18 kg)	Child (19–22 kg)	Large Child (24–30 kg)	Adult (≥32 kg)
Resuscitation bag	Infant	Child	Child	Child	Child	Child	Child/adult	Adult
O$_2$ mask	Newborn	Newborn	Pediatric	Pediatric	Pediatric	Pediatric	Adult	Adult
Oral airway	Infant/Small child	Infant/Small child	Small child	Child	Child	Child/Small adult	Child/Small adult	Medium adult
Laryngoscope blade (size)	0–1 straight	1 straight	1 straight	2 straight	2 straight or curved	2 straight or curved	2–3 straight or curved	3 straight or curved
Tracheal tube (mm)	Premature infant 2.5 term infant 3.0–3.5 uncuffed	3.5 uncuffed	4.0 uncuffed	4.5 uncuffed	5.0 uncuffed	5.5 uncuffed	6.0 cuffed	6.5 cuffed
Tracheal tube length (cm at tip)	10–10.5	10–10.5	11–12	12.5–13.5	14–15	15.5–16.5	17–18	18.5–19.5
Stylet (F)	6	6	6	6	6	14	14	14
Suction Catheter (F)	6–8	8	8–10	10	10	10	10	12
BP Cuff	Newborn/Infant	Newborn/Infant	Infant/Child	Child	Child	Child	Child/Adult	Adult
IV catheter (G)	22–24	22–24	20–24	18–22	18–22	18–20	18–20	16–20
Butterfly (G)	23–25	23–25	23–25	21–23	21–23	21–23	21–22	18–21
Nasogastric tube (F)	5–8	5–8	8–10	10	10–12	12–14	14–18	18
Urinary catheter (F)	5–8	5–8	8–10	10	10–12	10–12	12	12
Defibrillation/ Cardioversion external paddles	Infant paddles	Infant paddles until 1 year or 10 kg	Adult paddles when ≥1 year or ≥10 kg	Adult paddles	Adult paddles	Adult paddles	Adult paddles	Adult paddles
Chest tube (F)	10–12	10–12	16–20	20–24	20–24	24–32	28–32	32–40

Source: Adapted from the Broselow pediatric resuscitation tape.

KEY POINTS

- Begin your initial assessment by CBC then continue with the ABCDEs
- Begin management based on the CBC and ABCDs
- Focused history using SAMPLE
- Once child is stabilized, do a detailed physical examination
- Perform ongoing assessment throughout the stay
- For etiology, plan the required laboratory tests and imaging.

INTRODUCTION

Febrile seizures usually occur between 6 months and 6 years of age with a peak incidence between 12 and 18 months. It is usually a single episode of seizure, which is associated with fever. An active central nervous system (CNS) infection or a developmental delay should be ruled out before making this diagnosis. Febrile seizures occur on the 1st day of illness in most children. In some cases, a febrile seizure may be the first manifestation of the illness.

- Risk factors for febrile seizures
  - A positive family history of febrile seizures
  - High fever
  - Electrolyte abnormalities (hyponatremia and hypernatremia)
  - Recent immunization [measles, mumps and rubella (MMR), diphtheria, pertussis (whooping cough), and tetanus (DPT), and tetanus toxoid (TT)]
- *Simple febrile seizures*: This is the most common type. Characterized by one episode of generalized tonic-clonic seizures (GTCS) lasting <15 minutes without recurrence.
- *Complex febrile seizures*: Seizures may be of focal type, may recur and last longer (>15 min).

Investigations: Complete blood count (CBC) profile, electrolytes, random blood sugar (RBS), calcium, urinalysis, lumbar puncture, CT/MRI brain.

MANAGEMENT

- Assess airway, breathing and circulation. Maintain and protect the airway, including the use of a nasopharyngeal airway, if needed. Protect the patient from self injury during this time
- Hypoglycemia and hypocalcemia are common metabolic causes of seizures, especially in infants. Check RBS and Calcium and correct, if indicated.
- Administer an antiepileptic either through the buccal, rectal intramuscular or intravenous route route (**Table 1**).
- *Prophylaxis*: For simple febrile seizures, clobazam prophylaxis 1 mg/kg PO divided in two doses × 2 days may be given with the next episode of fever.

TABLE 1: Antiepileptics, route and dose for febrile seizures.

Antiepileptic	Route	Dose
Midazolam	Buccal	0.2 mg/kg (max: 10 mg)
	Intranasal	0.2 mg/kg (max: 5 mg/nare)
	Intramuscular	0.1–0.2 mg/kg (max: 10 mg)
	Intravenous	0.15 mg/kg (max: 10 mg)
Lorazepam	Buccal	0.1 mg/kg (max: 4 mg)
	Rectal	0.1 mg/kg (max: 4 mg)
Diazepam	Rectal	0.5 mg/kg (max: 20 mg)

Complications

- The postictal phase can be associated with confusion or agitation and drowsiness. Prolonged drowsiness is unusual.
- Transient hemiparesis (Todd's paresis), usually of complex or focal type, is seen in 0.4–2% of cases.
- Febrile status epilepticus.

CHAPTER 123

Acute Asthma and Status Asthmaticus

INTRODUCTION

Acute exacerbation of asthma is a very common emergency among children.

If a severe acute exacerbation of asthma does not respond to initial treatment with steroids and bronchodilators, it is termed "status asthmaticus". The classification of asthma based on severity of the episode as shown in **Table 1**.

TABLE 1: Severity score: Classification of mild, moderate, and severe asthma.

Parameter*	Mild	Moderate	Severe	Respiratory arrest imminent
Activity	Normal or dyspnea on exertion	Decreased activity. (Infants may have softer, shorter cry; difficulty feeding)	Decreased activity (Infants stop feeding). Hunched forward	Unable to eat
Speech	Normal	Phrases	Words	Not able to speak
Alertness	Alert	Might look agitated	Usually agitated	Drowsy or confused
Respiratory rate	Increased	Increased	Often >30 breaths/min	
	Age <2 months 2–12 months 1–5 years 6–8 years	Normal rate <60 breaths/min <50 breaths/min <40 breaths/min <30 breaths/min		
Accessory muscles and suprasternal retractions	Minimal intercostal retractions	Intercostal and substernal retractions	Significant respiratory distress. All accessory muscles usually involved	Marked respiratory distress. Paradoxical thoraco-abdominal movement
Wheeze	Moderate, often only end-expiration	Loud	Usually loud	Absent

Continued

Continued

Parameter*	Mild	Moderate	Severe	Respiratory arrest imminent
PEF after initial broncho-dilator % predicted or personal best	>80%	Approximately 60–80%	<60% predicted or personal best (<100 L/ min adults) or response lasts <2 h	Not able to perform
SpO$_2$%	>94%	91–94%	<90%	<90%

*The presence of several parameters, but not necessarily all, indicates the general classification of the attack.

(PEF: peak expiratory flow)

MANAGEMENT OF ACUTE ASTHMA

- *Mild-to-moderate*:
  - Administer humidified O$_2$ at high concentration, keep O$_2$ saturation ≥94%
  - Administer salbutamol by a metered-dose inhaler (MDI) or nebulizer solution
  - Administer oral corticosteroids.
- *Moderate-to-severe*:
  - Administer humidified O$_2$ at high concentrations to keep O$_2$ saturation ≥94%. Use a nonrebreathing mask, if needed.
  - Administer salbutamol by MDI (with spacer) or nebulizer solution. If not responding, try continuous salbutamol administration.
  - Administer ipratropium bromide by nebulizer solution. Salbutamol and ipratropium may be mixed for nebulization.
  - Administer corticosteroids PO/IV.
  - Consider administering magnesium sulfate by slow (15–30 min) IV bolus infusion while monitoring heart rate and blood pressure.
- *Impending respiratory failure*:
  - In addition to the above therapies, the following are indicated:
    - Administer O$_2$ at high concentrations
    - Administer salbutamol by continuous nebulizer
    - Administer corticosteroids IV if not already given.
    - Consider giving terbutaline subcutaneously or by continuous infusion
    - Consider subcutaneous or IM epinephrine as an alternative
    - Consider bilevel positive airway pressure (noninvasive positive-pressure ventilation), especially in alert, cooperative children
    - Consider endotracheal intubation for children with refractory hypoxemia (low O$_2$ saturation), worsening clinical condition (e.g.,

decreasing level of consciousness and irregular breathing), or both despite the aggressive medical management described above. Intubation in an asthmatic child carries significant risk for respiratory and circulatory complications. Consider using a cuffed endotracheal (ET) tube.

KEY POINTS

- Recognize asthma since all the wheezes are not asthma.
- Determine severity of the asthmatic exacerbation on arrival.
- *Primary treatment of asthma exacerbation*: Oxygen, inhaled salbutamol, and systemic corticosteroids.
- *In severe exacerbations, consider*: Anticholinergic agents, IV magnesium sulfate, and IV terbutaline.

At discharge, prescribe: MDI salbutamol, oral prednisolone × 3–5 days, and consider initiating inhaled corticosteroids to prevent future exacerbations.

ACUTE STRIDOR

Introduction

Stridor is a high-pitch harsh inspiratory sound produced due to airflow through a narrowed or obstructed airway (oropharynx, subglottis or trachea). In severe obstruction, stridor may occur during expiration also.

Causes of stridor are shown in **Table 1**. The most common cause is acute laryngotracheobronchitis or croup.

Laryngotracheobronchitis is an acute viral infection of the larynx and subglottic region and is caused by parainfluenza virus type 1. It is insidious in onset and presents with hoarseness of voice, stridor, and a peculiar brassy cough.

Stridor is an acute medical emergency. The emergency department management is shown in **Table 2**.

Note:

- Give dexamethasone 0.6 mg/kg IV/oral stat. Most of the time for Grade-1 and -2 stridor, one dose is sufficient. Alternatively, oral prednisolone 1 mg/kg may be used.
- Dexamethasone 0.15 mg/kg/dose 12 hourly can be continued if stridor persists.
- *Nebulized adrenaline*: For Grade III and IV croup—0.5 mL/kg up to maximum 5 mg of 1 in 1,000 adrenaline solution via nebulizer. Constitute the solution to 4 mL for nebulization. Can be repeated 0.5–1 hourly, if necessary.

TABLE 1: Causes of stridor.

Infectious	Congenital	Acquired	Allergic
<ul><li>Laryngotracheitis</li><li>Acute epiglottitis</li><li>Bacterial tracheitis</li><li>Retropharyngeal abscess</li></ul>	<ul><li>Laryngomalacia</li><li>Vocal cord paralysis</li><li>Congenital subglottic stenosis</li><li>Vascular ring</li></ul>	<ul><li>Laryngeal granuloma</li><li>Foreign body</li><li>Neoplasms</li></ul>	<ul><li>Acute angioneurotic edema</li></ul>

TABLE 2: Classification of stridor at arrival and management in the emergency department.

Grade I	Grade II	Grade III	Grade IV
• No stridor at rest • Stridor only on crying	• Stridor at rest without sternal and chest wall retractions and no distress	• Stridor at rest with sternal and chest wall retractions	• Marked respiratory distress • Tachycardia • Sweating, pallor/cyanosis
Management Algorithm of Acute Laryngotracheobronchitis/Croup			
• Do not upset the child • Gentle handling • Oral prednisolone/dexamethasone stat and observe in ED	• Dexamethasone IV/oral stat • Dexamethasone q12h can be continued if stridor persists	• Oxygen and IV fluid • Dexamethasone IV stat and prn • Maintenance dexamethasone • Nebulized adrenaline	• Oxygen and IV fluids • Dexamethasone IV stat abd prn • Maintenance dexamethasone • Nebulized adrenaline • ICU admission • If needed consider—BMV and RSI • Call for ENT help for tracheostomy if required

(BMV: bag-mask ventilation; ED: emergency department; RSI: rapid sequence intubation)

ACUTE EPIGLOTTITIS

Introduction

Acute epiglottitis is a life-threatening inflammation of the supraglottic structures (arytenoids, aryepiglottic folds, and epiglottis) that may be complicated by severe laryngospasm, stridor, and irreversible airway obstruction. It has become a very rare occurrence after introduction of the *H. influenzae* vaccine.

Etiology

- *S. pyogenes, S. pneumoniae, S. aureus,* and *H. influenzae.*
- *H. influenzae* was responsible for most of the cases in the preimmunization era.

Clinical Features

Acute onset fever, throat pain and discomfort, excessive drooling and stridor. Symptoms may progress rapidly (few hours) or subacutely (1–2 days). Cough is usually not a typical feature.

The child appears sick and typically assumes the "tripod position" or "sniffing position" in which the chin is pushed forward with the neck slightly extended.

Diagnosis

Diagnosis is mainly clinical. Lateral X-ray soft tissue of the neck (neck extended during inspiration) may show the characteristic "thumb sign" of the swollen epiglottis.

Management

- Assess and protect the airway. Ensure that facilities to provide a surgical airway are readily available, if intubation is difficult.
- Adrenaline nebulizations and steroid (budesonide) nebulizations are helpful in relieving the edema.
- *Antibiotics*: Second or third generation cephalosporins for 7–10 days.

RESPIRATORY INFECTIONS AND PNEUMONIA IN CHILDREN

Pneumonia: It may be classified as lobar pneumonia, bronchopneumonia, or interstitial pneumonia.

Clinical Assessment

- Check temperature, respiratory rate, and the type of cough
- Chest in drawing, low saturation, and cyanosis
- Stridor, wheeze, crepitations, and bronchial breath sounds
- Assess the sensorium of the child
- Assess the nutritional status

Investigations

- Complete blood count, blood culture
- Chest X-ray for severe pneumonia and very severe disease.

Criteria for Hospitalization

- Children less than 3 months of age irrespective of severity of pneumonia
- Moderate-to-severe respiratory distress
- Respiratory failure, hypoxemia $SpO_2 < 90\%$ on room air
- Dehydration or inability to feed orally
- Recurrent pneumonia
- Toxic appearance
- *Underlying conditions that may predispose to serious course of pneumonia*: Cardiac conditions, genetic syndromes, neurocognitive disorders, immuno-compromised host, and metabolic conditions
- Complications (effusion/empyema)
- Failure of outpatient therapy.

The classification of illness and the ED management of patients with pneumonia are shown in **Table 1**.

TABLE 1: Classification of illness and management.

Severity	Features	Management

No pneumonia	• *Respiratory rate:*
	  ○ <2 months: <60 breaths/min
	  ○ 2–12 months: <50 breaths/min
	  ○ 1–5 years: <40 breaths/min
		Symptomatic management

Pneumonia not severe	• Fast breathing without chest in drawing
	• *Respiratory rate:*
	  ○ <2 months: >60 breaths/min
	  ○ 2–12 months: >50 breaths/min
	  ○ 1–5 years: >40 breaths/min
		• Amoxicillin 50–100 mg/kg/day PO in three divided doses × 5–7 days
		• Ensure that the child receives adequate fluids
		• Encourage breastfeeding and oral fluids

Severe pneumonia	• Fast breathing with chest indrawing • Nasal flaring • Grunting	• Crystalline penicillin IV 200,000 units/kg/day q6h • OR Ampicillin IV 100–150 mg/kg/day q6h • OR Co-amoxiclav 25–40 mg/kg/day PO (of Amoxicillin) three divided doses × 5–7 days • Intravenous fluid: ± • Monitor and ensure oxygen saturation >94% • Suspecting *S. aureus*: Add injection Cloxacillin 100–200 mg/ kg/day IV in four divided doses
Very severe disease	• Vomiting or unable to drink • Convulsions • Stridor • Malnutrition • Central cyanosis • Head nodding	• Ceftriaxone 100 mg/kg IV once a day (may give IM if no IV access) OR • Cefuroxime-axetil 75–100 mg/kg/day IV in three doses (change to oral Cefuroxime at dose of 20–30 mg/kg/day when child improves) • IV fluids • Monitor and ensure oxygen saturation >94% • *Suspecting S. aureus*: Add injection Cloxacillin 100–200 mg/kg/day IV in four divided doses

INDICATIONS OF INTENSIVE CARE

- Signs of impending respiratory failure (lethargy, increased work of breathing, hypercarbia, saturation <90% with 100% FiO_2).
- Recurrent apnea or slow irregular respiration, altered mental status
- Cardiovascular compromise with progressive tachycardia and hypotension
- *Need for ventilatory support*: Individualized based on clinical, laboratory and radiological findings.

KEYPOINTS

- Tachypnea is the most reliable predictor for lower respiratory tract infection (LRTI)
- Drug of choice for uncomplicated pneumonia: Amoxicillin
- If hypoxia persists despite 100% FiO_2, consider respiratory failure
- Do not perform a routine chest X-ray to confirm uncomplicated pneumonia.

Acute Otitis Media and Otitis Externa

ACUTE OTITIS MEDIA

Introduction

Acute otitis media refers to inflammation of the middle ear and is characterized by ear pain, discharge, fever, irritability, vomiting, and anorexia.

Etiology

- *Bacteria*: *S. pneumoniae* (40–50%), *H. influenzae* (30–40%), *M. catarrhalis* (10–15%), *S. aureus* and *C. pneumoniae* (1–2%).

Clinical features: Ear discharge, otalgia, headache, fever, and anorexia.

Management

- *Antibiotics*: Syrup Amoxicillin × 7–10 days
- *Nasal decongestants*:
  - Xylometazoline nasal drops (3 drops q8h) × 3 days
  - Normal saline nasal drops (3 drops q6h) × 7 days
  - Syrup Chlorpheniramine + Phenylephrine (T-Minic) 1–2 mg/mL
    - *2–5 years*: 1 mL PO q6h
    - *>6 years*: 2 mL PO q6h
- *Keep the ear dry*: Advice the patient to keep cotton soaked in vaseline in the ears while having a bath.

ACUTE OTITIS EXTERNA

Introduction

Acute otitis externa, also referred to as Swimmer's ear, is an inflammation of the external auditory meatus. Children exposed to water for long periods are at risk.

- *Symptoms*: Ear pain, aural fullness, and itching.
- *Signs*: Tragal tenderness, diffuse aural canal edema, erythema, and ear discharge.
- *Etiology*: *Staphylococcus aureus* is the usual organism. Malignant otitis externa is caused by *P. aeruginosa*.

Management

- Ear canal cleaning
- *Antibiotics*: Syrup/Tablet Cloxacillin q6h × 7 days
- *Keep the ear dry*: Advice the patient to keep cotton soaked in vaseline in the ears while having a bath.

INTRODUCTION

The term "acute gastroenteritis" denotes infections of the gastrointestinal tract caused by bacterial, viral, or parasitic pathogens.

Bloody diarrhea with visible blood and mucus is called dysentery and is usually bacterial in etiology.

When a child presents to the emergency department, assess the hydration status of the child to classify the severity of diarrhea (**Table 1**).

TABLE 1: Classification of dehydration.			
	No dehydration	*Some dehydration*	*Severe dehydration*
Appearance	Well and alert	Restless/irritable	Lethargic/unconscious/floppy
Thirst	Drinks normally	Thirsty	Unable to drink
Skin pinch	Goes back quickly	Goes back slowly	Goes back very slowly
Tongue	Moist	Dry	Very dry
Eyes	Normal	Sunken	Sunken
Vital signs	Normal	Tachycardia, may have delayed CRT	Tachycardia, weak peripheral pulses, delayed CRT, cold peripheries, with or without hypotension

(CRT: capillary refill time)

COMMON PATHOGEN CAUSING ACUTE GASTROENTERITIS IN CHILDREN

- *Viruses (70%)*: Rotaviruses, adenovirus, calicivirus, astrovirus, and enterovirus.
- *Bacteria (10–20%)*: *Campylobacter*, *E. coli*, *Shigella*, *V. cholerae*, *Yersinia*, *S. typhi*, and *S. paratyphi*.
- *Protozoa (<10%)*: *Giardia*, *E. histolytica*, and *Cryptosporidium*.

MANAGEMENT

- Fluid resuscitation with ORS or IV/IO fluids should be initiated immediately (**Table 2**).
- *Zinc supplementation*: Zinc supplementation is shown to reduce duration and severity of diarrhea.

TABLE 2: Management of acute watery diarrhea.

No dehydration: Plan-A	Some dehydration: Plan-B	Severe dehydration: Plan-C

Exclusively breastfed (give ORS in addition to breast milk)
 	
• <2 years: 50–100 mL with each loose stool
 	
• >2 years: 100–200 mL with each loose stool, or
 	
• 10 mL/kg ORS with each loose stool
	• The approximate amount of ORS: 75 mL/kg over 4 h
	
	• After 4 h, reassess the child and classify the child for dehydration
		• Start IV/IO fluids immediately
		
		• If central pulse weak—give 20 mL/kg fluid of RS/NS over 20 min
		
		• Then, give 100 mL/kg RL or normal saline divided as follows:
		
		  ○ *Age <12 months*: 30 mL/kg over 1 h, then 70 mL/kg over 5 h
		
		  ○ *Age >12 months*: 30 mL/kg over 1/2 h, then 70 mL/kg over 2.5 h
		
		Reassess the patient after 6 h. As soon as child can drink, give ORS, usually after 3–4 h for infants and 1–2 h for older children

-   ○ *Children 2–6 months*: 10 mg/day of elemental zinc for 14 days.
-   ○ *Children >6 months*: 20 mg/day of elemental zinc for 14 days.
- *Antibiotics*:
  - ○ Diarrhea in children is mostly of viral etiology and hence does not warrant antibiotics.
  - ○ Administer antibiotics only if the child has the following symptoms
    - – Bloody diarrhea with visible blood and mucus
    - – High fever with suspected sepsis
    - – Traveler's diarrhea.
  - ○ *Antibiotic of choice*: Syrup Cefixime 8 mg/kg/day in two divided doses for 5 days.

Special Instructions to the Mother

- Recommend longer duration of breastfeeding to the mother at each feed
- Teach the mother how to prepare and give ORS. If the child vomits, tell her to wait for 5–10 minutes and then retry giving ORS slowly. Tell her to give more ORS if the child wants more.
- In addition to ORS, food-based fluids like soup or rice water may be given to children who are not exclusively breastfed.
- Older children can be encouraged to continue to take their usual diet.

CHAPTER 128

Drugs and Dosages in Pediatric Emergencies

INTRODUCTION

The wide spectrum of drug dosages based on age is a challenge in the emergency department. Commonly used drugs in pediatric emergencies and their dosage are given in **Table 1**.

TABLE 1: Drugs and dosages in pediatric emergencies.

Drug	Route	Recommended pediatric dosage
Activated charcoal	NG	• *Up to 1 year*: 10–25 g or 0.5–1 g/kg • *1–12 years*: 25–50 g or 0.5–1 g/kg • *Adolescents and adults*: 25–100 g
Acyclovir	IV	HSV infection, encephalitis: 10 mg/kg/dose q8h • *Max dose*: 1,500 mg/m²/day
	Oral	• *<2 years*: 100 mg five times a day • *2–18 years*: 200 mg five times daily
Adenosine	IV	• *Neonate*: 0.05 mg/kg • *Infant/child*: 0.1 mg/kg (maximum 1st dose 6 mg, by rapid bolus) followed by 0.2 mg/kg/dose (maximum 12 mg)

Adrenaline	IV, IM, ET, IO, SC	• *IV*: 0.1 mL/kg 1:10,000 dilution
		• *ET*: 0.1 mL/kg 1:1,000 dilution
		• *IM*: For anaphylaxis 1:1,000 dilution
		  ○ *<6 years*: 150 µg (0.15 mL)
		  ○ *6–12 years*: 300 µg (0.3 mL)
		  ○ *>12 years*: 500 µg (0.5 mL)

Albendazole	PO	• *1–2 years*: 200 mg single dose • *>2 years*: 400 mg single dose Repeat dose after 2 weeks for roundworms
Amikacin	IV, IM	• *Preterm*: 7.5 mg/kg IV OD • *Neonates*: 10 mg/kg/day IV OD • *Infant and child*: IV/IM: 15–22.5 mg/kg/day q8h
Amiodarone	IV	• *For pulseless VF/VT*: 5 mg/kg IV/IO by rapid bolus (can repeat 5 mg/kg bolus to a total of 15 mg/kg/24 h) • Maximum single dose 300 mg • *For SVT/stable VT*: 5 mg/kg given over 60 min. Maximum total dose 15 mg/kg per 24 h

Continued

Continued

Drug	Route	Recommended pediatric dosage
Amoxicillin	PO	• *Standard dose*: 50 mg/kg/day in 2–3 divided doses • *High dose (resistant S. pneumoniae)*: 80–90 mg/kg/ day in 2–3 divided doses • *Maximum dose*: 2 g/day
Amoxicillin/ Clavulanic acid	IV/PO	45 mg/kg/day q8h

Ampicillin	IV	• *Neonates*:
		  ○ <7 days: 50 mg/kg/dose IV q12h
		  ○ 7–21 days: 50 mg/kg/dose IV q8h
		  ○ 21 days: 50 mg/kg/dose IV q6h
		For suspected meningitis with group B Steptococcal infection: 100 mg/kg/dose
		• *Infant/child*: 25 mg/kg/dose (maximum: 1 g) IV q6h
		  ○ *1 month–2 years*: 12.5 mg/kg/dose PO q6h
		  ○ *2–12 years*: 250 mg/dose PO q6h
		  ○ *12–18 years*: 500 mg/dose PO q6h

Aminophylline	IV	For bronchospasm: 5 mg/kg IV loading dose over 20–30 min
Atropine	IV, ET, IO	• *ET*: 0.02 mg/kg/dose, q5 min × 2–3 doses • *Maximum single dose*: 0.5 mg • *Minimum dose*: 0.1 mg

Azithromycin	PO/IV	• *6 months–12 years*: 10 mg/kg/day PO od
		• *Maximum dose*:
		  ○ *3–7 years*: 200 mg
		  ○ *8–11 years*: 300 mg
		  ○ *12–14 years*: 400 mg
		  ○ *>14 years*: 500 mg
		• *Enteric fever*: IV/oral: 20 mg/kg/day q12h

Benzathine Penicillin	IM	For rheumatic fever prophylaxis: • *<27 kg*: 6 lakh units IM single dose after test dose • *>27 kg*: 12 lakh units IM single dose after test dose
Calcium gluconate 10%	IV	• *Hyperkalemia*: 1 mL/kg with equal volume of water slow IV over 10 min • *Hypocalcemia*: 2 mL/kg with equal volume of water for slow IV over 10 min *Stop injection if symptomatic bradycardia occurs. Extravascular administration can result in severe skin injury. • Maximum 10 mL as a stat dose

Continued

Continued

Drug	Route	Recommended pediatric dosage
Cefoperazone	IV	50–200 mg/kg/day q8H
Cefazolin	IV	25–100 mg/kg/day divided every 6–8 h • *Maximum*: 6 g daily
Cefixime	PO	• *Infant and child*: 8 mg/kg/day in 2 divided doses • *Adolescents*: 400 mg/day in 1–2 divided doses

Cefotaxime	IV, IM	• *Neonates*: IV/IM 150 mg/kg/day q8h
		• *Infant and child*:
		  ○ *Sepsis*:100 mg/kg/day IV q6h
		  ○ *Meningitis*: 200 mg/kg/day IV q6h
		• *Maximum dose*: 12 g/24 h

Ceftazidime	IV	100–150 mg/kg/day IV q8h
Ceftriaxone	IV, IM	• *Mild-to-moderate infection*: 50–75 mg/kg/dose once daily; maximum daily dose: 1,000 mg • *Severe infection*: 100 mg/kg/day divided every 12–24 h; maximum daily dose: 4,000 mg

Cefuroxime	IV, PO	• *Neonate*: 50–100 mg/kg/24 h IVq12h
		• *Child*:
		  ○ *Mild-to-moderate infection*:
		    – *Oral*: 20–30 mg/kg/day divided twice daily; maximum single dose: 500 mg
		    – *IM, IV*: 75–100 mg/kg/day divided in 3 doses; maximum single dose: 1,500 mg
		  ○ *Severe infection*: IM, IV: 100–200 mg/kg/day divided in 3–4 doses; maximum single dose: 1,500 mg

Cefoperazone + Sulbactam	IV	40–80 mg/kg/day in 2–4 divided doses • *Maximum*: 160 mg/kg/day
Cephalexin	PO	25–100 mg/kg/day q6h
Chloramphenicol	IV	• *Neonates <14 days*: 12.5 mg/kg/dose IV q12h • *Neonates >14 days*: 12.5 mg/kg/dose IV 2–4 times • *Children*: 50 mg/kg/day in 4 divided doses (double dose for meningitis and septicemia) • *Maximum dose*: 1 g/day
Ciprofloxacin	PO, IV	• *Neonates*: 10 mg/kg PO/IV q12h • *Children*: 15–30 mg/kg/day IV/PO q12h • *Maximum dose*: 800 mg/24 h
Clindamycin	IV	• *Neonates*: 15–20 mg/kg/day IM/IV divided q6–8h • *Infants, children, and adolescents*: 20–40 mg/kg/day IM/IV divided q6–8h • *Maximum dose*: 450 mg/dose

Continued

Continued

Drug	Route	Recommended pediatric dosage
Clobazam	PO	0.5–1 mg/kg/day q12h
Cloxacillin	PO, IV	• 50–100 mg/kg/day q6h • High dose 200 mg/kg/day q6h
Cotrimoxazole	IV, PO	• 6–20 mg TMP/kg/day PO q12h • 15–20 mg TMP/kg/day IV q12h
Crystalline Penicillin	IV	• *Neonates*: 1 lakh unit/kg/dose IV q12h • *Infant and child*: 50,000 units/kg/dose IV q6h
Dexamethasone	IV	• *Croup*: 0.6 mg/kg/dose • *Meningitis*: 0.15 mg/kg/dose
Digoxin	Oral IV	• *Maintenance dose*: 0.01 mg/kg/day, once a day, 5/7 • *Atrial fibrillation (rate control)*: Total digitalizing dose (TDD): 8–12 µg/kg IV; administer half of TDD over 5 min with the remaining portion as 25% fractions at 4–8 h intervals
Dobutamine	IV	Infusion 15 mg/kg in 50 mL NS (1 mL: 5 µg/kg/min)
Dopamine	OV	Infusion 15 mg/kg in 50 mL NS (1 mL: 5 µg/kg/min)
Doxycycline	PO	• *Cholera*: Oral 6 mg/kg/dose stat • *Rickettsial infection*: 4 mg/kg/day q12h • *Maximum dose*: 300 mg/day
Erythromycin	PO	• *0–7 days*: 20 mg/kg/day q12h • *>7 days*: 30 mg/kg/day q8h • *Infant–child*: 30–50 mg/kg/day q6h • *Maximum dose*: 4 g/24 h
Fentanyl	IV	1–2 µg/kg/dose
Fluconazole	Oral	• *Mucosal candidiasis*: 3-6 mg/kg/day PO od • *Systemic candidiasis/Cryptococcosis*: 6–12 mg/kg/day PO od
Furosemide (Lasix)	IV	• 0.5–1 mg/kg/dose • *For infusion*: 3–4 mg/kg/day in 24 mL of NS, at 1 mL/h
Gentamicin	IV, IM	• *Neonates <7 days*: 2.5 mg/kg IV/IM q12h • *Neonates >7 days*: 2.5 mg/kg IV/IM q8h • *Children <12 years*: 7.5 mg/kg/day IV/IM in 3 divided doses • *12–18 years*: 3–6 mg/kg/day IV/IM in 3 divided doses
Hydrocortisone	IV	• *Infants*: 10–25 mg IV stat followed by 10–25 mg/day in divided doses q6h • *Children <5 years*: 25–50 mg IV stat followed by 25–50 mg/day in divided doses q6h • *Children ≥5 years*: 50–100 mg IV stat followed by 50 mg/day in divided doses q6h • *Adolescents*: 100 mg IV stat followed by 100 mg/day in divided doses q6h

Continued

Continued

Drug	Route	Recommended pediatric dosage

Hydroxyzine (Atarax)	Oral	• *Pruritus:*
		  ○ *6 months–6 years*: 5–15 mg PO hsod
		  ○ *7–12 years*: 10–15 mg PO hsod
		  ○ *12–18 years*: 25 mg PO hsod
		• *Anxiety:*
		  ○ <6 years: 50 mg/day PO in 3–4 divided doses
		  ○ >6 years: 100 mg/day PO in 3–4 divided doses

Hyoscine (Buscopan)	PO, IM, IV	• *PO*: 5–12 years: 10 mg/dose, 12–18 years: 20 mg/dose 3–4 times/day • *IM/IV*: <6 years: 5 mg/dose, 6–12 years: 5–10 mg/dose, >12 years: 20 mg/dose 3–4 times/day • *Maximum dose*: 1.2 mg/kg/day
Kayexalate (Sodium polystyrene sulfonate)	PO, rectal	• *PO*: 1 g/kg every 6 h • *Rectal*: 1 g/kg/dose every 2–6 h
KCl	PO	2–5 mEq/kg/day in divided doses; not to exceed 1–2 mEq/kg as a single dose
Ketamine	IM, IV	*IV*: 1–2 mg/kg/dose
Lidocaine	IV	1 mg/kg/dose
Lorazepam	IM, IV	0.1 mg/kg/dose
Levetiracetam	IV, PO	10–20 mg/kg/dose stat, followed by 10 mg/kg/dose bd for 1 week, then increase by 10 mg/kg/day up to maximum of 60 mg/kg/day
Mannitol (20%)	IV	2.5 mL/kg (0.5 g/kg given over 15 min)
Magnesium sulfate		0.1 mL/kg of 50% $MgSO_4$ as slow infusion with NS over 30 min

Meropenem	IV	• *Neonates:*
		  ○ *Sepsis*: 20 mg/kg/dose q12h
		  ○ *Meningitis*: 40 mg/kg/dose q12h
		• *Children:*
		  ○ *Moderate infection*: 20 mg/kg/dose IV q8h
		  ○ *Meningitis*: 40 mg/kg/dose IV q8h
		• *Maximum dose:*
		  ○ *Moderate infection*: 3 g/day
		  ○ *Severe infection*: 6 g/day

Continued

Continued

Drug	Route	Recommended pediatric dosage

Metronidazole	IV, PO	• *Neonates:*
		  ○ *Loading dose*: 15 mg/kg
		  ○ *Maintenance:*
		    – 7.5 mg/kg/dose q24h for VLBW
		    – 7.5 mg/kg/dose q12h for weeks 1–4
		    – 7.5 mg/kg/dose q8h over 4 weeks
		• *Child*: 7.5 mg/kg/dose IV/PO q8h
		* Maintenance dose should begin 48 h after loading dose for VLBW and 24 h after loading dose for term babies

Midazolam	IV, IM	*IV/IM*: 0.1 mg/kg/dose • *For infusion*: 0.5 mg/kg in 50 mL NS • *Seizure dose infusion*: 3 mg/kg in 50 mL NS: Start at 1 mL/h
Morphine	IV, IM, SC	0.1–0.2 mg/kg/dose
Nifedipine	Oral	• *HT urgency*: 0.1–0.25 mg/kg/dose. Can be repeated every 4–6 h • *Chronic treatment*: 0.25–0.5 mg/kg/day in 1 or 2 divided doses • *Maximum single dose*: 10 mg
Noradrenaline	IV	Add 0.3 mg/kg in 50 mL NS, 1 mL/h = 0.1 µg/kg/min, 2 mL/h = 0.2 µg/kg/min
Pancuronium	IV	• *Neonates*: 0.05–0.10 mg/kg/dose • *Children*: 0.05–0.15 mg/kg/dose
Pantoprazole	IV/oral	1 mg/kg/dose od • *Maximum dose*: 40 mg/day
Pheniramine maleate (Avil)	IM, IV, PO	0.5 mg/kg/day q8h
Phenobarbitone	IV	20 mg/kg loading dose slow IV over 20 min followed by 5 mg/kg/day in 2 divided doses • *Maximum dose*: 30 mg/kg/day
Phenytoin sodium	IV	*Loading* 15–20 mg/kg in 50–100 mL NS slow infusion over 20 min and then 3–4 mg/kg/day in 2 divided doses in neonates and 5–6 mg/kg/day in 2 divided doses in children
Piperacillin-Tazobactam	IV	• *Infant*: 300 mg/kg/day in 3 divided doses • *Child*: 400 mg/kg/day in 3 divided doses • *Maximum single dose*: 4.5 g
Propranolol	IV, oral	• *Oral*: 0.5–1 mg/kg/day q6–12h • *IV*: 0.15–0.25 mg/kg/dose slow IV push (TOF)

Continued

Continued

Drug	Route	Recommended pediatric dosage
Ranitidine	IV, PO	1 mg/kg/dose q8h
Salbutamol	PO	0.1 mg/kg/dose q8h
Sodium bicarbonate	IV	1 mEq/kg/dose or 0.3 × kg × base deficit
Spironolactone	PO	1–3 mg/kg/day in 2 divided doses
Succinylcholine	IV	1–2 mg/kg/dose * Increases ICP, contraindicated in burns, massive trauma, hyperkalemia
Thiopental	IV	1–5 mg/kg/dose
Tranexamic acid	PO, IV	10 mg/kg/dose
Tramadol	IM, IV	1–2 mg/kg/dose 6th hourly • *Maximum single dose*: 100 mg
UDCA	PO	5–10 mg/kg/dose twice a day
Valproate	PO, IV	• *IV*: 20 mg/kg loading dose followed by 5–10 mg/ kg/dose • *Maximum dose*: 60 mg/kg/day

Vancomycin	IV	• *Neonates*: 15 mg/kg/dose IV
		  ○ <28 weeks: Once daily
		  ○ 29–35 weeks: Twice daily
		  ○ >35 weeks: Thrice daily
		• *Children*: 15 mg/kg loading dose followed by 10 mg/kg/dose q6h
		• *Maximum dose*: 2 g/day

Vecuronium	IV	0.1 mg/kg/dose
Vitamin K1	IM, SC, IV	• *Infant and child*: 2.5–5 mg/24 h, PO od • *Infant and child*: 1–2 mg/dose, IM, SC, IV, od • *Adolescent and adult*: 10 mg/dose, PO, SC, IV, IM, od
Ipravent (Neb)		• <12 years: 250 µg/dose, q20 min × 3 then q6–8h • >12 years: 500 µg/dose, q30 min × 3 then q6–8h
Salbutamol (Neb)		• *<2 years*: 0.3 mL in 3 mL of NS • *2–5 years*: 0.5 mL in 3 mL of NS • *>5 years*: 1 mL in 3 mL of NS

Adrenaline (Neb)		0.5 mL/kg 1 in 1,000, diluted in 3 mL of NS
		• *Maximum dose*:
		  ○ <4 years 2.5 mL/dose
		  ○ >4 years 5 mL/dose

(HSV: herpes simplex virus; ICP: intracranial pressure; NS: normal saline; SVT: supraventricular tachycardia; TOF: tetralogy of Fallot; UDCA: ursodeoxycholic acid; VF/VT: ventricular fibrillation/ventricular tachycardia; VLBW: very low birth weight baby)

Section **18**

Disaster Management

DISASTER MANAGEMENT: HOSPITAL PREPAREDNESS

Disaster, mass casualty, and catastrophe have all become household terms in this 21st century by virtue of the global change in environment and lifestyle. The impact of these disasters not only imply on life but also on the functional status of the individual and the society. Disaster management is no more a topic of discussion but a field of specialty called disaster medicine and nursing. This chapter focuses on the hospital preparedness and response for disaster and mass casualties.

Objectives of Hospital Preparedness

To ensure that the healthcare team is able to:
- Be prepared in disaster risk reduction (DRR)
- Respond appropriately to mass casualty/disaster management
- Document the response toward disaster management.

Definitions of Terminology Used in Hospital Disaster Management Center for Research on the Epidemiology of Disasters (CRED)

- *Disaster*: A situation or event, which overwhelms local capacity, necessitating a request to national or international level for external assistance [definition considered in emergency events database (EM-DAT)]; an unforeseen and often sudden event that causes great damage, destruction, and human suffering. Though often caused by nature, disasters can have human origins (EM-DAT).
- *Hazard*: Threatening event, or probability of occurrence of a potentially damaging phenomenon within a given time period and area.
- *Risk*: Expected loss (of lives, persons injured, property damaged, and economic activity disrupted) due to a particular hazard for a given area and reference period. Based on mathematical calculations, risk is the product of hazard and vulnerability.
- *Transport accident*: Disaster type term used in EM-DAT to describe technological transport accidents involving mechanized modes of transport.
- *Vulnerability*: Degree of loss (0–100%) resulting from a potential damaging phenomenon.

Classification of Hospital Disasters

- *Internal disasters*: Events that result in loss of resources used for regular hospital activities.
  Examples: Fire, earthquake, loss of utilities, worker strikes, release of chemicals, or radiation.
- *External disasters*: Events that occur in the community outside the hospital that may affect the hospital's ability to carry out regular activities.
  Examples: Road, rail accidents, and technological hazards.

> This chapter focuses on the response of the emergency department toward external disaster, which means, response to mass casualty incidents reporting to the hospital.

MASS CASUALTIES IN THE EMERGENCY DEPARTMENT

A mass casualty incident (MCI) is any incident in which emergency medical services resources, such as personnel and equipment, are overwhelmed by the number and severity of casualties. The mass casualty management (MCM) depends upon the policy of the institution and is based on the capacity and the resources.

The success of MCM system depends on the following:
- Pre-established procedures, to be used in daily emergency activities and to be adapted to meet demands of a major incident, such as an event in which there may be large number of patients reporting to the ED at the same time (Disaster plan).
- Optimal use of existing resources (Logistics).
- Multidimensional preparation and response (Capacity building).
- Strong preplanned and tested coordination (Mock drill).

Management of a MCI in the ED of CMC, Vellore (Flowchart 1)

Step 1: Verification of the MCI: On receiving information/arrival of first patient of an MCI, the ED registrar and nurse in-charge should confirm the authenticity of the information from the public relations officer (PRO) or the administration.

Step 2: Notification of MCI: The ED registrar or nurse should inform the on-call trauma coordinator (TC) and trauma nurse coordinator (TNC). The TC and TNC should inform the head of the department and arrive in the ED within 5–10 minutes.

Step 3: Activation of the MCM team: This is done by the TC and TNC through telephone exchange (Ph. No. 2500). The TC is the incident commander of the MCM team.

Step 4: Team members reporting to the ED: All team members should report to the ED at the earliest and perform their roles as described.

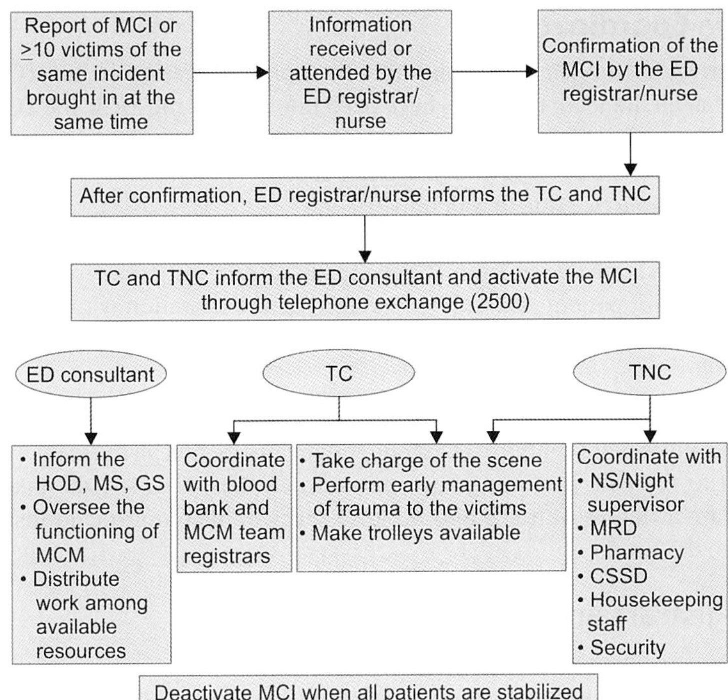

(ED: emergency department; TC: trauma coordinator; TNC: trauma nurse coordinator; HOD: head of the department; MS: medical superintendent; GS: general superintendent; MCM: mass casualty management; MRD: medical records department; CSSD: central sterilization and supply department; NS: nursing superintendent)

FLOWCHART 1: Mass casualty management (MCI) protocol at CMC, Vellore.

Step 5: Deactivation of MCI: This is done when all the patients are attended to and stabilized.

The MCM Team Members Responding to an MCI in CMC

- *Emergency department:* TC, TNC, additional doctors and nurses, paramedics, social worker, and housekeeping staff.
- *Other departments:* Medical superintendent (MS), general superintendent (GS), nursing superintendent (NS), orthopedics, neurosurgery, general medicine, general surgery, pharmacist, medical records, central sterile supply department, PRO, additional security, blood bank, ICU, and chaplain.

JOB DESCRIPTION OF THE TEAM MEMBERS

The TC and TNC should wear color-coded aprons for easy identification.

Trauma Coordinator

Upon arrival in the ED, the TC should take charge of the scene. The TC should ensure that all the team members have been informed of the MCI. The TC should make trolleys available by:
- Transferring the existing patients, if needed
- Making stable patients to wait outside, and
- Discharging the patients.

In case of a large disaster, the TC should identify the surge capacity area in the Trauma Bay. All patients should be managed in collaboration with the involved specialties.

Trauma Nurse Coordinator

The TNC, after taking charge of the scene should ensure that all the team members respond to the call. In coordination with the TC, the TNC should ensure that trolleys are available at triage and nondisaster patients requiring admission are shifted to the wards.

ED Registrars and Nurses

They have to ensure continuity of care of patients in their bays and quickly discharge or shift out stable patients to priority 3. At least three trolleys should be made available in each bay for receiving MCI patients. They have to take up the area of management as advised by TC and TNC.

Others

- The pharmacist should report in person within the department with the stipulated drugs needed for MCM.
- The medical records person should bring patient charts with predesignated hospital numbers so that investigations may be sent without waiting for registration.
- The PRO coordinates with the Head of ED, MS, and GS to update the press. The PRO also provides needed support to the relatives through volunteers.
- A minimum of five security officers, including two sergeants report to the TC for crowd control. They take charge of patient's valuables in prelabeled MCM bags and look after the safety of the hospital staff involved in patient care.
- Attenders and housekeeping staff support the medical and nursing staff to mobilize patients to the wards and to priority 3 and arrange equipment as needed in consultation with TNC.

A debriefing of the MCM should be done by the head of the ED on the next working day.

Medicolegal Cases

CHAPTER 130

Medicolegal Cases

INTRODUCTION

A medicolegal case (MLC) is any case of injury or ailment, etc., in which investigations by the law-enforcing agencies are essential to fix the responsibility regarding the causation of the injury or ailment. An MLC has not been explicitly defined anywhere in the law. It depends more or less upon the judgment of the doctors.

LIST OF COMMON MEDICOLEGAL CASE

The following are the common MLCs for which an incident report has to be filed:
- All vehicular, railway, airplane, ship, boat accidents, or other unnatural accidents where there is likelihood of death or grievous hurt
- All thermal and electrical injuries
- All workplace injuries/accidents
- All deliberate self-harm attempts (Indian Penal Code, IPC: 309)
- Suspected or evident sexual assaults
- Suspected or evident criminal abortion
- Suspected or evident homicide attempt (assault)
- Drowning/hanging/strangulation
- Domestic violence causing grievous injury
- Unconscious cases where the cause is not natural or not clear
- Animal-related injuries
- Snake bite (only when requested by relatives for claiming compensation)
- Dead on arrival cases where an unnatural cause is suspected
- Any other case not falling under the above mentioned category but has legal implications.

GRIEVOUS AND NONGRIEVOUS INJURIES

Section 320 in the IPC defines grievous hurt. The punishment is enhanced when the injury is grievous. The wound certificate issued should include the grievous or nongrievous nature of injury; the following are the guidelines to designate an injury as grievous:
- Emasculation
- Permanent privation of the sight of either eye
- Permanent privation of the hearing of either ear
- Privation of any member or joint

- Destruction or permanent impairing of the powers of any member or joint
- Permanent disfiguration of the head or face
- Fracture or dislocation of a bone or tooth
- Any injury which endangers life or which causes the sufferer to be during the space of 20 days in severe bodily pain, or unable to follow his ordinary pursuits
- Any intra-abdominal injury can be considered as grievous.

INCIDENT REPORTING

All MLCs who present to the hospital should be directly reported to the police. If a patient has been treated elsewhere and referred, it is the responsibility of the referring doctor to inform the police. However, in our ED, we report all MLC that present acutely after the incident (<48 h). The incident report has to be filled online through the ED module. The report will be sent to the police station through the Medical Superintendent office.

DEATH OF AN MEDICOLEGAL CASE

In case of a brought dead MLC, the nearest police station has to be informed immediately through the "brought dead MLC form". The body may be kept in mortuary for the investigation to take place. However, if the relatives are aggressive and insist on releasing the body, to ensure safety of the healthcare workers first, the police should first be informed and the body may be released after taking informed signed con sent from the relatives on the "release of body" form.

Section **20**

Triage

INTRODUCTION

Triaging is a process by which victims are classified according to the severity and nature of their injuries. The purpose of triage is to ensure prioritization so that the "right patient gets the right treatment at the right time". When more than one victim is brought into the emergency department (ED), it is essential to assess and identify those who require immediate care. This process of prioritizing the patient facilitates appropriate care. The primary objectives of triage are:
- Identification of immediate life-threatening situations
- Reducing severity of the condition by ensuring immediate intervention
- Reducing delay in the treatment.

The commonly used color coding of triage categories are as follows:
- *Red*: Priority 1, most urgent
- *Yellow*: Priority 2, urgent
- *Green*: Priority 3, nonurgent
- *Black*: Dead

Many different triaging systems are used across the World with 3–5 triage categories. Some of the commonly used ones are Australasian Triage System (5 categories), Canadian Triage and Acuity scale (5 categories), Manchester Triage Scale (5 categories) and the Emergency Severity Index (5 categories). Though triaging is based on physiological parameters of the patient at presentation, it is better to incorporate common regional medical and surgical emergencies into the triaging criteria. This is the strength of the 4-category CMC Vellore triage guidelines which were the first triage system developed in India in 1999. This has been further revised every 2 years with the latest revision in January, 2021 (**Tables 1** to **4**).

TABLE 1: CMC Triage guidelines (Revised edition, January 2021: Priority I).

Trauma	Non-trauma
ABC compromised	ABC compromised
GCS ≤ 8	GCS ≤ 8/altered sensorium
Penetrating ocular trauma	RR < 12 or > 40/min or SpO_2 < 94%
Hemodynamically unstable abdominal and pelvic injuries	HR < 50/min or >150/min Palpitations with HR > 150/min Hemodynamically unstable SBP < 80 mm Hg

Continued

Continued

Trauma	Non-trauma
Limb injuries with vascular compromise	Acute onset fever with altered sensorium
Obvious dyspnea with chest pain (post-trauma) with any of the following: • RR < 12 or > 30/min • SpO_2 < 94% • Subcutaneous emphysema • Open pneumothorax • Penetrating chest/neck wound	Hypertensive emergency: SBP > 180 mm Hg and/or DBP > 120 mm Hg with evidence of end organ failure like altered sensorium, chest pain, breathing difficulty, visual disturbance, and oliguria
Hypovolemic shock (SBP < 90 mm Hg or HR > 130/min)	Poisoning with h/o consumption < 2 h or GCS < 13 or hemodynamically unstable
	Active seizures
	Cerebrovascular accidents < 4.5 h
	Chest pain < 8 h (back, shoulder, and epigastric pain)

(ABC: airway, breathing, and circulation; GCS: Glasgow coma scale; RR: respiration rate; HR: heart rate; SBP: systolic blood pressure; DBP: diastolic blood pressure)

TABLE 2: CMC Triage guidelines (Revised edition, January 2021: Priority II).

Trauma	Non-trauma
ABC not compromised	ABC not compromised
• RR: 12–30/min • SpO_2 >94% • GCS ≥9 • All dislocations • Ear, nose, and throat (ENT) bleed • All long bone fractures with no vascular compromise • Treated and referred open fractures • Compartment syndrome • Foreign body in the eyes • Subcutaneous emphysema with no dyspnea • Hemodynamically stable abdomen and pelvic injuries • Pregnant women with stable vital signs (following trauma)	• Dyspnea with RR 28–40/min, SpO_2 > 94%, use of accessory muscles, and comorbid conditions • Hemoptysis or hematemesis within 24 h. • Chest pain more than 8 h or ongoing chest pain >24 h • Palpitations with HR < 150/min and hemodynamically stable • Acute gastroenteritis with HR > 120/min • High sugars with acetone positive • High sugars with acetone negative but with dehydration and fever • Severe pain which requires immediate attention or analgesics including acute abdominal pain • Poisoning without ABC compromise and normal sensorium • Scorpion sting/bee sting/unknown bite/ snake bite • Hematological illness with active bleeding • Giddiness with associated features

Continued

Continued

Trauma	Non-trauma
	• Altered sensorium of any cause with vitals stable
	• Hyperemesis gravidarum with urinary ketones positive
	• Pregnant patient with bleeding per vaginal (PV)/abdomen pain/spotting PV
	• Acute deep vein thrombosis
	• Fever ≥ 103°F
	• Fever with vomiting and not tolerating orally and dehydration
	• Fever with neck stiffness

(ABC: airway, breathing, and circulation; GCS: Glasgow coma scale)

TABLE 3: CMC Triage guidelines: Revised edition, January 2021: Priority III (Patients with acute problems and stable vital signs).

Trauma	Non-trauma
• GCS 15/15 with no loss of consciousness (LOC), stable vital signs, and no history of vomiting	• Mild abdominal pain, passed stool, and flatus
• Isolated closed forearm fractures without neurovascular deficit	• Acute gastroenteritis with stable vitals
• Lacerations with no active bleed	• Acute urinary retention (fast track)
• Hand injury (fast track)	• Fever without high-risk factors and no features of sepsis
• Closed ankle and foot injuries (fast track)	• Localized cellulitis
• Burns <9% and peripheral in location	• Isolated facial palsy
• Trauma in children without vomiting, LOC, and child being active	• Toothache
• Any patient in pain (fast track)	• Dog bite
	• Patients with incidentally detected high blood sugars
	• Giddiness with no associated illness
	• Any patient in pain (fast track)

TABLE 4: CMC Triage guidelines: Revised edition, January 2021: Priority IV

Trauma	Nontrauma
Patients with chronic trauma with no acute worsening	Patients with chronic problems with no acute worsening

Miscellaneous

Heat-related Illnesses

INTRODUCTION

Heat-related illnesses have a spectrum of severity.
- *Heat cramps*: Core temperature is between 37°C and 39°C. Characterized by brief cramps usually after exertion. Mental function is normal.
- *Heat exhaustion*: Core temperature is between 37°C and 40°C. Symptoms include weakness, fatigue, headache, vertigo, nausea, vomiting, giddiness, and syncope. Mental status remains normal. Most patients recover with adequate rest and fluid replacement.
- *Heat stroke*: Core temperature is more than 40°C (104°F). Many patients with heat-related illnesses may have a core temperature greater than 104°F. However, only patients with central nervous system (CNS) dysfunction (irritability, confusion, hallucinations, ataxia, seizures, focal deficits, or coma) are classified as having a heat stroke. All thermoregulatory function is lost.

DIAGNOSIS

The diagnosis of classic (non-exertional) heat stroke is made clinically with the following triad:
- An elevated core body temperature (generally > 40°C/104°F)
- CNS dysfunction (e.g., altered mental status)
- Exposure to severe environmental heat. This should be determined through history of type of house, place of work, and availability of cooling facilities like air conditioning.

There are two types of heat stroke:
1. *Classic (nonexertional) heat stroke*: Usually, affects the elderly with underlying chronic medical conditions. Bedbound patients left in a hot environment at home and patients on anticholinergics are especially vulnerable.
2. *Exertional heat stroke*: Young healthy people like athletes, military training recruits who perform rigorous exercises in a hot and humid environment may develop exertional heat stroke.

DIFFERENTIAL DIAGNOSIS

Consider the following as the differentials; otherwise you may miss the diagnosis:
- *Infections*: Cerebral malaria, leptospirosis, septic shock, CNS infections
- *Noninfectious causes*: Neuroleptic malignant syndrome (NMS), malignant hyperthermia, thyroid storm, serotonin syndrome.

INVESTIGATIONS TO BE SENT

Complete blood count, liver function tests, electrolytes, creatinine, Urea, prothrombin time, activated partial thromboplastin time, creatine phosphokinase, blood c/s, arterial blood gas, ECG, chest X-ray, urinalysis.

MANAGEMENT

- Secure circulation, airway, and breathing
- *Fluid resuscitation*: IV crystalloids to be rushed in
- *Cooling measures*: The target of cooling at the end of the golden hour (1st hour) should be a core body temperature of 39°C.
  - Move to a cool environment
  - Start internal cooling via cold NS, nasogastric tube ice cold saline/water
  - *Evaporative cooling*: Undress the patient, spray tepid water (not cold) and cool by fans blowing parallel to the body to maximize evaporative heat loss
  - Keep ice packs in the axilla, groin, head and neck (**Fig. 1**)
  - Apply wet sheets loosely over the patient.
- Correct electrolyte abnormalities
- Control shivering with injection promethazine (phenergan) 12.5–50 mg IV
- Anti-epileptic of choice for seizures is phenobarbitone. Avoid phenytoin.
- Identify and treat complications (e.g., CNS dysfunction, rhabdomyolysis, acute kidney injury, acute liver failure, disseminated intravascular coagulation). Monitor sugars for hypoglycemia.

Drugs to be avoided: Anticholinergics, antipyretics (will not help), α adrenergics (increases peripheral resistance), salicylates (may worsen platelet dysfunction), large dose of paracetamol (may worsen hepatic injury).

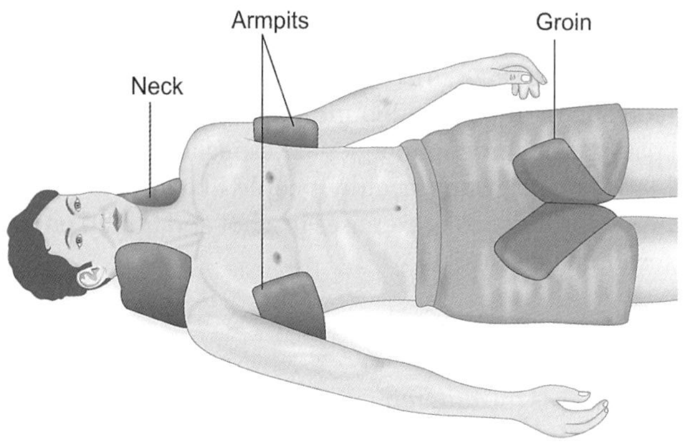

FIG. 1: Ice pack application.

INTRODUCTION

Malignant hyperthermia (MH) is a rare inherited life-threatening condition characterized by excessive oxidative metabolism in the skeletal muscles resulting in hyperpyrexia, circulatory collapse, and even death upon exposure to certain drugs. It usually occurs in the operating theater or during the immediate post-operative period.

Susceptible patients have genetic skeletal muscle receptor abnormalities (abnormal RYR1 or DHP receptors) that allow excessive myoplasmic calcium to accumulate when exposed to certain anesthetic triggering agents. This leads to unregulated passage of calcium from the sarcoplasmic reticulum into the intracellular space, resulting in sustained muscle contraction, change to anaerobic metabolism, rhabdomyolysis, and hyperthermia.

DRUGS IMPLICATED AS POTENTIAL TRIGGERS

These are:
- Halothane
- Isoflurane
- Enflurane
- Sevoflurane
- Desflurane
- Succinylcholine.

CLINICAL PRESENTATION

The earliest sign is an increase in end-tidal carbon dioxide ($ETCO_2$)
- *Early signs*: Sinus tachycardia, masseter muscle rigidity, generalized muscle rigidity
- *Late signs*: Hyperthermia, ECG changes of hyperkalemia, ventricular fibrillation/ventricular tachycardia (VF/VT), myoglobinuria, bleeding.

DIAGNOSIS

The diagnosis must be considered in all patients receiving triggering agents. An increased $ETCO_2$, generalized muscle rigidity, hyperkalemia (K > 6 mEq/L), arterial blood gas pH <7.25, base excess (BE) < –8 mEq/L, creatine phosphokinase >20,000 IU and myoglobinuria strongly suggest the diagnosis.

MANAGEMENT

It includes:

- Stabilize airway and breathing. Optimize oxygenation and ventilation
- *Circulation*: Ensure adequate hydration by administering cold crystalloids
- Discontinue triggering agents
- Dantrolene bolus dose of 2.5 mg/kg IV followed by boluses every 5 minutes of 1 mg/kg IV until acute symptoms abate. Dantrolene binds to the RYR1 receptor and inhibits release of calcium from the sarcoplasmic reticulum; thus reversing the negative cascade of effects
- Monitor and treat hyperkalemia
- *Cooling measures*:
  - Move to a cool environment
  - Start internal cooling via cold normal saline (NS), nasogastric (NG) ice cold saline or water
  - *Evaporative cooling*: Undress the patient, spray tepid water and cool by fans blowing parallel to the body to maximize evaporative heat loss.
- *For ventricular dysrhythmias*: Procainamide loading dose 20–50 mg/min or 100 mg every 5 minutes until arrhythmia is controlled or hypotension occurs.

Neuroleptic Malignant Syndrome

INTRODUCTION

Neuroleptic malignant syndrome (NMS) is a life-threatening emergency caused by an adverse reaction to certain neuroleptic agents. It is characterized by hyperthermia, generalized muscular rigidity, altered sensorium, and autonomic dysfunction.

Drugs that can cause NMS:

- *Neuroleptic agents*:
  - *Highly potent neuroleptics*: Haloperidol, fluphenazine, and prochlorperazine
  - *Low potency neuroleptics*: Chlorpromazine and promethazine
  - *Newer "atypical" antipsychotics*: Clozapine, risperidone, and olanzapine.
- *Antiemetic agents*: Domperidone and metoclopramide.

CLINICAL MANIFESTATIONS

The classical tetrad of NMS symptoms usually evolve over 1–3 days.

- Mental status change in the form of an agitated delirium with confusion or pyschosis is seen in the majority of patients
- Generalized muscular rigidity characterized by "lead pipe rigidity"
- Hyperthermia >38°C
- Autonomic instability in the form of tachycardia, labile or high BP, tachypnea, dysrhythmias, or diaphoresis.

DIAGNOSIS

There is no diagnostic test for NMS. Diagnosis is purely clinical. The differential diagnosis for NMS includes heat stroke, malignant hyperthermia, and severe sepsis. Laboratory abnormalities include leucocytosis (10,000–40,000/cumm), elevated creatine phosphokinase (CPK), electrolyte abnormalities (hypo/hypernatremia, hyperkalemia, hypocalcemia, hypomagnesemia), hepatic transaminitis, and myoglobinuria.

MANAGEMENT

- Discontinue any neuroleptic agent or precipitating drug
- Obtain IV access and start fluid resuscitation. Ensure adequate hydration
- Maintain cardiorespiratory stability

- *Cooling measures*:
  - Move to a cool environment
  - Start internal cooling via cold normal saline (NS), nasogastric (NG) ice cold saline or water
  - *Evaporative cooling*: Undress the patient, spray tepid water and cool by fans blowing parallel to the body to maximize evaporative heat loss.
- Benzodiazepines (lorazepam 0.5–1.0 mg) may be needed to control agitation.
- *Specific therapy*:
  - *Dantrolene*: A direct-acting skeletal muscle relaxant. Doses of 1–2.5 mg/kg IV is typically used in adults and can be repeated every 5–10 minutes to a maximum dose of 10 mg/kg/day, or
  - *Bromocriptine*: A dopamine agonist. Doses of 2.5 mg (through nasogastric tube) q6-8h and titrate up to a maximum dose of 40 mg/day, or
  - *Amantadine*: It has dopaminergic and anticholinergic effects. Initial dose is 100 mg orally.

Electrical Injuries

INTRODUCTION

An electric shock may cause cardiac or respiratory arrest. Thermal injury from the electrical current can result in burns and muscle damage. Muscle spasms from a shock may result in dislocations or fractures or precipitate a fall causing major trauma.

- An electrical short circuit near a person may cause sudden vaporization of metal and deposition of a thin layer of hot metal on the skin, without any electricity passing through the body. These are often superficial and heal uneventfully.
- In contrast, an electrical arcing through the body produces high temperatures and may cause deep dermal or full-thickness burns, especially if clothing catches fire.

CLINICAL PRESENTATION

- If electricity passed through the patient, there are usually two or more entry or exit wounds that are typically painless, gray to yellow depressed areas. Tissue damage will be more extensive than the visible burns.
- Myoglobinuria and renal failure may be caused by damage to deeper layers of skeletal muscles.
- Cardiac injury may result in arrhythmias in up to 30% of victims. Low voltage alternating current (AC) may trigger ventricular fibrillation, while high voltage AC or direct current (DC) are likely to induce transient ventricular asystole.
- Neurological effects, seen in up to 50% of patients include transient loss of consciousness, seizures, coma, headache, transient paralysis, and peripheral neuropathy.
- Other common injuries include spinal cord injuries (due to vertebral fractures), orthopedic injuries (due to associated falls or tetanic muscle contractures), blast injuries, inhalation injuries, ocular injuries (cataract, retinal detachment, corneal burns, intraocular hemorrhage), auditory injuries, and disseminated intravascular coagulation.

INVESTIGATIONS

Complete blood count (CBC), electrolytes, creatinine, urea, serum myoglobin, creatine kinase, urinalysis, ECG, chest X-ray.

MANAGEMENT

- Assess and stabilize airway, breathing, and circulation.
- Examine thoroughly for head, chest, abdomen, and skeletal injuries.
- Examine all over for skin entry or exit burns. Cleanse the skin, and dress the burns with silver sulfadiazine or mafenide acetate.
- Monitor ECG for arrhythmias, conduction defects, and ST and T wave changes. Continuous cardiac monitoring should be instituted for all high-voltage injuries.
- Begin fluid resuscitation with crystalloids (NS/RL). Administer an initial fluid volume of 20–40 mL/kg over the first 1 hour and titrate to urine output of 0.5–1 mL/kg/h in patients with significant burns or myoglobinuria.
- Extremities with significant burns should be splinted in a functional position (35–45-degree extension at the wrist, 80–90-degree flexion at the metacarpophalangeal, and full extension of the proximal interphalangeal and distal interphalangeal joints) to minimize edema and contracture formation.
- Check for compartment syndrome locally. Perform a fasciotomy if needed and debride necrotic tissue.

When to Refer

- Asymptomatic patients with minor low-voltage burns, normal ECG, no palpitations, and no myoglobinuria may be observed for 6–8 hours and discharged.
- All patients with electrical burn injuries need to be referred to plastic surgery.
- Patients with no or minimal external burns but having arrhythmias or renal failure need to be referred to medicine.

INTRODUCTION

Burns is a traumatic injury to the skin cause by excessive heat. They may be caused by heat (flames, hot liquid, steam or hot solid objects), electrical discharge, friction, chemicals (acid/alkali) or radiation.

The severity of burns is determined by the burned surface area, depth of burns (**Table 1**) and presence of co-morbidities. The 'Rule of 9's' is commonly used to estimate the burned surface area in adults and in children (**Table 2** and **Fig. 1**).

- If there is no airway compromise and burns area is greater than 20%, refer to plastic surgery immediately for admission to the burns unit.
- If there is airway compromise or if the burns area is less than 20, admit the patient in the ED and initiate resuscitation as described below.

TABLE 1: Evaluation of depth of burns.

	Superficial burn	Partial thickness burn		Full-thickness burn
		Superficial	Deep	
Appearance	Pink or small blisters	Red to white large blisters	Red and mottled blisters	Waxy, leathery, charred
Sensation	Painful	Pinprick feels sharp	Pinprick feels dull	Anesthetic
Capillary return	Present	Delayed	Absent	Absent
Spontaneous healing	5–10 days	10–14 days	14–21 days	Requires grafting

TABLE 2: Percentage of burns by rule of 9 in adults and children.

	Adults	Children
Upper limbs	9% each (18%)	9% each (18%)
Lower limbs	18% each (36%)	14% each (28%)
Back of trunk	18%	18%
Front of trunk	18%	18%
Head and neck	9%	18%
Perineum	1%	0

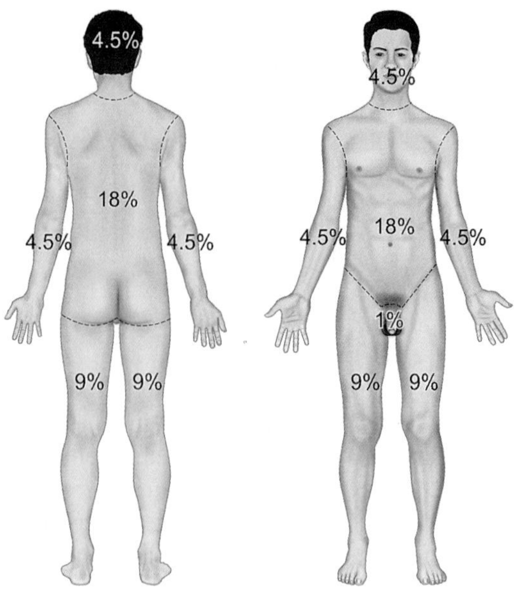

FIG. 1: Rule of 9 in adults.

EMERGENCY DEPARTMENT MANAGEMENT OF BURNS

1. *Maintain airway*: Look for inhalational or facial injuries. Suspect airway compromise and secure the airway.
2. *Secure venous access*: Start 2 large bore (16-G or 18-G) IV lines and send sample for complete blood count (CBC), urea, creatinine, electrolytes, creatine phosphokinase, and liver function test.
3. *Start IV fluids based on modified Parkland formula.*

> *Initial 24 hours:* NS/RL 2–4 mL/kg/% burn (adults)
>
> *Next 24 hours:* Begin colloid infusion of 5% albumin 0.3–1 mL/kg/% burn/16/h

During the first period of 8 hours since the incident, give one half of the above volume. During the second period of 16 hours, give the other half of the total volume.

4. *Provide pain relief*:
   - Injection morphine 0.1 mg/kg IV in small boluses
   - Injection paracetamol 1 g in 100 mL NS
   - Avoid nonsteroidal anti-inflammatory drugs.
5. *Antibiotics*: Prophylactic antibiotics are not indicated in the early postburns period.
6. *Wound management*:
   - Administer diphtheria tetanus (dT) toxoid
   - Debride large blisters and just puncture the small ones with a 25-G needle

- Apply sterile dressings if other unit registrar is going to open the wound initially to allow for repeat examination
- If no further review is required and the wound is clean and dry, apply occlusive dressing which is to be removed after a week.
- *Do not use Paraffin gauze or Sofra-tulle.*
- Silver sulfadiazine (SSD):
    - To be used only in full-thickness and in infected burns
    - Do not use SSD for partial thickness burns
    - Do not wrap SSD dressings circumferentially. Apply them longitudinally.

Admission Criteria/Referral to Plastic Surgery

- More than 15% burns in children
- More than 20% burns in adults
- Involvement of face, hands, feet, genitalia, perineum, and major joints
- Electric burns
- Chemical burns
- Suspected inhalational injury
- Circumferential burns
- Burns in the extreme age groups.

CHAPTER 137

Drowning or Submersion Injuries

INTRODUCTION

In nonfatal drowning, the victim survives at least temporarily after being immersed or submersed in a liquid medium. Drowning may be classified as wet and dry drowning.

- *Wet nonfatal drowning*: Aspiration of fluid into the lungs occurs resulting in pulmonary edema.
- *Dry nonfatal drowning*: No aspiration occurs but patient has a period of asphyxia due to severe persistent laryngospasm. This is triggered by a small amount of water entering the larynx and results in asphyxia with immediate outpouring of thick mucus and froth.

END-ORGAN EFFECTS

- *Pulmonary*: Fluid aspiration may result in varying degrees of asphyxia. Both salt water and fresh water wash out the surfactant in the lungs causing acute respiratory distress syndrome or noncardiogenic pulmonary edema. Some patients may develop dry drowning as described earlier.
- *Cardiovascular*: Arrhythmias may occur secondary to hypothermia and hypoxemia.
- *Neurological*: Hypoxemia and ischemia cause neuronal damage, which may cause cerebral edema and raised intracranial pressure.
- *Metabolic*: A metabolic and/or respiratory acidosis is a common finding.
- *Renal*: Usually due to acute tubular necrosis resulting from hypoxemia, shock, hemoglobinuria, or myoglobinuria.
- Other injuries and disorders that are associated with submersion injuries are spinal cord injuries, hypothermia, panic, seizures and worsening of premorbid conditions.

MANAGEMENT

- Maintain the airway. Remove regurgitated fluid or debris by suction. If the patient is apneic or gag reflex is absent, ventilate with bag and mask and proceed with early endotracheal intubation.
- Ensure adequate ventilation and correct hypoxia with supplemental oxygen.
- Keep the patient on continuous cardiac monitoring. Ventricular dysrhythmias (ventricular tachycardia/ventricular fibrillation), bradycardia, and asystole may occur as a result of acidosis and hypoxemia rather than electrolyte imbalance.

- If patient has a cardiac arrest, commence cardiopulmonary resuscitation. Begin mouth to mouth assisted ventilation at the earliest, even before the victim is extricated from the water. Manoeuvres such as Heimlich and Patrick to remove water from the lungs are ineffective and increase the risk of aspiration. As such, these manoeuvres are not recommended unless airway occlusion by a foreign body is suspected.
- Remove all wet clothing. Check core body temperature and correct hypothermia with with rapid core rewarming techniques (warmed IV fluid infusion, warming adjuncts like blankets and other devices). Defibrillation will not be effective unless hypothermia is corrected and core body temperature is >30°C.
- Insert nasogastric tube to relieve gastric distension.
- Consider the possibility of alcohol or drug overdose.
- Prophylactic antibiotics (carbapenems/piperacillin-tazobactam) may be warranted, if the incident occurred in contaminated water.
- Inhaled particles may have to be removed by bronchoscopy.

Remember that cervical spine trauma may be present in any victim of shallow or rocky water immersion injury. Apply a cervical collar till C spine injury is ruled out.

Alcohol-related Emergencies

ALCOHOL WITHDRAWAL

Alcohol withdrawal symptoms may occur with stopping alcohol consumption or even with decreasing in the daily dose in chronic alcohol consumers. Genetic predisposition may have a role in the fact that some patients develop much severe withdrawal symptoms than others.

Minor withdrawal symptoms: Symptoms include insomnia, tremors, anxiety, gastrointestinal upset, anorexia, headache, diaphoresis, palpitations, and occur due to central nervous system (CNS) hyperactivity.

Withdrawal seizures: These are generalized tonic-clonic seizures that typically occur within 12–48 hours after the last drink, but may occur after only 2 hours of abstinence.

DELIRIUM TREMENS

- Occurs in some alcoholics who undergo withdrawal and carries significant mortality.
- Symptoms of delirium tremens (DT) include hallucinations, disorientation, agitation, hypertension, hyperthermia, tachycardia, and diaphoresis in the setting of acute reduction or abstinence from alcohol.
- Delirium tremens usually manifests between 48 to 96 hours after the last drink and symptoms may last up to 5 days.
- Death occurs from arrhythmias, infection, seizures, or cardiovascular collapse.

WERNICKE'S ENCEPHALOPATHY

This is an acute syndrome that occurs in chronic alcohol consumers who are thiamine deficient. It is characterized by degenerative changes surrounding the third ventricle, aqueduct, and mammillary bodies.

The classic triad of Wernicke's encephalopathy (WE) includes:
- *Encephalopathy*: Profound disorientation, indifference, and inattentiveness
- *Oculomotor dysfunction*: Nystagmus, lateral rectus palsy, and conjugate gaze palsies
- *Gait ataxia*: Ataxia typically affects the trunk and lower extremities.

KORSAKOFF'S PSYCHOSIS

This refers to a chronic neurologic condition that usually occurs as a consequence of thiamine deficiency. Patients suffer from severe impairment of memory (profound retrograde and anterograde amnesia) with relative preservation of other intellectual abilities.

MANAGEMENT OF ALCOHOL WITHDRAWAL/WE/DT

- *Rule out alternative diagnoses*: Metabolic causes, infections, and CNS bleed.
- *Supportive care*: Intravenous (IV) fluids, nutritional supplementation, and frequent clinical reassessment. Thiamine and glucose should be administered in order to prevent or treat WE:
    - Parenteral thiamine 500 mg infused in 1 pint NS over 30 minutes. This can be repeated three times daily. Alternatively, 1 ampoule of multivitamin infusion can be added to dextrose normal saline in each subsequent maintenance fluid.
    - The notion that thiamine must be given prior to dextrose to avoid precipitating WE is largely unsupported.
    - In the ED, do not withhold administration of dextrose for hypoglycemia, if thiamine is not available. However, do not forget to administer thiamine at the earliest.
- *Symptom control*: Benzodiazepines are used to decrease psychomotor agitation. IV lorazepam (2–4 mg IV every 15–20 min) or diazepam (5–10 mg IV every 5–10 min) until the appropriate level of sedation is achieved. Oral chlordiazepoxide (25–100 mg q1h) may also be given till agitation is controlled.
- Patients with severe withdrawal symptoms need admission.
- Patient with mild-to-moderate symptoms may be discharged after controlling agitation on the following medications.
    - *If no liver failure*: Chlordiazepoxide 25 mg PO q6-8h for 5 days and taper.
    - *In patients with chronic liver disease*: Lorazepam 2 mg PO q8h for 5 days and taper.
- Oral thiamine replacement (100 mg od) should continue along with multivitamin supplementation for the next 6 months.
- Refer to psychiatry for further rehabilitation.

INTRODUCTION

- Acute transient visual loss is defined as a sudden onset of visual loss in one or both eyes lasting less than 24 hours. It is caused by a transient vascular occlusion in the circulation to the eye or visual cortex, or by neuronal depression after a seizure or migraine.
  - *Amaurosis fugax*: Unilateral temporary loss of vision within a few seconds to minutes. The cause is a small embolus to the retinal, ophthalmic or ciliary artery and the patient describes it as "a curtain coming down". There is complete recovery.
- Acute persistent visual loss may be defined as visual loss lasting at least 24 hours and is typically not caused by transient ischemia. This can be divided into three categories:
  i. *Media problems*: Keratitis, corneal edema, hyphema, lens changes, vitreous hemorrhage, and uveitis.
  ii. *Retina problems*: Vascular occlusion, retinal detachment, and acute maculopathy.
  iii. *Visual pathway problems*: Optic nerve disease, chiasmal, and retro-chiasmal visual pathway pathology.

COMMON CAUSES OF SUDDEN ONSET PERSISTENT PAINLESS LOSS OF VISION

- *Central retinal artery occlusion (CRAO)*:
  - Due to arterial emboli. There may be a history of amaurosis fugax
  - Look for atrial fibrillation (AF), murmurs or carotid bruit
  - Examination of the eye shows a sluggish or absent direct pupil reaction and a normal consensual reaction (afferent pupillary defect)
  - Fundoscopy shows pale retina with swollen optic disk and "cherry red macula spot".
  - *Treatment*:
    - Gentle digital massage for 5–15 seconds may dislodge the emboli.
    - Acetazolamide 500 mg IV stat (to decrease intraocular pressure).
- *Central retinal vein occlusion*:
  - More frequent cause of painless visual loss than CRAO
  - *Risk factors*: Diabetes mellitus (DM), hypertension (HT), old age, chronic glaucoma, and hyperviscosity syndromes

- Examination shows decreased visual acuity and afferent pupillary defect
- Fundoscopy shows a "stormy sunset appearance" (hyperemia, flame-shaped hemorrhages)
- Outcome is variable. There is no specific treatment refer to ophthalmology to salvage the other eye.
- *Temporal arteritis*:
  - Seen in those aged more than 50 years and is associated with polymyalgia rheumatica
  - Visual loss may be preceded by headaches, jaw claudication, malaise and myalgia
  - Fundoscopy shows a pale disk
  - *Pathology*: Inflammation of the posterior ciliary artery causing optic neuritis
  - If suspected, give 200 mg hydrocortisone IV stat.
- *Vitreous hemorrhage*:
  - *Risk factors*: DM, patients with bleeding disorders
  - Small bleeds may cause vitreous floaters with little visual loss, large bleeds cause visual loss
  - Elevate the head end of the bed to allow blood to collect inferiorly.
- *Retinal detachment*:
  - Occurs in myopes, diabetics, post-trauma and in the elderly
  - Patients may report premonitory flashing lights or a "snow storm" before developing clouding of vision
  - Retina is dark and opalescent but may be difficult to visualize by fundoscopy.
- *Optic neuritis*:
  - Optic nerve inflammation causing visual loss occurs over a few days Usually occurs in young women
  - Most recover untreated, some develop multiple sclerosis.
- *Other causes*: Methanol poisoning, quinine overdose, optic atrophy, and cataract.

APPROACH TO A PATIENT WITH SUDDEN PAINLESS LOSS OF VISION

- Consider ophthalmological pathology and refer to ophthalmologist, if any obvious cause is found.
  - *Examine*: Visual acuity, pupillary reactions, eye movements, fundoscopy.
- Consider and rule out a central cause of blindness:
  - History of recurrent headaches (temporal arteritis), risk factors for an occipital infarct (smoking, DM, HT, etc.), and history of substance abuse (methanol poisoning).

- *Examination*:
    - Palpate temporal artery for tenderness (temporal arteritis)
    - Look for any obvious source of emboli: AF, cardiac murmurs or carotid bruit
    - Look for cortical blindness (patient is aware of his/her blindness and does not deny it) or
    - Anton syndrome (patient is unaware of being blind and denies the problem even when it is pointed out).
- *Investigations*: CT brain or MRI brain and other routine tests.
- *Treatment*:
    - If an occipital infarct is found, give aspirin and statins
    - If temporal arteritis is suspected, give steroids and refer to medicine
    - If no obvious central cause is found refer the patient to ophthalmology.

INTRODUCTION

Acute red eye is a common presentation to the emergency department (ED). The common causes include:
- Foreign body
- *Conjunctivitis*: Allergic, chemical, viral, or bacterial
- Subconjunctival hemorrhage
- Corneal ulceration
- Acute angle closure glaucoma
- Iritis, episcleritis, uveitis.

History

Ask for history of unilateral/bilateral involvement, trauma, visual changes, amount and type of discharge, pain, photophobia, use of contact lens, and presence of systemic disease.

Examination

- Assess vision and visual fields
- Evert the eyelids and inspect the undersurface
- Check pupil size and reflexes
- Examine the cornea, conjunctiva, and iris using a slit lamp, if available.

CHEMICAL OCULAR INJURY

Chemicals including acids and alkalis can cause severe ocular injury and requires immediate intervention right at the site of the incident. These incidents typically occur in industrial settings.
- Irrigate the eye with at least 2 L of normal saline (NS) or ringer lactate (RL). Use an intravenous infusion line to direct a steady controlled flow of NS or RL on to the ocular surface, for atleast 10–15 minutes.
- The goal of irrigation is to remove the offending chemical and restore physiological pH. Monitor the pH using a litmus paper till the target of 7–7.4 is achieved.
- Continue irrigation with up to 8–10 L of NS or RL depending on the chemical and till target pH is achieved.
- Topical cycloplegic (homatropine 5% or cyclopentolate) to alleviate ciliary spasm.
- Topical erythromycin ointment 0.5% every 1–2 hours.

The clinical features and management of common causes of acute red eye is shown in **Table 1**.

TABLE 1: Clinical features and management of acute red eye.		
Etiology	*Clinical features*	*Management*
Conjunctival foreign body	Feeling of foreign body sensation	• Eye irrigation • Evert the eyelid and use a sterile cotton bud to remove the foreign body
Allergic conjunctivitis	Itching, watery discharge, chemosis, history of allergy	• Remove inciting agent • Artificial drops 5–6 times per day • Antihistamine (pheniramine) eye drops 4 times daily • Lubricant (hydroxypropyl methylcellulose) eye drops 4 times daily in both eyes • *In severe cases*: Steroid (fluorometholone) eye drops 4 times daily • Cold compress 4 times daily
Viral conjunctivitis	• Watery discharge, chemosis, conjunctival inflammation • May have viral respiratory symptoms	• Antihistamine (Pheniramine) eye drops 4 times daily • Steroid (fluorometholone) eye drops 4 times daily • Lubricant (hydroxypropyl methylcellulose) eye drops 4 times daily in both eyes • Cold compress 4 times daily
Bacterial conjunctivitis	Mucopurulent discharge, eyelash matting, conjunctival inflammation	• *Antibiotic eye drops*: Chloramphenicol or lomefloxacin or ofloxacin or ciprofloxacin eye drops 4–6 times daily in both the eyes • Antibiotic ointment should be applied on the lower fornix and smeared along the lids at bed time. This prevents the eyelids from sticking together • Lubricant (hydroxypropyl methylcellulose) eye drops 4 times daily in both eyes
Glaucoma (Acute angle closure glaucoma)	Eye pain, headache, cloudy vision, visual halos, vomiting, conjunctival injection, fixed mid-dilated pupil, corneal clouding, raised intraocular pressure	• Refer urgently to ophthalmology • Acetazolamide 500 mg PO stat • Topical timolol 0.5% • Topical pilocarpine 1% 1 drop q15 min for 2 doses • If intraocular pressure does not decrease and vision does not improve, start mannitol IV 100 mL IV stat

URTICARIA

Urticaria (hives) is a common allergic cutaneous reaction characterized by pruritic, erythematous fleeting wheals of various sizes. Angioedema is a similar but more severe edematous reaction involving deeper dermis of the face, neck, and extremities.

Management

- Identify and immediately remove the offending agent
- Antihistamines (Tablet levocetirizine 5-10 mg od × 3-5 days plus tablet ranitidine 150 mg bd × 3-5 days) with or without steroids are the mainstay of treatment
- Advice the patient to apply cold compresses and calamine lotion locally for soothing effect

ERYTHEMA MULTIFORME

- This is an acute self-limited condition characterized by sudden appearance of erythematous or violaceous macules, papules, vesicles, or bullae, distributed in a symmetrical pattern on the palms, soles and back of the hands, arms, legs, or feet.
- Characteristic skin lesions include "target lesions" with three zones of color (a central dark papule or vesicle, surrounded by a pale zone and an erythematous halo)
- Common precipitants include infections (mycoplasma, herpes simplex virus), drugs (antibiotics, anticonvulsants), and malignancies.
- This condition may remain localized to the skin or may evolve into a multi-system disease with mucosal involvement into Stevens–Johnson syndrome (SJS), which could be fatal.

Management

- The most important step is identification and immediate discontinuation of the offending agent
- Supportive care includes fluid and electrolyte replacement, maintenance of thermal regulation, maximizing protein nutrition, meticulous wound care, and aggressive infection control.
- Mild forms may resolve spontaneously in 2-3 weeks. Severe cases with systemic involvement may require a short course of systemic steroids (prednisolone 60–80 mg in divided doses for 3-5 days)
  - Blisters and bullous lesions may be treated with cool, wet soaks of 1:16,000 solution of $KMnO_4$ or 5% aluminum acetate.

Stevens–Johnson Syndrome/Toxic Epidermal Necrolysis

- Stevens-Johnson syndrome/Toxic epidermal necrolysis (TEN) represents opposite ends of a spectrum of the same rare life-threatening mucocutaneous reaction characterized by erythema, epidermal necrosis, and desquamation.
- The percentage of body surface area (BSA) affected determines whether the reaction is classified as SJS or TEN. In SJS <10% BSA is involved, whereas 10–30% BSA is involved in SJS/TEN overlap and >30% BSA epidermal detachment is seen in TEN.
- Common medications responsible for SJS/TEN are allopurinol, NSAIDs, sulfonamide antibiotics, and anticonvulsants (phenytoin, phenobarbitone, and carbamazepine).
- SJS/TEN usually occurs 1–3 weeks after starting the causative drug. Initial manifestations are typically nonspecific. There may be a prodrome of fever, malaise, sore throat, skin tenderness, followed by development of dusky erythematous macules that may progress to flaccid blisters. Buccal, genital and ocular mucosa are commonly involved. Epidermal detachment may result in massive fluid loss and electrolyte imbalance, while severe ocular involvement may result in permanent scarring and visual loss.
- *Management:*
  - The most important step is identification and immediate discontinuation of the offending agent
  - Supportive care includes fluid and electrolyte replacement, maintenance of thermal regulation, maximizing protein nutrition, meticulous wound care, and aggressive infection control.

BULLOUS DISEASES

- Pemphigus vulgaris is a generalized, autoimmune, mucocutaneous eruption common in the 40–60-year age group.
- The typical skin lesions are small, flaccid bullae that break easily forming superficial erosions and crusted ulcerations, which heal slowly and are prone to secondary infections.
- Nikolsky sign (easy dislodgment of the superficial epidermis from the dermal–epidermal junction by a lateral shearing force) is a characteristic finding of this condition
- Bullous pemphigoid is a generalized mucocutaneous blistering disease of the elderly (average age: 70 years) with deeper blisters (below the epidermal basement membrane), better prognosis and more rapid response to therapy than pemphigus vulgaris.
- *Management:*
  - Local wound care and pain control are essential components of management.
  - Refer to dermatology for initiation of steroid therapy or other immuno-suppressants.

INTRODUCTION

Needle stick injuries refer to penetration of the skin by a sharp object, usually hypodermic needles that has been in contact with blood, tissue or other body fluids before the exposure. These injuries increase the risk of blood borne infections and hence extreme caution must be exercised during venesection and while performing major and minor surgical procedures.

Potentially Infectious Exposures

- A percutaneous injury (hollow needles are more infectious than solid needles)
- Contact of mucous membrane or nonintact skin.
  The rate of transmission of HIV, HCV, and HBV through needle-stick injuries (NSI) is 0.3%, 10%, and 30%, respectively.

Body Fluids of Concern

- *Body fluids definitely proven to be infective*: Blood, semen, and vaginal secretions.
- *Potentially infectious fluids of undetermined risk*: Cerebrospinal fluid, synovial, pleural, peritoneal, pericardial, and amniotic fluids.
- *Fluids that are NOT considered infectious*: Tears, saliva, nasal secretions, gastric secretions, sweat, urine, vomitus, and feces.

When to Test for HIV after Exposure?

With or without prophylaxis, testing must be done at baseline, 6 weeks, 3 months, and 6 months.

POSTEXPOSURE PROPHYLAXIS: GENERAL MEASURES

- *Needle-stick injuries:* Wash for 10 minutes with soap and water. Small wounds and punctures can be washed with alcohol (alcohol is virucidal to HIV, hepatitis B virus, and hepatitis C virus).
- *Mucosal exposure*: If eye is involved, irrigate with 500 mL of running NS over 10 minutes with the eye being held open by another person.

PROTOCOL FOR PEP FOR HIV

- Healthcare worker with percutaneous, mucous membrane or non-intact skin exposure to body fluids of concern from a known HIV patient: Follow post exposure prophylaxis (PEP) as shown in **Table 1**.

TABLE 1: Categorization of exposure and recommended prophylaxis.

Exposure	Features	Recommended PEP
Low risk	Solid needles, superficial wound, and low-risk source	Tenofovir 300 mg + Emtricitabine 200 mg × 4 weeks
Mucocutaneous	Small volume	Same as low-risk PEP
High risk	Hollow needle, device with visible blood, needle from artery or vein of the source and high-risk patient	Tenofovir 300 mg + Emtricitabine 200 mg + (Lopinavir 400 mg + Ritonavir 100 mg) × 4 weeks

(PEP: postexposure prophylaxis)

- Healthcare worker with exposure from a source with unknown HIV status. The source should be tested for HIV and PEP can be stopped if the test is negative unless the source is suspected to have acute HIV infection.
- Contamination from an unknown source.

  PEP for HIV should be started as soon as possible. Those who started PEP should complete a full 4-week course of the drugs.

PROTOCOL FOR PEP FOR HEPATITIS B

After exposure to hepatitis B virus, timely prophylaxis can prevent acute infection and development of chronic complications. The mainstay of prophylaxis against hepatitis B is the hepatitis B vaccine and in certain situations, hepatitis B immune globulin for added protection.

Infants born to HBV-positive mothers should be given hepatitis B vaccine and hepatitis B immunoglobulin within 12 hours of birth.

The protocol for PEP for hepatitis B is shown in **Table 2**.

- If the patient presents after 72 hours, administer only hepatitis B virus vaccine (0, 1, and 2 months).
- Check hepatitis B surface antigen status after 6 months and 12 months.

PROTOCOL FOR PEP FOR HEPATITIS C

- Hepatitis C is a major infectious cause of cirrhosis and is associated with high morbidity and mortality.
- Wash the affected area thoroughly (refer general measures for PEP).
- Though many directly acting anti-HCV antiviral (DAA) regimens are currently available, there is insufficient evidence to recommend them as PEP.
- Immunoglobulin is not effective.

TABLE 2: Protocol for PEP for hepatitis B (when presenting within 72 hours of exposure).

Exposed person	Exposure source		
	HBsAg positive	*HBsAg negative*	*Status unknown*
Unvaccinated	Administer HBIG 0.06 mL/kg intramuscularly and initiate the HBV vaccine	Initiate the HBV vaccine	Initiate the HBV vaccine
Vaccinated	Check anti HBs titer, if available: • >100 million IU: No therapy • 10–100 million IU: Administer 1 dose of HBV vaccine • <10 million IU: Administer HBIG + 1 dose of HBV vaccine	No PEP recommended	Check anti-HBs titer, if available: • >100 million IU: No therapy • 10–100 million IU: Administer 1 dose of HBV vaccine • <10 million IU: Give 1 dose of HBV vaccine

(HBsAg: hepatitis B surface antigen; HBIG: hepatitis B immune globulin; HBV: hepatitis B virus; PEP: postexposure prophylaxis)

Drugs in Pregnancy

143

SAFETY RATING OF DRUGS IN PREGNANCY AND LACTATION (TABLE 1)

- *Category A*: Controlled studies in women did not show any risk to the fetus in the first trimester or later. Drugs can be used freely in pregnant and lactating mothers.
- *Category B*: Animal reproduction studies have not demonstrated a fetal risk but there are no controlled studies in pregnant women. Drugs can be used freely in pregnant and lactating mothers.
- *Category C*: Animal studies revealed adverse effects on the fetus. There are no controlled studies among women. Drugs can be administered only if the potential benefit justifies the potential harm to the fetus.
- *Category D*: Evidence of human fetal risk has been demonstrated. However, benefit to the mother from usage in pregnancy significantly outweighs the risk to the fetus. To be used only in life-threatening situations.
- *Category X*: Studies in humans and animals have demonstrated fetal abnormalities and the risks clearly outweigh any possible benefits. These drugs are contraindicated in women who are or may become pregnant.

TABLE 1: List of drugs and their safety during pregnancy.

	Pregnancy	Lactation
Antibiotics		
Amoxicillin, ampicillin, penicillin	Yes (A)	Yes
Augmentin (amoxicillin + clavulanate)	Yes (A)	Yes
Azithromycin	Yes (B)	Yes
Ceftriaxone, cephalexin, cefazolin, ceftazidime	Yes (A)	Yes
Metronidazole	Yes (B)	Yes
Clindamycin	Yes (A)	Yes
Acyclovir, valacyclovir	Yes (B)	Yes
Amikacin	Avoid (D)	Yes
Ciprofloxacin, levofloxacin	Avoid (B)	Yes
Piperacillin-Tazobactam	Yes (B)	Avoid

Continued

Continued

	Pregnancy	Lactation
Ertapenem, imipenem, meropenem	Yes (B)	Yes
Trimethoprim/sulfamethoxazole	Avoid (C)	Yes
Doxycycline	Avoid (D)	No
Albendazole	Avoid (D)	No
Linezolid	Yes (B)	Caution
Rifampicin	Yes (C)	Yes
Chloroquine	Yes (D). Do not withhold in malaria	Yes
Artemether	No data. Do not withhold in malaria	Yes
Antacids		
Ranitidine, omeprazole, pantoprazole	Yes (A)	Yes
Antiemetics		
Doxylamine, metoclopramide, ondansetron, promethazine (phenergan)	Yes (A)	Yes
Antihistamines/nasal decongestants		
Chlorpheniramine (Avil), diphenhydramine (Benadryl), fexofenadine (Allegra)	Yes (A)	Yes
Cetirizine, loratadine	Yes (B)	Yes
Oxymetazoline, phenylephrine	Avoid (D)	Avoid
Antiepileptics		
Phenytoin, phenobarbitone	Yes (D)	Yes
Sodium valproate	Avoid	Avoid
Carbamazepine	Yes (D)	Yes
Levetiracetam, clobazam	Yes (B)	Yes
Antihypertensives		
Amlodipine, nifedipine	Yes (C)	Yes
Diltiazem, verapamil	Yes (C)	Yes
Enalapril, losartan	Avoid (D)	Yes
Hydrochlorothiazide	Yes (C)	Avoid
Metoprolol, atenolol, propranolol	Yes (C)	Yes
Prazosin	Yes (B)	Yes

Continued

Continued

	Pregnancy	Lactation
Others		
Warfarin	Avoid (D)	Yes
Statins	No (C)	Avoid
Enoxaparin	Yes (C)	Yes
Gabapentin	Yes (B)	Yes
Methotrexate	Avoid (D)	Avoid
Ibuprofen, naproxen, diclofenac	Yes (C)	Yes
Ketamine	Yes (B)	Avoid

ACUTE MONOARTHRITIS

Presentation

Acute monoarthritis presents as a hot, swollen red joint, joint line tenderness, decreased range of movements, and systemic symptoms (fever and malaise).

Examination

Look for evidence of a multisystem disease (rash, ocular involvement, orogenital ulcers, and gastrointestinal symptoms).

Causes

- *Traumatic*: Fracture and hemarthrosis (hemophilia)
- *Infective*: Septic arthritis
- *Crystal arthropathy*: Uric acid (gout), calcium pyrophosphate (pseudogout), and hydroxyapatite.

Synovial fluid analysis: This is done to confirm the diagnosis. Send the aspirate for:
- Synovial fluid white blood cells (WBC)
- Synovial fluid gram smear and culture (if frank pus aspirated)
- Polarized microscopy for crystals.

SEPTIC ARTHRITIS

It is due to direct invasion of joint space by various microorganisms. Common pathogens are *Staphylococcus aureus*, *Neisseria gonorrhoeae*, *Streptococcus* and gram-negative bacteria. Most septic joints have a synovial fluid WBC count more than 50,000/μL, with more than 75% neutrophils.

Management

- Strict bed rest. No weight bearing on the joint
- Administer adequate analgesia [opioids and nonsteroidal anti-inflammatory drugs (NSAIDs)]
- *Antibiotics*: (Injection cefazolin 1 g IV stat or injection cloxacillin 1 g IV stat). Continue for 2–4 weeks
- Refer to Orthopedics.

GOUT

Gout refers to deposition of monosodium urate (MSU) crystals in joints, most commonly the great toe, tarsal bones, ankles, knees. Though hyperuricemia is associated, diagnosis can only be confirmed from aspiration of strongly birefringent needle shaped MSU crystals from the inflamed joints or tophi.

- Prompt administration of analgesics is helpful. NSAIDs are the first choice.
- Tablet colchicine is an alternative for acute episodes. Give 1 mg initially followed by 0.5 mg every 4 hours until pain is relieved or vomiting or diarrhea occurs.
- Intra-articular steroid injections may be given to those who cannot take NSAIDs or colchicine.
- Systemic steroids (prednisolone 20–40 mg) for 1–2 days may be given in severe cases.
- Allopurinol and probenecid are not useful for acute attacks of gout.

ACUTE POLYARTHRITIS

Polyarthritis that resolves within 6 weeks is generally associated with viral infections. If symptoms last >6 weeks, it is classified as chronic polyarthritis and warrants a detailed evaluation. Common causes are rheumatoid arthritis, seronegative arthritis (psoriatic arthropathy, ankylosing spondylitis, enteropathic arthritis, and reactive arthritis), systemic lupus erythematosus, crystal arthropathy, and infections.

REACTIVE ARTHRITIS (REITER SYNDROME)

It comprises a triad of:
- Seronegative arthritis
- Nonspecific urethritis
- Conjunctivitis.

It has been associated with:
- Gastrointestinal infections, caused by *Shigella, Salmonella, Yersinia, Campylobacter*, and others
- Genitourinary infections, caused by *Chlamydia trachomatis*.

  The arthritis begins about 2 weeks after infection and the lower limb joints are most commonly affected. Joint involvement is usually asymmetrical and resolves over months. NSAIDs are the mainstay of therapy.

INTRODUCTION

- Procedural sedation involves the use of short-acting analgesic and sedatives to perform procedures effectively, while monitoring for potential adverse effects.
- Propofol, benzodiazepines (midazolam), etomidate, ketamine, fentanyl, and ketofol (ketamine + propofol) are usually used.

KETAMINE

It provides sedation, analgesia, and amnesia.

Dissociative anesthesia: Acts by causing dissociation between the thalamocortical and limbic systems. It provides analgesia and amnesia without loss of consciousness.

Contraindications:
- Raised intracranial pressure (ICP)
- Severe systemic hypertension
- Raised intraocular pressure
- History of seizures or psychosis
  Onset of action is 1–2 minutes and duration of action is 10–20 minutes.

Dose:
- Usual induction dose is 1–2 mg/kg over 1–2 minutes
- Doses of 0.25–0.5 mg/kg may be repeated every 5–10 minutes thereafter.

Side effects: Tachycardia, hypertension, laryngospasm, emergence reactions (disorientation, hallucinations, nightmares), hypersalivation, nausea, and vomiting.
- Glycopyrrolate (5 µg/kg) or atropine (0.5–1 mg) may be given for hypersalivation.
- Midazolam 1–2 mg may be used for treating or preventing emergence reactions.
- *Laryngospasm*: If a patient develops laryngospasm, attempt to break it by applying a painful inward and anterior pressure at the "Larson's point"/"laryngospasm notch", which is located near the top of the ramus of the mandible (**Fig. 1**). Also consider deepening the sedation with a low dose of propofol to reduce laryngospasm.

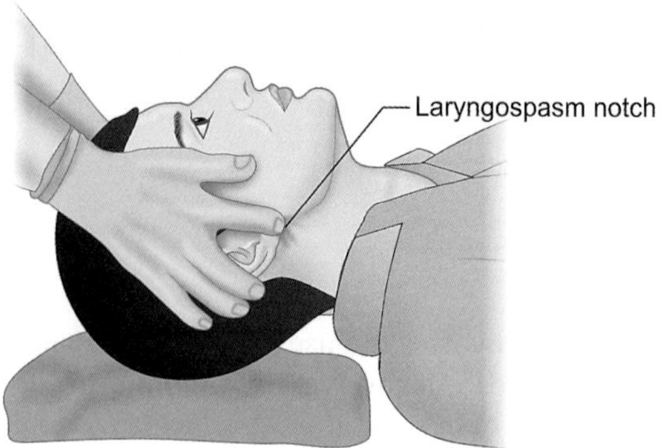

FIG. 1: Larson's point/laryngospasm notch.

MIDAZOLAM

Midazolam is a short acting benzodiazepine that provides anxiolysis and amnesia. No analgesia.

Dose:
- 0.02–0.03 mg/kg slow intravenous (IV) bolus
- Repeat doses may be given every 2–5 minutes as necessary
- Maximum single dose is 2.5 mg and maximum cumulative dose is 5 mg.
- Onset of action is 1–2 minutes and duration of action is 30–60 minutes.

Side effects: Respiratory depression and hypotension. Action reversed by flumazenil.

FENTANYL

It is a synthetic short-acting opioid that has 75–125 times the potency of morphine. It provides analgesia. No amnesia or anxiolysis.
- Onset of action is 1–2 minutes and duration of action is 30–60 minutes.

Dose:
- 0.5–1 µg/kg slow IV push every 2 minutes, until an appropriate level of sedation and analgesia is achieved
- The maximum total dose is 5 µg/kg or approximately 250 µg.

Side effects: Respiratory depression and hypotension (rare). Naloxone may be used to reverse respiratory depression.

Section **22**

Procedures

INTRODUCTION

Nerve blocks should be administered to all patients requiring emergency procedures such as debridement, dressing, fracture reduction, and wound wash with or without procedural sedation. Digital nerve block, wrist block, and ankle block are the most commonly administered blocks and do not require ultrasound guidance.

- The choice of the local anesthetic (LA) depends on the desired duration of the block. 2% lignocaine is used for shorter duration of blockade, while 0.5% bupivacaine is used for longer blockade (**Table 1**).
- Ensure IV access, monitoring, and full resuscitation facilities are available prior to the procedure, due to possibility of anaphylaxis/systemic toxicity.

TABLE 1: Characteristics of local anesthetics.

Local anesthetic	Onset of action (minutes)	Anesthesia (hours)	Analgesia (hours)
2% lignocaine	10–20	2–5	3–8
0.5% bupivacaine	15–30	5–15	6–30

DIGITAL NERVE BLOCK (FINGER WEB SPACE BLOCK)

This is administered for conditions like finger or toe lacerations, nail bed injuries, paronychia drainage, and nail avulsion.

Contraindications

- Infection at the site of block
- Allergy to the anesthetic agent
- Compromised digit circulation.

Techniques (Fig. 1)

- Prepare the area with chlorhexidine solution
- Place the hand flat with palmar side down on a sterile drape.
- Inject 2 mL of 2% lignocaine or 0.5% bupivacaine into the subcutaneous tissue of web space at the base of finger just distal to metacarpophalangeal joint using a 26-G hypodermic needle

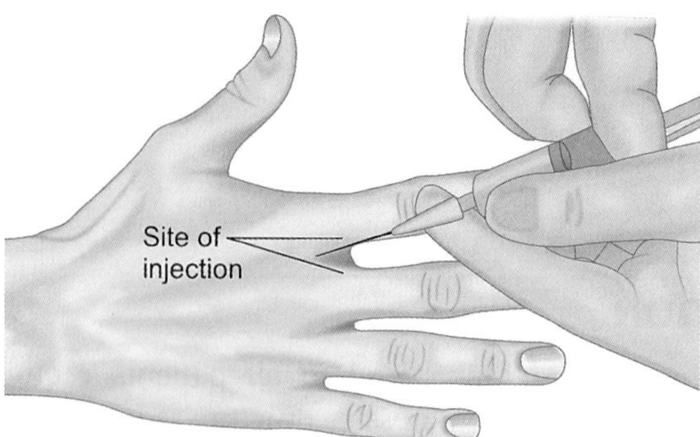

FIG. 1: Web space block.

- Withdraw the needle completely and repeat the procedure on the web space of the opposite side of the finger.

Precautions

- Avoid using an anesthetic with adrenaline for webspace blocks
- Aspirate before injecting the drug to rule out intravascular injection
- Avoid injecting directly into the nerves.

WRIST BLOCK

A wrist block is a procedure by which the terminal branches of the ulnar nerve, median nerve, and radial nerve are blocked separately by administering an LA.

Indications

Surgeries of the hand and finger, carpal tunnel.

Contraindications

- Infection at the site of block
- Allergy to the drug.

Radial Nerve Block

Anatomy

Radial nerve emerges between the brachioradialis tendon and the radius just proximal to the styloid process and becomes superficial to supply the dorsum of hand. Because the radial nerve has a less predictable anatomic location and divides into multiple smaller cutaneous branches, a more extensive infiltration is required.

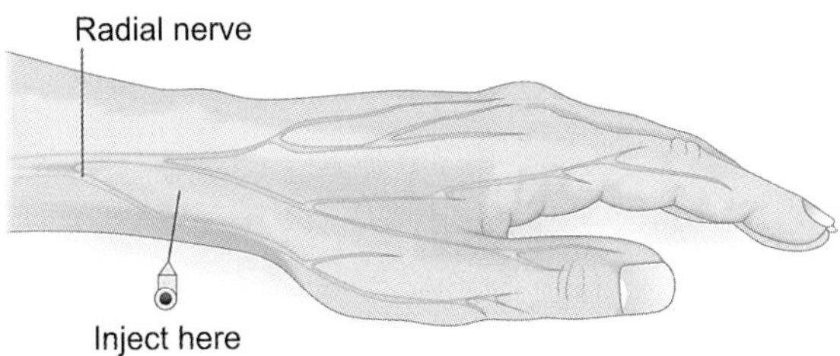

FIG. 2: Radial nerve block.

Procedure (Fig. 2)

- Position: With the patient supine or sitting, keep the arm abducted, fore arm pronated, and wrist in slight dorsiflexion.
- Insert a 26-G needle just proximal to the styloid process of the radius in the anatomical snuff box and aim medially
- After negative aspiration, inject about 3 mL of 2% lignocaine
- After that, direct the needle laterally and inject an additional 3 mL of LA subcutaneously in a fan-shaped manner.

Median Nerve Block

Anatomy

Median nerve is located in the flexor retinaculum between tendons of palmaris longus and flexor carpi radialis. The palmaris longus can be identified by asking the patient to oppose the thumb and the little finger.

Procedure (Fig. 3)

- Insert a 26-G needle between the tendons of palmaris longus and flexor carpi radialis until it hits the bone.
- Withdraw the needle slightly and inject about 3–5 mL of LA after ruling out intravascular injection by negative aspiration.

Ulnar Nerve Block

Anatomy

The ulnar nerve runs between the ulnar artery and the flexor carpi ulnaris tendon (the most medial tendon palpable).

Procedure (Fig. 3)

- Insert a 26-G needle under the flexor carpi ulnaris tendon and advance about 5–10 mm laterally
- After negative aspiration, inject about 3 mL of LA.
  The cutaneous nerve supply of the hand is shown in **Figure 4**.

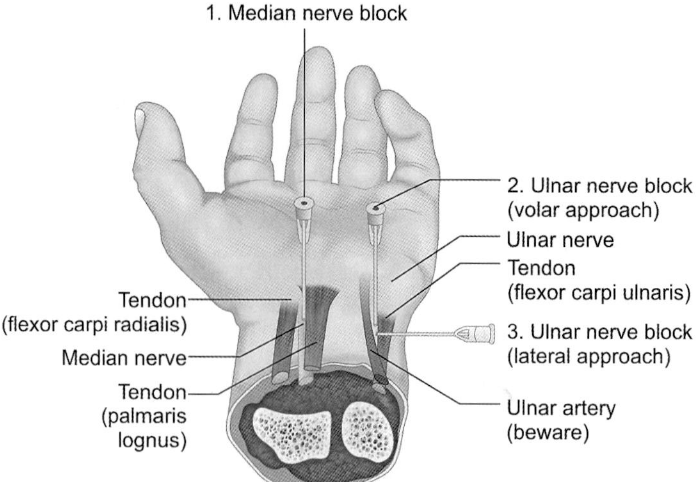

FIG. 3: Median and ulnar nerve blocks.

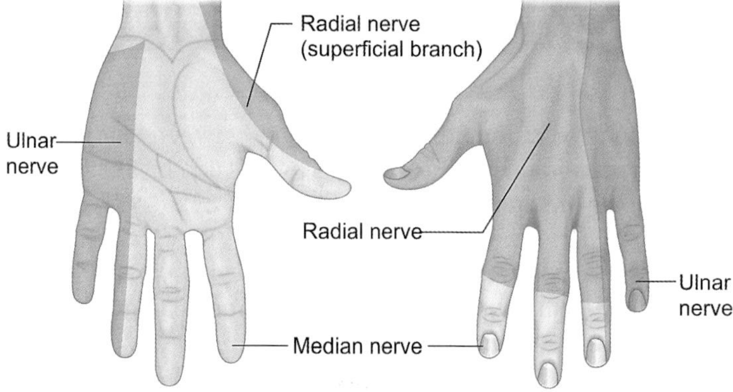

FIG. 4: Cutaneous nerve supply of the hand.

ANKLE BLOCK

The ankle block is used for surgery of the foot and toes and is a purely sensory block. It consists of separate blocks of five nerves (**Figs. 5** to **7**):

1. Four branches of the sciatic nerve
   i. Superficial peroneal (fibular) nerve
   ii. Deep peroneal (fibular) nerve
   iii. Tibial nerve
   iv. Sural nerve
2. One cutaneous branch of the femoral nerve
   i. Saphenous nerve.

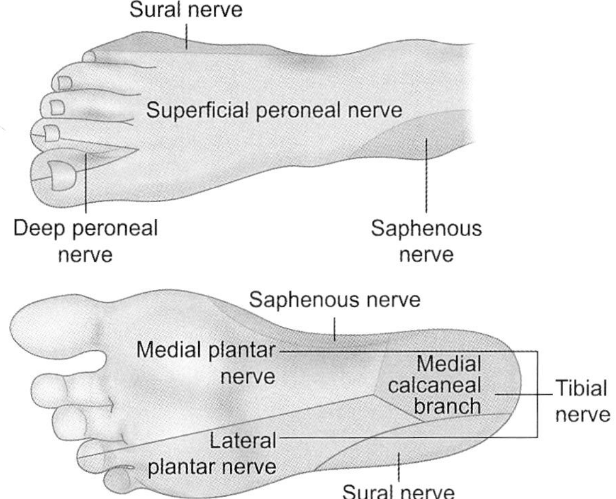

FIG. 5: Cutaneous nerve supply of the foot.

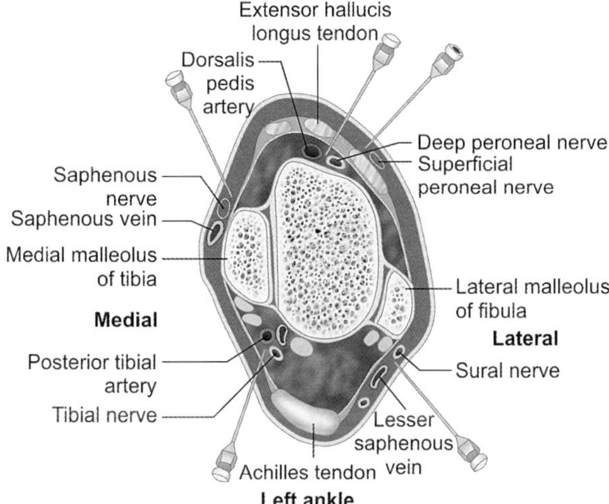

FIG. 6: Axial view showing the plane of the nerves at the level of the ankle.

Positioning

Position the patient supine, with the foot elevated and supported on blankets or pillows, and the ankle is rotated as necessary for needle placement.

Deep Peroneal Nerve Block

- Palpate the dorsalis pedis artery between the tendons of extensor hallucis longus and extensor digitorum longus. Extensor hallucis tendon can be identified by having the patient extend the great toe.

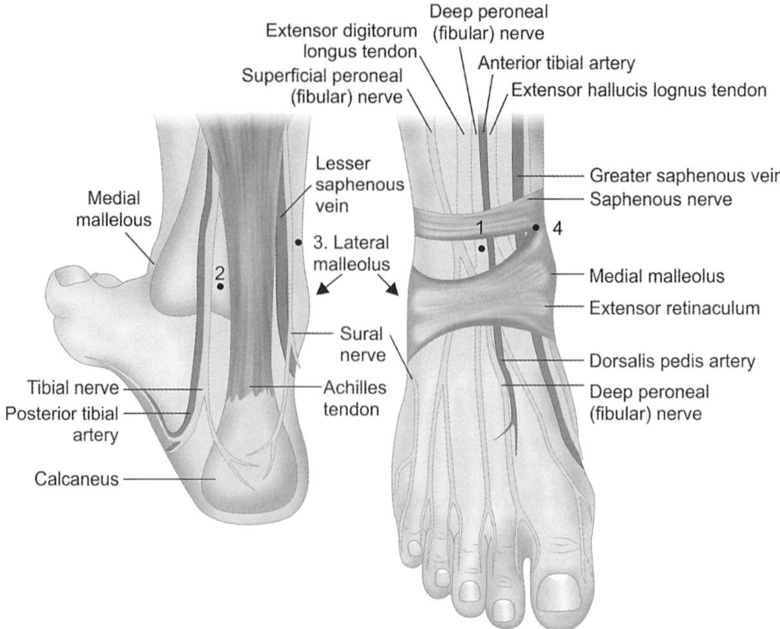

FIG. 7: Nerves around the ankle and ankle block injection sites.

- At the mid-tarsal portion of the foot, insert the needle just lateral to the extensor hallucis tendon and advance until bone is encountered.
- Inject 2–3 mL of LA in the deep plane as the needle is slowly withdrawn.

Superficial Peroneal Nerve Block

- The superficial peroneal nerve innervates the dorsum of the foot and is blocked by subcutaneous infiltration of LA.
- Insert the needle at the injection site for deep peroneal nerve block.
- Inject about of 5–10 mL of LA subcutaneously over the dorsum of the foot medially and then laterally from the site of needle insertion to the level of the malleoli.

Posterior Tibial Nerve Block

- The distal tibial nerve provides sensation to the calcaneus and plantar surface (sole) of the foot and is blocked at the level of the medial malleolus
- Palpate the posterior tibial artery behind the medial malleolus
- Insert the needle posterior to the artery, and advance until the bone is reached while aiming toward the malleolus at a 45 degree angle
- After negative aspiration, inject 2–3 mL of LA
- To increase the success rate of the block, inject an additional 1–2 mL of LA using a fan technique, medially and laterally.

Sural Nerve Block

- The sural nerve innervates the lateral ankle and foot, as well as the fifth toe. It runs within the subcutaneous tissues behind the lateral malleolus
- Insert the needle subcutaneously just behind the lateral malleolus
- Inject 2–3 mL of LA behind the lateral malleolus directed toward the Achilles tendon as a subcutaneous wheal.

Saphenous Nerve Block

- The saphenous nerve innervates the medial aspect of the ankle and foot. It is blocked at the ankle using anatomic landmarks
- Insert the needle medial and superior to the medial malleolus and direct it posteriorly toward the Achilles tendon
- After negative aspiration, inject 2–3 mL of LA as a subcutaneous wheal.

> Deep peroneal nerve and posterior tibial nerves lie deep and need to be injected deep for nerve block.
>
> Superficial peroneal nerve, sural nerve and saphenous nerve lie superficially and need to be injected subcutaneously for nerve block.

SYSTEMIC TOXICITY OF LOCAL ANESTHETICS (BUPIVACAINE/LIGNOCAINE)

While generally safe, local anesthetic agents can be toxic. The toxicity of local and infiltration anesthetics can be local or systemic. Systemic toxicity of anesthetics most often involves the central nervous system (CNS) or the cardiovascular system (CVS). Manifestations of local anesthetic toxicity typically appear 1–5 minutes after the injection, but onset may range from 30 seconds to as long as 60 minutes.

- *CNS manifestations*: Systemic toxicity begins with symptoms of CNS excitement (circumoral and/or tongue numbness, metallic taste, lightheadedness, dizziness, muscle twitching, convulsions, etc.) followed by CNS depression (unconsciousness, coma, respiratory depression, and arrest)
- *Cardiovascular manifestations*: Chest pain, shortness of breath, palpitations, diaphoresis, hypotension, syncope
- *Hematologic manifestations*: Methemoglobinemia (benzocaine, lidocaine, prilocaine, etc.)
- *Allergic manifestations*: Rash, urticaria, anaphylaxis (very rare), etc.

Management of Systemic Toxicity

Treatment of local anesthetic toxicity includes the following:
- Stop injecting more local anesthetic
- Stabilize airway

- *Seizure suppression*: Benzodiazepines/barbiturates for seizures
- *Management of cardiac dysrhythmias*: Look for prolonged PR, QRS, and QT intervals potentiating reentrant tachycardias with aberrant conduction, which may herald CVS toxicity. Follow advanced cardiac life support (ACLS) guidelines for management of arrhythmias.
- Use Amiodarone as first line drug for arrhythmias in usual doses.
- *Lipid emulsion therapy*: Cardiac resuscitation may be difficult and prolonged (>30 min) because some anesthetics are very lipid soluble and require a long time for redistribution. Lipid emulsion therapy is performed with an intravenous (IV) infusion of a 20% solution.
  - Administer a bolus of 1.5 mL/kg over 1 minute. (If patient >70 kg then give a maximum dose of 100 mL IV bolus)
  - Then convert to an infusion at a rate of 0.25 mL/kg/min for 30–60 minutes or until hemodynamic stability is restored
  - After that, the infusion should be continued for at least 10 minutes longer.
  - Repeat the bolus dose and double the rate of infusion in case of persistent or recurrent cardiovascular collapse.
  - Maximum dose of lipid emulsion: 12 mL/kg
- *Treatment of allergic reactions*: Antihistamines or epinephrine as needed.

SUBCLAVIAN LINE

- It is associated with the lowest rate of thrombosis.
- Position a sheet roll between the shoulder blades and keep the head down.
- If the patient is on a chest tube, insert the line on the same side.
- Site of insertion of the needle: 2 cm inferior to the junction of the middle and medial third of the clavicle.
- Advance the needle under and along the inferior border of the clavicle toward the suprasternal notch until the vein is entered.
- Fix the line at 14 cm for females and 16 cm for males.
- Postprocedure X-ray check is mandatory and should be followed up by the person inserting the central line.

INTERNAL JUGULAR LINE

- Place the patient in Trendelenburg position with the head down.
- *Site of insertion of the needle*: Locate the apex of the triangle formed by the sternal and clavicular heads of the sternocleidomastoid (SCM) muscle and the clavicle. The internal jugular vein (IJV) lies 1 cm lateral to the internal carotid artery.
- Insert the needle at the apex of this triangle, lateral to the carotid pulsation and directed toward the ipsilateral nipple at an angle of 30–45 degree to the skin.
- The IJV should be reached no deeper than 2.5 cm.
- Ensure good dilatation of the SCM before inserting the central venous catheter.
- Postprocedure X-ray check is mandatory and should be followed up by the person inserting the central line.

FEMORAL LINE

- Consider this in a patient with bleeding risk, and bleeding parameters not available. It is the safest site to start a central line.
- This is also the route of choice for an inexperienced person in an emergency
- The point of insertion is 1 cm below the inguinal ligament and 1 cm medial to the pulsating femoral artery.
- Drawback of a femoral approach is an increased incidence of venous thrombosis.

Technique of Insertion of a Central Line

- Seldinger technique is used for placement of the central venous catheter.
- Clean and drape the site of catheter insertion. Identify the target vessel and anesthetize the site with lignocaine by creating a subcutaneous wheal.
- Connect a wide bore introducer needle in the central venous set to a 5 cc disposable syringe. Insert the needle at the anesthetized site and advance gradually with negative pressure on the syringe to aspirate venous blood. Disconnect the syringe once there is free flow of venous blood and occlude the needle hub to avoid air being drawn by the negative intrathoracic pressure.
- Then, insert the blunt tipped guidewire through the introducer needle and remove the introducer needle while holding the guidewire in place.
- Enlarge the insertion site with a stab using 11-size blade or using a dilator. Thread the dilator over the guidewire while holding the guidewire in place during insertion and removal of the dilator.
- Then thread the central venous catheter over the guidewire while withdrawing the guidewire until it protrudes from the infusion port of the catheter. Hold the guidewire firmly and place the catheter at the desired depth. Remove the guidewire.
- Aspirate and confirm free flow of blood from all lumens, secure the catheter with appropriate sutures.

SURGICAL PEARLS

- Wear appropriate PPE including mask, cap, gown, and gloves.
- Make sure that all the required equipment is in place, sterile area secured, towels clamped, all lines flushed and guidewire ready for access before starting the procedure.
- Anesthetize the suture site as well as the insertion site.
- Watch out for ectopic beats on the monitor while inserting guidewire during IJV and subclavian cannulation, readjust guidewire to prevent arrhythmias.
- Look out for a return of red pulsatile blood, which indicates that the needle is in an artery. Remove the needle immediately and apply firm pressure for at least 2 minutes or longer, if required to prevent hematoma formation.

Chest Tube Insertion

148

REQUIREMENT

- 1% or 2% lidocaine with epinephrine
- Syringes and needle for local
- Blade No. 10 or No. 11
- Large and medium Kelly clamps
- Large straight suture scissors
- Chest tube of appropriate size
  - *Adult male*: 28–32F
  - *Adult female*: 24–28F
  - *Child*: 12–28F
  - *Infant*: 12–16F
  - *Neonate*: 10–12F.
- Silk or nylon suture, 0 or 1-0 needle holder
- Chest tube drainage device with water seal.
- Personal protective equipment (PPE)
- Sterile drapes, sponges, gauze and elastic tape.

PROCEDURE

- The arm on the affected side should be abducted and externally rotated, simulating a position in which the palm of the hand is behind the patient's head.
- Identify "safe triangle" formed (**Fig. 1**):
  - Anteriorly by the lateral border of the pectoralis major
  - Laterally by the lateral border of the latissimus dorsi
  - Inferiorly by the line of the fifth intercostal space
  - Superiorly by the base of the axilla.
- Make a 1-cm skin incision in between the midaxillary and anterior axillary lines over the lower rib in the fifth intercostal space.
- Direct the drain track over the top of the lower rib to avoid the intercostal vessels lying below each rib. The incision should easily accommodate the operator's finger.
- Using a curved clamp, deepen the track by blunt dissection only. Insert the clamp into muscle tissue and spread to split the fibers. The track should be developed with the operator's finger.
- Once the track comes onto the rib, angle the clamp just over the rib and continue dissection until the pleura is entered by puncturing it.

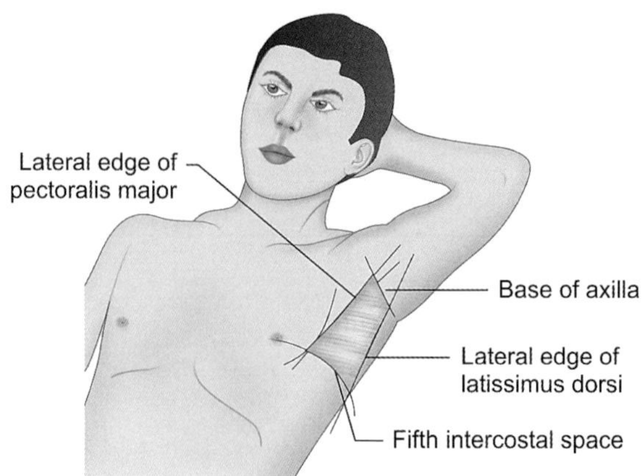

FIG. 1: Site of chest tube insertion (safe triangle).

- Insert a finger into the pleural cavity and explore the area for pleural adhesions.
- Mount the appropriate size chest tube on the clamp and pass it along the track into the pleural cavity. Direct the tube superiorly for pneumothorax and inferiorly for pleural effusion/hemothorax.
- Connect the tube to an underwater seal and suture or secure it in place.
- Reexamine the chest to confirm effect.
- Perform a chest X-ray (CXR) to confirm the placement and position.

COMPLICATIONS

- *Improper placement*: Make sure that all the holes in the chest tube are inside the pleural cavity. Subcutaneous position of the holes may cause subcutaneous emphysema.
- *Bleeding*: Local bleeding usually responds to direct pressure. Intercostal artery injury might require thoracotomy.
- *Hemoperitoneum (liver or spleen injury)*: This may require urgent laparotomy.
- Tube dislodgement.
- *Infection*: Local (site of insertion) or empyema.

INTRODUCTION

An intraosseous (IO) line is as effective as an intravenous (IV) route for emergency drugs and fluid administration. It can be inserted much faster than a peripheral line in patients in shock or cardiac arrest in whom IV access may be difficult. Fluids and drugs should be administered under pressure using a syringe and stopcock manually, using pressure bag or infusion pumps

PROCEDURE

- Palpate the tibial tuberosity. Locate one finger's breadth below and medial to the tuberosity. (The bone can be felt under the skin at this site).
- Clean the skin over and surrounding the site with an antiseptic solution.
- Stabilize the proximal tibia with the left hand by grasping the thigh and knee above and lateral to the cannulation site, with the fingers and thumb wrapped around the knee but not directly behind the insertion site (**Fig. 1**).
- Insert the needle at a 90-degree angle with the bevel pointing toward the foot. Advance the needle using a gentle but firm, twisting, or drilling motion.
- Stop advancing the needle when you feel a sudden decrease in resistance.
- Aspirate 1 mL of the marrow contents (looks like blood); using a 5 mL syringe, to confirm that the needle is in the marrow cavity.

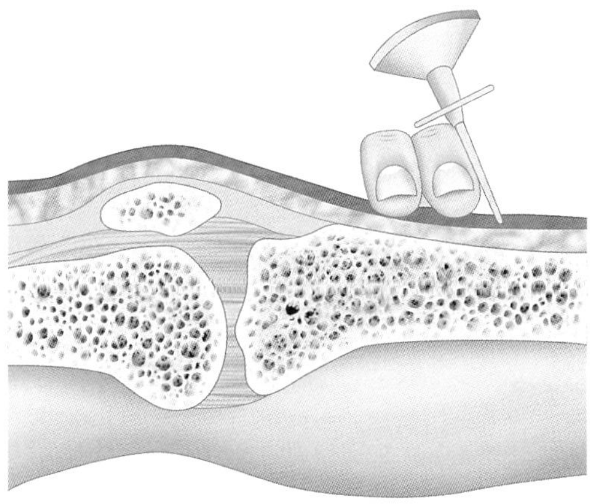

FIG. 1: Intraosseous needle insertion.

- Attach a 5 mL syringe filled with normal saline. Stabilize the needle and slowly inject 3 mL while palpating the area for any leakage under the skin. If no such infiltration is seen, start the infusion.
- Apply dressings and secure the needle in its place.

Note: IO infusions should not continue for >24 hours. It is usually removed within 8 hours once a central venous access is established.

COMPLICATIONS

- *Incomplete penetration of the bony cortex*: This happens if the needle is not well fixed; infiltration occurs under the skin. Push in the needle further to overcome this problem.
- *Penetration of the posterior bone cortex (more common)*: Suspect this if infiltration occurs (calf becomes tense), with the needle well fixed. Remove the needle and repeat at another site. This problem may be avoided by placing the index finger against the skin to prevent the needle from going in too deeply.
- *Blockage of the needle by marrow*: Suspect this if the infusion stops. The line must then be flushed by 5 mL of normal saline.
- *Infection*: This is rare if the infusion is left for less than 24 hours, osteomyelitis is very rare. Cellulitis may be seen at the site of the infusion. Remove the IO needle unless it is essential; give local skin care and antibiotic treatment.
- *Necrosis and sloughing of the skin at the site of the infusion*: This occurs particularly when drugs such as adrenaline or sodium bicarbonate pass into the tissues. Avoid by infusing gently and not under pressure.

INTRODUCTION

Cricothyroidotomy is performed as a last resort in cases of airway compromise where intubation is impossible. This procedure is easier and quicker to perform than tracheostomy, does not require manipulation of the cervical spine, and is associated with fewer complications.

INDICATIONS

- Facial and oropharyngeal swelling from severe trauma, or due to inhalational burns
- Angioneurotic edema
- Foreign body obstruction
- Facial, oropharyngeal, and laryngeal edema from anaphylaxis (insect bites, bee stings, drugs, etc.)
- Infection (epiglottitis).

ANATOMY OF THE CRICOTHYROID MEMBRANE

The cricothyroid membrane, as the name suggests, is bounded by the cricoid cartilage inferiorly and the thyroid cartilage superiorly. The key anatomic landmarks are hyoid cartilage, thyroid cartilage, cricothyroid membrane, cricoid cartilage, and the tracheal rings.

- In adults, the laryngeal prominence at the upper border of the thyroid cartilage is easily felt. The thyroid cartilage can then be followed inferiorly to locate the cricothyroid membrane.
- In children, the laryngeal prominence is not developed, making it difficult to identify the thyroid cartilage. Instead, it is easier to follow the tracheal rings superiorly to locate the prominence of the cricoid cartilage.

The cricothyroid arteries and veins usually overlie the apical portion of the membrane and proceed from the sides, anastomosing in the midline. Hence, cricothyroidotomy should be performed in the central, lower portion of the membrane.

NEEDLE CRICOTHYROIDOTOMY (FIG. 1)

This is a temporary measure, to be adapted when surgical cricothyroidotomy cannot be performed due to lack of equipment or experience. It may be performed on patients of any age but is considered to be preferable to surgical

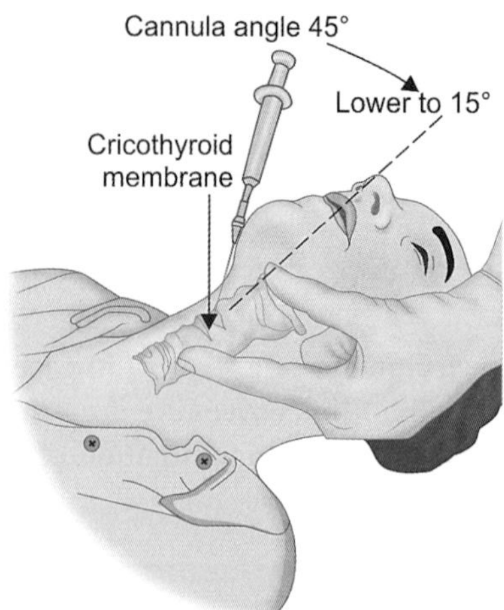

FIG. 1: Needle cricothyroidotomy.

cricothyroidotomy in children up to 12 years of age because of less potential damage to the larynx and surrounding structures. It is important to remember that effective ventilation cannot be established by this maneuver, since it provides very limited airflow.

Equipment: 12G or 14G intravenous (IV) cannula, 2 mL syringe.
- Fix a 2 mL syringe with 1 mL of saline or water for injection in it, on the end of the wide bore IV cannula.
- Identify the cricothyroid membrane
- Introduce the cannula through the cricothyroid membrane at 90 degree with the needle pointing inferiorly.
- Aspirate gently as the cannula is introduced. Bubbles of air escape through the saline in the syringe.
- Advance the cannula forward off the needle until its hub is at the skin surface and then remove the needle.
- Take the plunger out of the 2 mL syringe and then force the oxygen tubing down the end of the barrel of the 2 mL syringe and connect to the oxygen source.
- The patient can be adequately oxygenated for about 45 minutes. Because of inadequate exhalation, there will be progressive accumulation of carbon dioxide.
- Establish more definite airway.

SURGICAL CRICOTHYROIDOTOMY (FIG. 2)

Equipment needed: Scalpel with no. 10 blade, bougie and cuffed tracheostomy tube size 6.

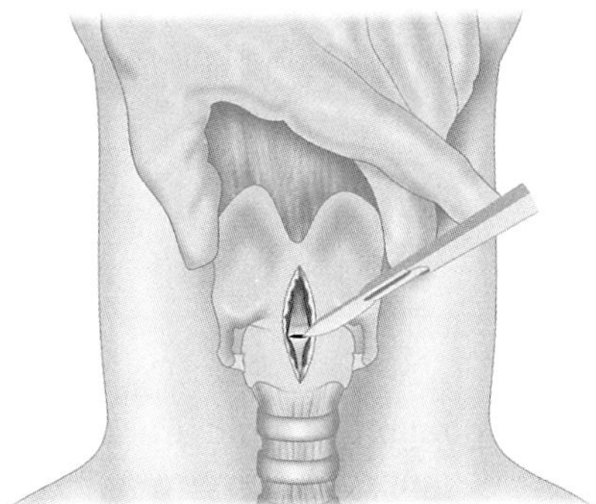

FIG. 2: Surgical cricothyroidotomy.

- Stand on right side of the patient if you are right-handed. Stabilize the larynx with the left hand by using thumb and middle finger over the thyroid cartilage. Identify the cricothyroid membrane by palpation using the index finger.
- Make a 4 cm vertical incision over the skin in the midline at the level of the membrane and use blunt dissection till the membrane. Make a horizontal stab in the membrane using the blade and rotate the blade by 90-degree (sharp end caudally) to create a stoma.
- Use blade to stent the opening and insert the bougie. Direct the bougie caudally and feel for tracheal clicks or resistance if the carina is reached to confirm position into the trachea. Avoid forcing the bougie.
- Insert the tracheostomy tube or size 6 endotracheal tube over the bougie into the trachea and remove the bougie

Complications of surgical cricothyroidotomy:
- Bleeding
- Placement of the tube anterior to the trachea in the subcutaneous plane resulting in a subcutaneous emphysema.

INTRODUCTION

Pericardiocentesis is the aspiration of fluid from the pericardial space that surrounds the heart. In case of tamponade, even a small amount of fluid aspirated can cause a significant improvement to the hemodynamic status of the patient. The classic Becks triad of cardiac tamponade includes distended neck veins, muffled heart sounds, and hypotension. Most patients will have at least one of these signs; all three rarely appear simultaneously.

INDICATIONS

- *Emergency pericardiocentesis*: Suspected cardiac tamponade with life-threatening hemodynamic changes.
- *Nonemergency pericardiocentesis*: For diagnostic, palliative, or prophylactic reasons, performed under ultrasonography.

TECHNIQUE (FIG. 1)

- Subcostal (subxiphoid) approach
  - Prepare the skin by applying a chlorhexidine-based solution to the chest and upper abdomen and drape the region to maintain sterility
  - Anesthetize the puncture site and needle track in alert patients via infiltration of local anesthetic

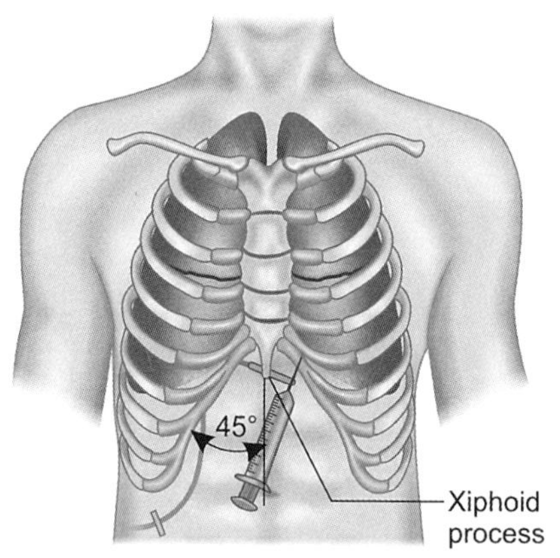

FIG. 1: Pericardiocentesis (subxiphoid approach).

- ○ Introduce the needle substernally 1 cm inferior to the left xiphocostal angle
- ○ Aim the needle toward the left shoulder at an angle of 30–45 degree to the chest wall and advance it slowly while continuously aspirating
- ○ If no fluid is aspirated, the needle should be withdrawn promptly and redirected. In the absence of ultrasound guidance, withdraw the needle to the skin and redirect it along a deeper posterior trajectory
- ○ In most cases, a 7–9 cm needle is adequate, but longer needles (up to 12 cm) may be needed for obese patients
- ○ When you strike blood, withdraw the stylet and leave the cannula behind
- ○ Observe for improvement in hemodynamic status. If cardiac tamponade is present, there is instant relief even with aspiration of 10 mL of blood.
- *Parasternal approach*: Insert the needle perpendicular to the skin and over the cephalad border of the fifth or sixth rib immediately adjacent to the sternal margin.
- *Apical approach*: Insertion site is at least 5 cm lateral to the parasternal approach within the 5th, 6th, or 7th intercostal space. Advance the needle over the cephalad border of the rib and towards the patient's right shoulder. There is a higher risk of pneumothorax with this approach.

COMPLICATIONS

- Cardiac dysrhythmia
- Cardiac puncture
- Pneumothorax
- Hemothorax
- Coronary vessel injury
- Left internal mammary artery injury
- Peritoneal puncture, liver or stomach injury, diaphragmatic injury (with the subxiphoid approach).

PROCEDURE

Site: Insert the needle midway between the spine and posterior axillary line in the 6th, 7th or 8th intercostal space based on fluid level, based on percussion. Direct the needle above the upper border of lower rib to avoid injury to neurovascular bundle that lies on the lower border.

INVESTIGATIONS TO BE SENT

- *Routine*: Pleural fluid TC, DC, protein, sugar, lactate dehydrogenase (LDH), etc.
- *Other tests in specific situations*: pH, triglycerides (chylothorax), amylase (pancreatic effusion), cytology, routine culture, acid-fast bacillus (AFB) culture, etc. Send serum protein (liver function test, LFT) and LDH along with other blood investigations.

INTERPRETING THE PLEURAL FLUID ANALYSIS: LIGHT'S CRITERIA

If any one of the following is present, the fluid is an exudate:
- Pleural fluid protein/serum protein >0.5
- Pleural fluid LDH/serum LDH >0.6
- Pleural fluid LDH >2/3 of the upper limit of normal serum range.

Note: This misclassifies 25% of transudates. If there is a mismatch between clinical and laboratory parameters, look at serum-pleural fluid protein and albumin gradient. If protein gradient is >3.1 g% or albumin gradient is >1.2 g% it indicates transudative fluid.

If the pleural fluid is hemorrhagic, consider malignancy or pulmonary embolism, tuberculosis, traumatic or catamenial.

If the pleural fluid is grossly hemorrhagic look at the pleural fluid hematocrit (Hct) *Pleural fluid Hct >50% of blood Hct suggests a hemothorax (refer to thoracic surgery).*

CHAPTER 153

Ascitic Tap (Paracentesis)

INTRODUCTION

Paracentesis is a procedure in which a needle or catheter is inserted into the peritoneal cavity to obtain ascitic fluid for diagnostic or therapeutic purposes.

INDICATIONS

- Diagnostic tap
    - New onset ascites to determine etiology, to differentiate portal hypertension versus other pathologies and to detect the presence of malignant cells
    - Suspected spontaneous or secondary bacterial peritonitis.
- Therapeutic tap
    - Respiratory compromise secondary to ascites
    - Abdominal pain or pressure secondary to ascites (tense ascites).

TECHNIQUE

Site of insertion of the needle: Right or left lower quadrant of abdomen. Two finger breadth above and medial to anterior superior iliac spine (ASIS). Left lower quadrant is preferred due to thinner abdominal wall and avoidance of cecum or appendicectomy scar as on right.

Insert the needle in an angle or using Z track technique (traction on skin during initial needle insertion) to create a displaced track which will help prevent leakage of fluid after procedure.

Note: Avoid scars on abdomen as bowel may be tethered. Avoid needle introduction medial to rectus muscle to prevent bleeding from injury to inferior epigastric artery.

THERAPEUTIC PARACENTESIS

There is no volume limit for paracentesis under monitoring. For practical purposes, remove 500 mL to 2 L of ascitic fluid, if indicated. If large volume is removed, give normal saline (NS) or albumin to replace intravascular volume loss.

INVESTIGATIONS TO BE SENT

Routine tests
- *Ascitic fluid TC, DC*: Neutrophil count ≥250 cells/mm^3 suggests spontaneous bacterial peritonitis (SBP).
- *Ascitic fluid culture*: In bactec medium (blood culture bottle)
- *Ascitic fluid albumin*: Send concomitant serum albumin to determine the serum ascites albumin gradient (SAAG)
  - SAAG >1.1 suggests portal hypertension as the etiology [chronic liver disease (CLD), Budd-Chiari syndrome, etc.]
  - SAAG <1.1 suggests peritoneal pathologies as the etiology [tuberculosis (TB), malignancy, pancreatitis, etc.].

OTHER TESTS DONE IN SPECIFIC SITUATIONS

- *Ascitic fluid lipase*: Elevated in pancreatitis.
- *Ascitic fluid acid-fast bacilli (AFB) culture*: If TB abdomen is suspected. Collect sample in a culture tube.
- *Ascitic fluid cytology for malignant cells*: Collect sample in a cytology bottle and send to the laboratory immediately for centrifugation and processing.
- *Ascitic fluid creatinine*: When a "urinoma" is suspected. A urinoma is a collection of extravasated urine in the peritoneal cavity or it may be encapsulated. Usually seen after a blunt trauma to the abdomen or after a laparotomy, if the ureter is injured.
  Ascites: Serum creatinine ratio of >1.0 is suggestive of intraperitoneal urinary leak/urinoma.
- *Ascitic fluid triglyceride*: Chylous ascites has triglyceride content more than 200 mg/dL.

Section **23**

Protocols

INTRODUCTION

- Rapid sequence intubation (RSI) is the standard of care in emergency airway management for intubations not anticipated to be difficult
- Rapid sequence intubation is the virtually simultaneous administration of a sedative and a neuromuscular blocking agent to render a patient rapidly unconscious and flaccid in order to facilitate urgent endotracheal intubation and to minimize the risk of aspiration.

RAPID SEQUENCE INTUBATION PROTOCOL (TABLE 1)

- Midazolam and fentanyl can cause hypotension and hence should be avoided in hemodynamically unstable patients.
- Succinylcholine induces rapid, complete, and predictable paralysis with spontaneous recovery in about 5 minutes. However, in certain situations, it causes potassium release from the muscles and can cause dangerous hyperkalemia, especially in patients with extensive burns and soft tissue injuries.
- Succinylcholine is contraindicated in patients with hyperkalemia. Avoid succinylcholine/check K before intubation in patients with the following conditions:
  - Known case of chronic kidney disease
  - Extensive burns (can be given if patient presents within 24 hours of incident)
  - Patients with spinal shock presenting 24 hours after the incident.
- If succinylcholine is absolutely contraindicated in hemodynamically unstable patients, a small dose of midazolam (2 mg) can be given during RSI.

TABLE 1: Rapid sequence intubation protocol.

Hemodynamically stable	Hemodynamically unstable
• Preoxygenate with 100% oxygen	• Preoxygenate with 100% oxygen
• Midazolam 5 mg (0.1 mg/kg)	• Ketamine 100 mg (1–2 mg/kg)
• Fentanyl 100 µg (2 µg/kg)	• Succinylcholine 100 mg (2 mg/kg)
• Succinylcholine 100 mg (2 mg/kg)	• Wait for 60 s, then intubate
• Wait for 60 s, then intubate	

Difficult Airway

For all intubations in the ED, be prepared for a difficult airway and seek help when needed. Refer Chapter 6 for Assessment of Airway.
- Plan A: Direct/video laryngoscopy
- Plan B: Bag and mask ventilation with/without viral filter /LMA
- Plan C: Surgery–cricothyroidotomy

Postintubation Checklist

- Confirm position by 5-point auscultation
- Check $ETCO_2$ and wave form capnography
- Check the cuff pressure (optimal range: 20-30 cm H_2O)
- Optimize ventilator settings
- Check blood pressure
- Monitor SpO_2

END-TIDAL CARBON DIOXIDE (ETCO₂)

The $ETCO_2$ measured by wave form capnography indicates the concentration of CO_2 at the end of expiration ('end-tidal'). Normal value is 35–45 mm Hg and correlates closely with $PaCO_2$.

Uses:
- Confirms tracheal placement of endo-tracheal tube
- Is a dynamic marker for chest compressions during CPR of intubated patients (should be >10 mm Hg)
- Is a reliable indicator of ROSC (>40 mm Hg)

Flat $ETCO_2$ trace: Esophageal intubation, ventilator disconnection, cardiac arrest.

Increased $ETCO_2$: Fever, increased cardiac output, increased BP, hypoventilation, bronchial intubation.

Decreased $ETCO_2$: Hypothermia, reduced cardiac output, hypotension, hyperventilation, pulmonary embolism, cardiac arrest.

CHAPTER 155

Investigations Protocol

Basic investigations to be sent by emergency department (ED) registrars for common conditions are shown in **Table 1**.

TABLE 1: Basic investigations to be sent by emergency department (ED) registrars for common conditions.

	General medicine	
Acute febrile illness	CBC, electrolytes, creatinine, LFT, blood c/s × 2, malarial parasite	If dysuria: Urinalysis, urine c/s If neck stiffness/altered sensorium: CT brain If cough/breathlessness: CXR
Poisonings	CBC, electrolytes, creatinine, LFT, ECG, CXR (if cough/breathlessness/ risk of aspiration)	Organophosphorous/unknown poison: Pseudocholinesterase Drug overdose: If known drug, phenytoin, phenobarbitone, valproate, paracetamol levels If fever/aspiration: Blood c/s
	Gastroenterology	
Acute pancreatitis	CBC, electrolytes, creatinine, LFT, amylase, lipase, CXR, ECG USG abdomen if LFT abnormal	If fever: Blood c/s If chest pain/ECG changes: Trop T
UGI bleed	CBC, electrolytes, creatinine, LFT, rapid BBVS, CXR, ECG, PT, aPTT	
DCLD with suspected SBP	CBC, electrolytes, creatinine, LFT, CXR, ECG, rapid BBVS (if not done before) Ascitic fluid TC, DC, c/s (protein and albumin if new case), PT, aPTT	
Corrosive poisoning	CBC, electrolytes, creatinine, LFT, ECG, rapid BBVS, PT, aPTT to be sent CXR, X ray neck soft tissue AP/ lateral	ENT consult for airway assessment

Continued

Continued

Neurology		
CVA/TIA	CBC, electrolytes, creatinine, ECG, CXR CT brain (Plain)/MRI stroke protocol (<4.5 h)	
Seizures	CBC, electrolytes, creatinine, CT brain (plain), CXR	
Surgery		
Abdominal pain	CBC, electrolytes, creatinine, LFT	Suspected ureteric colic: Urea, urinalysis, urine c/s, X-ray KUB, USG abdomen Suspected ovarian torsion: USG abdomen Suspected DU perforation: CXR erect, X-ray abdomen supine Suspected pancreatitis: Amylase, lipase If chest pain: ECG, Trop T If fever: Blood c/s
Cellulitis/ necrotizing fasciitis	CBC, electrolytes, creatinine, blood c/s	Consider X-ray of the limb, D-dimer If surgery required: CXR, ECG, PT, aPTT, rapid BBVS
Others		
COPD/asthma exacerbation	CBC, electrolytes, creatinine, ECG, CXR ABG (priority 1 and 2 patients)	If fever: Blood c/s If chest pain/ECG changes: Trop T
Febrile neutropenia	CBC, electrolytes, creatinine, LFT, blood c/s, MP, CXR, urinalysis	
CKD	CBC, electrolytes, creatinine, urea, urinalysis, ABG, ECG, CXR	If dialysis required: PT, aPTT, rapid BBVS (if not done before)
Suspected MI/ ACS	CBC, electrolytes, creatinine, Trop T, ECG, CXR	If abdominal pain: Amylase, lipase

(UGI: upper gastrointestinal; CBC: complete blood count; LFT: liver function test; CT: computed tomography; CXR: chest X-ray; ECG: electrocardiogram; ABG: arterial blood gases; USG: ultrasonography; BBVS: blood borne virus screen; PT: prothrombin time; aPTT: activated partial thromboplastin time; DCLD: decompensated chronic liver disease; SBP: spontaneous bacterial peritonitis; TC: total count; DC: differential count; AP: anteroposterior; ENT: ear, nose, and throat; CVA: cerebrovascular accident; MRI: magnetic resonance imaging; KUB: kidneys, ureters, bladder; DU: duodenal ulcer; COPD: chronic obstructive pulmonary disease; CKD: chronic kidney disease; MI: myocardial infarction; ACS: acute coronary syndrome).

SCALE TO ASSESS SEVERITY OF PAIN

- Verbal numeric rating scale (VNRS): 0–10.
- No pain-0. Worst pain-10.

The universal pain assessment tool is illustrated in **Figure 1**. Use the tool to assess pain score at admission and 30 minutes after administration of analgesics. Target pain score <4.

TIME TO ASSESS PAIN

- At the time of initial presentation to emergency department (ED) or respective bays or at acute change of character of pain.
- Every 30 minute after intravenous (IV) analgesic till target score is achieved.
- Then every 1 hour for 4 hours.

Analgesics

Be generous with administration of analgesics to trauma victims.

- *IV morphine*:
  - 0.1 mg/kg bolus.
  - 0.05 mg/kg every 30 minutes for a maximum of 3 doses.
  - Avoid in traumatic brain injury, biliary colic, and history of allergy.
  - *Watch for* sedation, decrease in respiratory rate, hypotension, and vomiting.
- *IV fentanyl*:
  - 1–2 µg/kg bolus
  - 1 µg/kg every 30 minutes for a maximum of 3 doses.

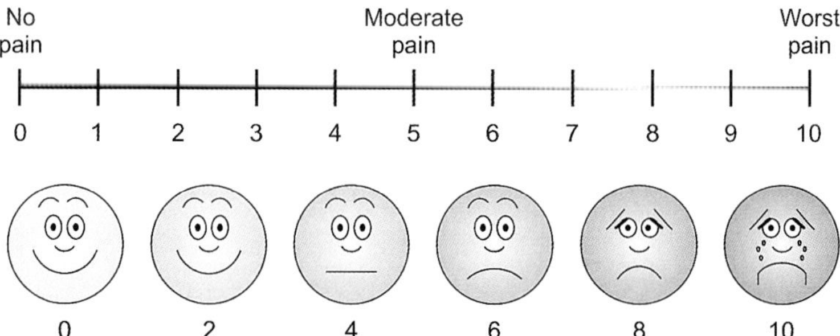

FIG. 1: Universal pain assessment tool.

- Avoid in traumatic brain injury, biliary colic, and history of allergy.
- *Watch for*: sedation, decrease in respiratory rate, and vomiting.
- *IV tramadol*:
  - 2–3 mg/kg bolus (maximum 150 mg)
  - Avoid in patients on antidepressants or with history of seizures, biliary colic, and history of allergy.
  - *Watch for*: Seizures and vomiting.
- *IV paracetamol*:
  - Use in *all* patients without *renal* and *hepatic* injury.
  - 15–20 mg/kg bolus in 100 mL normal saline (NS).
  - Dose to be repeated every 6 hours (without hepatic injury).
- *IV ketamine*:
  - Use for procedural analgesia with midazolam.
  - 0.5–1 mg/kg bolus.
- *Local anesthetic (lignocaine) infiltration*:
  - To be used for all procedures.
  - 1–60 mL (0.5–1% solution).

Always administer an antiemetic (ondansetron) along with any opioid.

Discharge Plan for Pain Relief

- *For adults*: Oral tramadol (50 mg) + paracetamol (500 mg) combination three times/day (if no contraindication to any of the drugs).
- If creatinine is normal, give a 3–5 day course of NSAIDs.

INTRODUCTION

Patients with polytrauma need urgent attention by many people (ED physician, paramedics, nurses, and the specialty registrars) in order to perform primary and secondary surveys and resuscitate at the same time. Hence, a polytrauma team should be activated through the telephone exchange.

Criteria to activate polytrauma team:

- Unexplained shock
- More than one system involvement
- Mass casualty incident, i.e., more than 10 patients with significant injuries from the same accident.

MEMBERS OF THE TRAUMA TEAM

- Senior registrars of general surgery, orthopedics, neurosurgery (trauma), radiology
- Duty radiographer
- Trauma coordinator (TC) of the ED
- Duty consultant of ED
- Duty chaplain

TRAUMA TEAM CALL OUT PROCEDURE

- Call telephone exchange (2,500) and say, "please activate the trauma team".
- The telephone exchange will activate trauma team members by a priority call.
- The team members should report to the resuscitation room (RR) of ED immediately in person. If they do not arrive within 20 minutes, the head of the respective departments should be contacted.

    Subspecialty consultation, i.e., thoracic surgery, plastic surgery, ENT, urology, etc., should be subsequently carried out by the TC, if necessary.
- All trauma victims below the age of 15 years should be assessed by the pediatric surgery team.
- If there is a delay or uncertainty in assuming primary responsibility by the clinical units, the ED on call consultant will decide the primary unit and admit the patient under that unit in the concerned ward/intensive care unit (ICU). This decision of the ED consultant is final and binding.

ROLE OF TRAUMA COORDINATOR

- The TC should take control of the situation and coordinate the trauma team in resuscitation.
- Documentation regarding progress in resuscitation and MLC should be done by the TC.
- The first two units of blood should be arranged. Call blood bank duty doctor and arrange crossmatched blood or Onegative blood, if patient is in shock.
- If necessary, the TC should activate massive transfusion protocol. (Refer Chapter 106)

CHAPTER 158

Prophylactic Antibiotic Protocol for Trauma Patients in the Emergency Department

INTRODUCTION

It is important to administer appropriate prophylactic antibiotic protocol for trauma patients in the emergency department. **Table 1** gives the prophylactic antibiotics protocol for trauma victims used in Christian Medical College (CMC), Vellore.

TABLE 1: Prophylactic antibiotics protocol for trauma patients in the Emergency department (ED).

Trauma sites		Antibiotics
1. Scalp	1a. Abrasion	Neosporin/Fusidic acid local application
	1b. Laceration (clean)	Daily cleaning and dressing, if needed
	1c. Laceration (contaminated)	Capsule cloxacillin 500 mg q6h × 3 days or Capsule cephalexin 500 mg q6h × 3 days + Tablet metronidazole 400 mg tid × 3 days (only if severely contaminated)
	1d. Laceration with underlying fracture of skull bones	Injection cloxacillin 1 g IV stat and q6h or Injection cefazolin 1 g IV stat and q8h or Injection cefuroxime 1.5 g stat and q8h + Injection metronidazole 500 mg IV stat and q8h (only if severely contaminated) If discharged from ED: Capsule cloxacillin 500 mg q6h × 3 days or Capsule cephalexin 500 mg q6h × 3 days + Tablet metronidazole 400 mg tid × 3 days (only if severely contaminated)

Continued

Continued

Trauma sites		Antibiotics
2. Face	*2a. Abrasion*	Neosporin/Fusidic acid local application
	2b. Superficial laceration (involves epidermis, dermis, and fascia)	Capsule cloxacillin 500 mg q6h × 3 days or Capsule cephalexin 500 mg q6h × 3 days
	2c. Superficial laceration involving dangerous area of face	Capsule cloxacillin 500 mg qid × 3 days
	2d. Superficial laceration involving dangerous area of face + intraoral laceration	Capsule cloxacillin 500 mg qid × 3 days + Tablet metronidazole 400 mg tid × 3 days
	2e. Deep laceration (involves epidermis, dermis fascia, and muscle)	Injection cloxacillin 1 g IV stat and q6h or Injection cefazolin 1g IV stat and q8h or Injection cefuroxime 1.5 g stat and q8h + Injection metronidazole 500 mg IV stat and q8h (*only if severely contaminated*)
	2f. Deep laceration with facial bone fractures	Injection cloxacillin 1 g IV stat and q6h or Injection cefazolin 1 g IV stat and q6h or Injection cefuroxime 1.5 g stat and q8h + Injection metronidazole 500 mg IV stat and q8h (only if severely contaminated) If discharged from ED: Capsule cloxacillin 500 mg q6h × 3 days or Capsule cephalexin 500 mg q6h × 3 days + Tablet metronidazole 400 mg tid × 3 days (*only if severely contaminated*)

Continued

Continued

Trauma sites		Antibiotics
	2g. Deep laceration + facial bone fractures + intraoral extension	Injection cloxacillin 500 mg IV stat and q6h or Injection cefazolin 1 g IV stat and q6h or Injection cefuroxime 1.5 g stat and q8h + Injection metronidazole 500 mg IV stat and q8h If discharged from ED: Capsule cloxacillin 500 mg q6h × 3 days or Capsule cephalexin 500 mg q6h × 3 days + Tablet metronidazole 400 mg tid × 3 days
3. Thorax, abdomen, back, and pelvis	*3a. Abrasion*	Neosporin/Fusidic acid L/A
	3b. Superficial laceration (involves epidermis, dermis, and fascia)	Capsule cloxacillin 500 mg q6h × 3 days or Capsule cephalexin 500 mg q6h × 3 days
	3c. Deep laceration (involves epidermis, dermis, fascia, and muscle)	Injection cloxacillin 1 g IV stat and q6h or Injection cefazolin 1 g IV stat and q6h or Injection cefuroxime 1.5 g stat and q8h + Injection metronidazole 500 mg IV stat and q8h *(only if severely contaminated)* If discharged from ED: Capsule cloxacillin 500 mg q6h × 3 days or Capsule cephalexin 500 mg q6h × 3 days + Tablet metronidazole 400 mg tid × 3 days *(only if severely contaminated)*
	3d. Penetrating injuries (stab entering parietal pleura or peritoneum)	Injection piperacillin-tazobactam 4.5 g IV stat and q8h

Continued

Continued

Trauma sites		Antibiotics
4. Animal/human bites	*4a. Human bite*	Tablet augmentin 625 mg tid × 3–5 days
	4b. Dog/cat/rat bite	Tablet augmentin 625 mg tid × 3–5 days
	4c. Bull gore injury (penetrating)	Injection piperacillin-tazobactam 4.5 g IV stat and q8h
5. Appendicular injuries Without fractures	*5a. Abrasion*	Neosporin/Fusidic acid local application
	5b. Superficial laceration (involves epidermis, dermis, and fascia)	Capsule cloxacillin 500 mg q6h × 3 days or Capsule cephalexin 500 mg q6h × 3 days
	5c. Deep laceration (involves epidermis, dermis, fascia, muscle, and tendon)	Injection cloxacillin 500 mg IV stat and q6h or Injection cefazolin 1g IV stat and q8h or Injection cefuroxime 1.5 g stat and q8h + Injection metronidazole 500 mg IV stat and q8h (only if severely contaminated) If discharged from ED: Capsule cloxacillin 500 mg q6h × 3 days or Capsule cephalexin 500 mg q6h × 3 days + Tablet metronidazole 400 mg tid × 3 days *(only if severely contaminated)*
Appendicular injuries with fractures	*5d. No or minimal contamination*	Injection cloxacillin 500 mg IV stat and q6h or Injection cefazolin 1 g IV stat and q8h or Injection cefuroxime 1.5 g stat and q8h
	5e. Heavily contaminated wound	Injection cefuroxime 1.5 g stat and q8h + Injection metronidazole 500 mg IV stat and q8h or Injection piperacillin-tazobactam 4.5 g IV stat and q8h

Index

Page numbers followed by *f* refer to figure, *fc* refer to flowchart, and *t* refer to table.

A

Abdomen 519
  examination of 343
  ultrasonography of 96, 321
Abruptio placenta 282, 386
Abscess 314
  intra-abdominal 72
  peritonsillar 298
  pilonidal 332
  retropharyngeal 297
Absolute neutrophil count 240
Absorbable suture materials 380
Acetaminophen 111
  overdose 111
Acid-base
  abnormalities 64
  disturbances 59, 66*fc*
Acid-fast bacillus 504
Acidosis 16, 56, 267
  metabolic 64, 80
  respiratory 45, 64
  severe metabolic 268
Acinetobacter 240
Activated charcoal 110, 426
  contraindications for 110
  multidose 110
Activated partial thromboplastin time 99, 233, 336, 347, 512
Acute angle closure glaucoma 470
Acute asthma 414
  classification of 180
  management of 180, 415
Acute coronary syndrome 22, 147, 154, 512
  spectrum of 147*fc*
Acute exacerbation 45, 182
  management of 183
Acute obstructive valve thrombus 170

Acute pancreatitis 227, 511
  etiology of 227
  modified Atlanta grading of severity of 227*t*
Acute red eye 469
  causes of 470
  management of 470*t*
Acute respiratory distress syndrome 80
Acyclovir 73, 426, 476
Adenomyosis 275
Adenosine 165, 426
Adenovirus 93
Adrenal disease, primary 264
Adrenal insufficiency 263
  causes 263
  clinical features 263
  diagnosis 264
  management 264
  primary 263
  secondary 263
Adrenaline 16-18, 33, 38, 426, 432
  infusion 36
  nebulized 417
Adrogue–Madias formula 55
Advanced cardiac life support 3
Aedes aegypti viral infection 75
Agitation 113
Air under diaphragm 316*f*, 362
Airway 3, 88, 111, 183, 191, 202, 392, 406, 446, 447
  assessment of 40
  management 40, 127, 388
  maneuvers 5
  oropharyngeal 7, 8*f*
Albendazole 71, 426, 477
Albumin 255
Alcohol 227
  withdrawal 464
    management of 465

Alkaline phosphatase 234
  levels, causes of 321
Alkalosis 56
  acute respiratory 59
  metabolic 64, 232
  respiratory 64
Allergic reaction 255
  mild 256
  treatment of 492
Allis technique 376, 376*f*
Alloimmunization 274
Alpha plus beta-blocker 155
Aluminum 122
  phosphide 121
Amantadine 456
Amaurosis fugax 466
Amenorrhea, history of 273
American Heart Association 3
Amikacin 106, 426, 476
Aminoglycosides 62
Aminophylline 427
Amiodarone 16, 161, 426
Amlodipine 114, 477
Amoxicillin 73, 74, 83, 103, 291, 297, 427, 476
Amphetamine 62, 135
Ampicillin 103, 427, 476
Amyl nitrite 142
Amylase 228
Anal fissure 331
Analgesia 379
Analgesics 279, 513
Anaphylactic reaction, severe 256
Anaphylaxis 29
  diagnosis of 29*t*
  management of 30
Androgens 263
Anemia 237
  cause of 237*t*, 238*t*
  evaluation of 239*fc*
  microangiopathic hemolytic 250
  pernicious 239
  severe 80, 245
Anesthesia, dissociative 481
Angina
  pectoris 147
  unstable 147, 153*t*
Angiography, interventional 192

Ankle 399, 490*f*
  block 488, 490*f*
  level of 489*f*
Ankylosing spondylitis 41, 480
Ankylostoma 71
Anorectal abscess 332
  location of 333*f*
  types of 332
Anorectal emergencies 331
Anorexia 317
Antacids 477
Anterior dislocation
  reduction of 357*f*
  temporomandibular joint 357*f*
Anterior glenohumeral dislocation 370
  types of 370*f*
Anterior hip dislocation 374, 375
  Epstein classification of 375*f*
Antibiotic 30, 103-106, 184, 191, 279, 291, 306, 423, 425, 460, 476
  doses 103
  empiric 83, 89
  protocol 71
  therapy 38, 81, 326
    indications for 230
Anticoagulants 88, 121, 247
  parenteral 248
Antidotes 111*t*, 124, 134
Antiemetic agents 455
Antiepileptics 204, 413*t*, 477
  drugs, doses of 210*t*
Anti-fibrinolytic activity 204, 285
Antigen-based rapid diagnostic tests 80
Antihistamines 30, 477
Antihypertensives 196
Antimalarial therapy 81
Antimicrobial spectrum 103, 103*t*, 104, 105, 106
Antiphospholipid syndrome 252
Antipsychotics, atypical 455
Antisnake venom 30, 128, 129
Antithrombin 255
  deficiency 252
Anton syndrome 468
Anxiolysis 482
Aortic aneurysm, abdominal 334
Aortic dissection 191, 334
Apathy 60, 62

Aplastic crisis 245
Apnea 47
Appendages, torsion of 304
Appendicitis 281, 301, 317, 318, 319*t*
Appendicular injuries 520
Areflexia 205
Arm 396
Arrhythmia 32, 33, 165
Artemesinin combination therapy 81
Artemether 477
Arterial blood gas 39, 46, 65, 84, 87, 325
Arteriovenous malformation 191, 214
Arteritis, temporal 215, 467, 468
Arthritis 41
 acute 479
 enteropathic 480
 reactive 480
 septic 73, 314, 479
Ascaris 71, 227
Ascites 506
Ascitic fluid
 acid-fast bacilli culture 506
 creatinine 506
 cytology 506
 lipase 506
 triglyceride 506
Ascitic tap 505
 indications 505
 technique 505
Asthma 179, 179*t*
 acute 180, 414
 bronchial 179
 life-threatening 180
 mild 414*t*
 moderate 414*t*
 refractory 181
 severe 414*t*
AstraZeneca 89
Ataxia 198, 205
Atenolol 477
Atrial fibrillation 159, 163, 164, 168
Atrial flutter 162, 162*f*, 162*t*
Atrioventricular nodal reentrant
 tachycardia 164
Atropine 16-19, 111, 117, 427
Atropinization targets 117

Attacks
 acute 213
 mild-to-moderate 213
 moderate-to-severe 214
Attitude 377
Augmentin 476
Automated external defibrillator 4, 5, 13
Aviator fracture 400
Avomine 296
Azathioprine 227
Azithromycin 71, 73, 74, 105, 279, 306,
 427, 476
Azotemia 84

B

Bacillary dysentery 71
Bacillus cereus 93, 94
Backfire fracture 397
Bacteremia 240
Bacteria 424
Bacteriology 233
Bacteriuria, asymptomatic 96
Bacteroides 297, 298
Bag-mask ventilation 8
Balloon mitral valvotomy 170
Bankart fracture 396
Barbiturates 113
Baricitinib 89
Barton fracture 396
Baseball finger 398
Basic life support 1, 3, 10, 10*fc*, 11, 14
 steps of 4*t*
Battle's sign 348
Bee and wasp stings 132
Bell's palsy 216
 differential diagnosis for 216
Bennett fracture 397
Benzathine penicillin 73, 427
Benzocaine 491
Benzodiazepines 111, 113, 131, 218,
 456, 465, 481
Benztropine 218
Bernard–Soulier syndrome 250
Beta-blocker 113, 155, 260
Betahistine 296

Bile acid sequestrants 260
Bile duct, common 233, 234
Bilevel positive airway pressure 45, 46
Biliary system, bacterial infection of 233
Biphasic defibrillator 12, 13
Bisphosphonates 59, 61
Bites 74, 520
Bladder 512
 rupture 362
Bleeding
 disorder 250
 gastrointestinal 225, 232
 intracranial 202
 normal regulation of 250
 per vagina 275
  etiology of 275
 postpartum 284
Blockade, shorter duration of 485
Blood
 ammonia concentration 232
 borne virus screen 233, 280, 318, 365,
  512
 components 255
 culture 233
 loss 225, 345*t*
 pressure 36, 76, 155, 161
  control 204
  diastolic 34, 154, 389, 446
  systolic 23, 34, 36, 38, 389, 393, 407,
   446
 products 255, 277
 transfusion 30, 255, 284
  complications of 255
  protocols 226
 urea nitrogen 54, 87
Body fluids 473
Bone 60, 353
 cortex, posterior 498
Bony cortex 498
Bosworth fracture 399
Botulism 206
Bowel perforation 72
Boxer's fracture 398
Bradyarrhythmias 14, 33
 management of 18
Bradycardia 20*fc*, 124, 125
 rhythms 17*t*
 symptomatic 14, 19*t*

Bradypnea 125
Brain
 abscess 98
 computed tomography of 200, 201,
  213
 function, abnormalities in 98
 injury, traumatic 348
 magnetic resonance imaging of 213
Break-dancer's thumb 398
Breast
 abscess 338
 disorders 338
 tissue 338
  acute inflammation of 338
Breathing 3, 88, 111, 183, 191, 202, 389,
 392, 406, 446, 447
Breathlessness 84, 86
Bromocriptine 456
Bronchiectasis 45, 190
Bronchiolitis 420
Bronchitis
 acute 73
 chronic 183
Bronchodilators 31
Bronchoscopy 191
Bronchospasm 134
Brudzinski's sign 99
Brugada sign 175*f*
Brugada syndrome 175
Bullous diseases 472
Bumper fracture 399
Bungarus caeruleus 128*t*
Bupivacaine 485, 491
Burns 32, 41, 459
 depth of 459*t*
 full-thickness 459
 management of 460
 partial thickness 459
 percentage of 459*t*
 superficial 459
Buscopan 302

C

Cairo–Bishop definition 243
Calcium 59, 228
 channel blockers 114
 gluconate 427

Campylobacter jejuni 94, 205
Canadian C-spine rules 351
Canakinumab 89
Candida 240, 314
Cannabis 134
Carbamates 111, 118, 120
Carbamazepine 210, 215, 477
Carbapenems 463
Carbon monoxide poisoning 140
Carcinoma, bronchogenic 190
Cardiac arrest 15*fc*, 23, 47
  management of 1, 14
  maternal 23, 24*fc*
Cardiac diseases 191
Cardiac dysrhythmias, management of 492
Cardiac tamponade 359, 360
Cardiomyopathy, restrictive 32
Cardiovascular system 29
Cardioversion 11
Carotid
  massage 165
  pulse check 5*f*
Cartilage 353
Casts 378
Catabolism 243
Catecholamine-secreting tumors 270
Cedell fracture 400
Cefalexin 104
Cefazolin 73, 104, 313, 428, 476, 479, 517, 518
Cefixime 104, 428
Cefoperazone 72, 103, 428
Cefotaxime 428
Ceftazidime 104, 428, 476
Ceftriaxone 71, 73, 74, 99, 104, 279, 291, 428, 476
Cefuroxime 72, 73, 104, 428, 517, 518, 520
Cells, shift out of 57
Cellulitis 72, 313
  investigations 313
  management 313
Centipede bite 132
Central nervous system 117, 134, 451
  dysfunction 259
  infection 98, 100*fc*, 412

Central retinal
  artery occlusion 466
  vein occlusion 466
Central venous
  access 493
  pressure 393
Cephalexin 72, 313, 338, 428, 476, 517, 520
Cerebra thevetia 124
Cerebral blood 199
Cerebral edema 204
  high-altitude 158
Cerebral function 98
Cerebral infarction 245
Cerebral venous thrombosis 199, 200*f*, 213
Cerebrospinal fluid 204
  analysis 79, 99, 206
Cerebrovascular accidents 195
Cervical spine 350
  injuries 350
  radiological evaluation of 351
  trauma 463
  X-ray
    interpretation of 352
    normal 353*f*
Cetirizine 477
CHADSVasc score 161*t*
Chance fracture 401
Charcot's triad 233
Chauffeur fracture 397
Chest
  compressions 3, 5
    technique of 6*f*, 11, 11*f*
  computed tomography of 86, 192
  crisis 245
  pain 125
    active ischemic 16, 21
  trauma 390
  tube insertion 495
    site of 496*f*
  wall injuries 392
  X-ray 84, 86, 87, 154, 187, 188, 228, 233, 335, 336
Chickenpox 73
Chlamydia
  pneumonia 82, 245
  trachomatis 279, 480

Chloramphenicol 71, 428
Chlordiazepoxide 465
Chlorinated hydrocarbon 118
Chloroquine 81, 477
Chlorpheniramine 477
Chlorpromazine 218, 455
Cholangiography, percutaneous
    transhepatic 234
Cholangitis 72, 233
Cholecystitis 72, 278, 320
    acalculous 320
Cholelithiasis 278
Cholera 71
Cholesteatoma 216
Cholinesterase reactivator 118
Chopart fracture 399
Chronic obstructive pulmonary disease
    44, 155, 179, 183, 188, 512
Chvostek's sign 60
Chylothorax 504
Cinnarizine 296
Ciprofloxacin 71, 105, 428, 476
Circulation 111, 183, 191, 202, 388, 389,
    393, 407, 446, 447
    spontaneous 22
Cisplatin 59
Clavulanate 73, 74, 83, 103, 291, 297,
    476
Clavulanic acid 427
Clay–Shoveler fracture 401
Cleistanthus collinus 124
Clindamycin 73, 81, 83, 106, 428, 476
Clobazam 210, 429, 477
Clonorchis sinensis 227
Clostridium 326
    botulinum 206
    perfringens 93
    tetani 101
Clotting disorder 250, 252
Cloxacillin 72, 73, 103, 313, 329, 338,
    429, 517, 518
Clozapine 455
Coagulation disorders, acquired 251
Coagulopathy 241, 276
Cobra bite 128
Cocaine 135
Colles fracture 366, 396
    reduction of 367*f*

Colonic malignancies 333
Coma 53, 62
Combustion, gas products of 140
Common drug overdose, specific
    management of 113*t*
Common medicolegal case, list of 441
Common thoracic injuries
    clinical features of 358*t*
    management of 358*t*
Compartment syndrome 383
    causes of 383
Complete blood count 78, 84, 87, 209,
    228, 229, 231, 233, 244, 336, 512
Computed tomography 86, 154, 192,
    200, 201, 209, 213
    pulmonary angiography 187
Confusion 38, 53, 60
Congestion, pharyngeal 84
Conjunctivitis 469
    allergic 470
    bacterial 470
    viral 470
Consciousness, level of 36
Constipation 232
Continuous positive airway pressure 45,
    47
Contusion, pulmonary 359
Convulsions 80
Copper sulfate 114
Coral reef snakes 128
Cord sign 201
Cormack and Lehane grading 42
Coronavirus disease-2019 86
Corpora cavernosa 309
Corrosive poisoning 137, 511
Corticosteroids 61, 88, 291
Coryza 84
Cotrimoxazole 71, 429
Cotton fracture 399
Cough 84
Countertraction method 373, 373*f*
Covaxin 89
COVID-19 86, 88
    management of 87*t*
Covishield 89
Coxsackie 98, 227
C-reactive protein 87
Creatine phosphokinase 384

Creatinine 78, 84, 228, 233, 336, 452, 457
Cricothyroid arteries 499
Cricothyroid membrane 499
  anatomy of 499
Cricothyroidotomy 499, 500
  indications 499
  surgical 500, 501*f*
Critical limb ischemia 335
Crohn's disease 333
Crush injury 327
Cryoprecipitate 255
Cryptosporidium 93
Crystal arthropathy 479
Crystalline penicillin 73, 83, 103, 429
Crystalloids, profile of 52*t*
C-spine
  assessment 352*fc*
  immobilization 350
  smart-D assessment of 351*t*
Cyanide
  poisoning 141
  sources of 141
Cyanosis, central 41
Cyclosporin 62
Cyst 214
Cystitis 95, 97
Cytomegalovirus 227
Cytotoxic damage 44

D

Daboia russelii 128
Dancer's fracture 401
Dantrolene 456
Datura 126
D-dimer 187
Deep neck space infections 297
Deep peroneal nerve block 489
Deep vein thrombosis, acute 337
Defibrillation 3, 11
Dehydration, classification of 424*t*
Delirium 62
  tremens 464
Dengue 75
  fever 75, 76
    management of 76
    warning signs in 76
  hemorrhagic fever 75, 76
  shock syndrome 75, 77

Denosumab 59
Dense triangle sign 201
Depression 60, 134
  respiratory 134
Desflurane 453
Dexamethasone 99, 264, 429
Dextrose
  infusion 264
  normal saline 52
Diabetes mellitus
  type 1 266
  type 2 266
Diabetic foot 72, 73
Diarrhea 32
  inflammatory 93
  noninflammatory 93
Diazepam 113, 413
Dichloro-diphenyl-trichloroethane 118
Diclofenac 478
Dicyclomine 279
Difficult airway assessment 40, 510
Difficult mask ventilation assessment 40
Digital nerve block 485
Digital subtraction angiography 204
Digitalis glycosides 111
Digitoxin 111
Digoxin 111, 114, 161, 429
  specific fab fragments 111
Diltiazem 114, 160, 477
Diphenhydramine 218, 477
Diphtheria 206
Diplopia 282
Direct cyanide binding 141
Direct thrombin inhibitors 247, 249
Disability 390, 393, 408
Disaster 435
  management 433, 435
Disc spaces 353
Disseminated intravascular coagulation
    80, 251, 386
Distal phalanx, fractures of 327
Diuretics 62
Diverticulitis 301
Dix–Hallpike maneuver 294
Dobutamine 33, 38, 429
Dog bite, management of 90
Domperidone 455
Dopamine 16, 18, 33, 429
  infusion 36

Dorsal-penile-nerve-block 309*f*
Doxycycline 71, 74, 81, 105, 306, 429, 477
Doxylamine 477
  succinate 278
Drowning 462
  management 462
Drugs 59
  list of 476*t*
  overdose 111
    general management of 111
  therapeutics 88
Dry nonfatal drowning 462
Ducts, biliary 233
Duodenal ulcer 512
  perforation 315
Dupuytren fracture 399
Duverney fracture 398
Dysentery 424
Dyspnea 86, 125
Dysrhythmias, ventricular 113
Dystonia
  acute 218
  drugs-induced 218
  reaction, acute 218

E

E-C clamp technique 9*f*, 9*t*
Echis carinatus 128
Echocardiography 187, 335, 393
Echovirus 98
Eclampsia 282, 283
Ectopic pregnancy 273, 278, 281
  clinical presentation 273
  diagnostic evaluation 273
  management 274
  ruptured 273
  unruptured 273
Edema
  acute pulmonary 16, 21
  cardiogenic pulmonary 45
  pulmonary 157
Electrical injuries 457
  clinical presentation 457
  investigations 457
  management 458

Electrocardiogram 87, 154, 159, 162, 165, 172*f*, 210, 228, 233
  basics of 171
Electrodiagnostic tests 205
Electrolyte 49, 53, 78, 84, 228, 233, 336, 452, 457
  abnormalities 268
  toxicity 256
Electromyography 205
Elevated ascitic fluid absolute neutrophil count 229
Embolectomy 325
Embolism, pulmonary 32, 186, 186*t*, 191
Emergency laparotomy, indications for 362
Emphysema 183
Empty delta sign 201
Empyema thoracis 83
Enalapril 477
Encephalitic rabies 90
Encephalitis 98, 99
  early feature of 98
Encephalopathy 199, 231, 464
Endocrine
  disorder 62
  emergencies 257
Endometritis 279
Endoscopic retrograde cholangiopancreaticography 228, 234
Endotracheal intubation 42
  indications for 47
Endotracheal tube 14, 191, 388
End-tidal carbon dioxide 510
Enflurane 453
Enoxaparin 88, 478
Entamoeba histolytica 93
Enterobacteriaceae anaerobes 72
Enteroviruses 98
Epididymitis 305
Epididymo-orchitis 304, 305
  clinical features 305
  etiology 305
  laboratory investigations 305
  management 306
Epiglottitis 73, 417, 418
Epilepsy 209

Epinephrine 31
Episcleritis 469
Episodic vertigo 296
Epistaxis 289
  anatomy 289
  anterior bleeds 289
  management 290
  nasal packing 290
  posterior bleeds 290
Epley's maneuver 294, 295*f*, 295*t*
Epstein–Barr virus 227
Ertapenem 72, 73, 106, 477
Erysipelas 313
Erythema multiforme 471
Erythromycin 429
Escherichia coli 229, 233, 240, 297
  enteropathogenic 71
  enterotoxigenic 71, 93
Esmolol 155
Essex–Lopresti fracture-dislocation 397
Estrogen therapy 276
Ethanol 111
  metabolism of 138*f*
Ethylene glycol 111
Ethylenediaminetetraacetic acid 256
Etomidate 481
Exacerbation, moderate 180
Expiratory phonation 41
Expiratory positive airway pressure 46
Extracellular fluid 52
Extremity
  examination of 344
  injuries 364

F

Face 402, 518
  mask 44, 88
Facial surgery, extensive 45
Factor V Leiden mutation 252
Fasciitis 314
  necrotizing 73, 313, 314
Fat embolism
  syndrome 378
  triad of 378
Fatigue 53
Febrile
  illness 71, 511
  neutropenia 240

reaction, mild 256
seizures 412, 413*t*
transfusion reaction 255
Felon 330
  drainage of 330*f*
  incision of 330*f*
Femoral line 493
Femur
  neck of 368
  shaft of 369
Fentanyl 429, 481, 482
Fetal monitoring 24
Fetor hepaticus 231
Fever 84
Fexofenadine 477
Fibrillation, ventricular 16, 166, 168, 168*f*, 432, 462
Fibrinogen 255
Finger's breadth 497
Fistula in Ano 333
Flail chest 359
Fluconazole 429
Fludrocortisone 264
Fluid 49
  compartments 51*f*
  replacement 228
  resuscitation 37, 267, 389
  therapy 51
Flumazenil 111
Flunarizine 296
Fluphenazine 218
Focal syndrome 199
Folic acid 278
Fomepizole 111
Fondaparinux 249
  dose of 249*t*
Food poisoning 93
  etiology of 94
Foot 400, 489*f*
Forearm 396
Foscarnet 59
Fosphenytoin 211
Fournier's gangrene 304, 314
Fractures 327, 364, 396
  intertrochanteric 368
  management of 365
Free thyroxine 259
Fresh frozen plasma 255, 347

Fungal infections 190, 240
Furosemide 429
Furunculosis 72
Fusobacterium 298

G

Gabapentin 478
Gait
    ataxia 464
    disturbances 53
Galeazzi fracture-dislocation 397
Gallstones 227
Gamekeeper's thumb 398
Gamma-glutamyl transpeptidase 321
Gangrene, spontaneous 326
Gardanella vaginalis 279
Gas gangrene 326
    clinical features 326
    diagnosis 326
    management 326
    traumatic 326
Gastric lavage 109, 124, 125
Gastroenteritis 51, 71, 93, 278, 424
Gastrointestinal
    disorder 62
    emergencies 223
    symptoms 125, 479
    system 29
    tract 123, 225, 321, 424
Gentamicin 106, 429
Geriatric trauma 392
Giardia lamblia 71, 93
Giardiasis 71
Glanzmann's thrombasthenia 250
Glasgow coma scale 45, 343, 348, 349*t*, 408, 446, 447
Glaucoma 470
Glenohumeral dislocation, posterior 370
Glucagon 31
Glucocorticoid 263
    metabolism 276
    therapy 38
Glucose-6-phosphate dehydrogenase 239
Glycopyrrolate 117
Golfer's elbow 397
Goodpasture syndrome 191

Goodsall's rule 333
Gosselin fracture 399
Gout 480
Graft-vs-host disease 256
Guillain–Barré syndrome 48, 90, 205
Gustilo and Anderson classification 364, 364*t*
Gynecological emergencies 271

H

H1N1 84
    influenza 245
Haemophilus influenzae 73, 82, 98, 245
Haloperidol 218
Halothane 453
Hand Doppler screening 336
Hand fractures 366
Hangman's fracture 401
Hazard 435
Head
    and face, examination of 343
    injury 348
    trauma 390
Headache 53, 213, 214, 282
Hearing loss 296
Heart
    block 124
        complete 18*f*
    disease, ischemic 285
    rate 14, 34, 35, 171, 446
Heat
    cramps 451
    exhaustion 451
    stroke 32, 451
        classic 451
        exertional 451
HELLP syndrome 284
Helminthiasis 71
Hematemesis 190*t*, 225
Hematochezia 225
Hematoma
    epidural 202
    extradural 202, 203
    mastoid 348
    subdural 202, 203
    subungual 327
Hemodynamics, unstable 45
Hemoglobin 209

Hemoglobinopathies 245
Hemolytic crisis 245
Hemolytic reaction, acute 255
Hemolytic-uremic syndrome 250
Hemoperitoneum 496
Hemophilia 253, 479
  A 253
  B 253
  investigations 253
  management 253
  mild-to-moderate 253
  severe 253
Hemoptysis 190, 190*t*
Hemorrhage 32, 284
  fetomaternal 387
  intracranial 202, 203*f*
  intraparenchymal 202, 203*f*, 204
  postpartum 284
  subarachnoid 202, 203, 219
  subconjunctival 469
  subdural 219
  vitreous 467
Hemorrhagic infarct 200*f*
Hemorrhoids 331
  external 331
  internal 331
Hemostasis 381
Hemothorax, massive 358, 359
Hemotoxic bite 129
Henoch–Schönlein purpura 304
Heparin, unfractionated 89, 246, 248
Hepatic encephalopathy, acute 232
Hepatitis 278
  B 473-475, 475*t*
  C 474
Hepato-renal syndrome 230
Herpes simplex virus 98, 216, 432
Herpes zoster
  oticus 293
  virus infection 216
High-flow nasal cannula 87, 88
Hill–Sachs fracture 396
Hip
  dislocation 374
    posterior 374, 375
    types of 374*t*
  fractures 368
Histidine-rich protein 2 80
Hoarseness 41

Holdsworth fracture 402
Holstein–Lewis fracture 396
Hormone
  adrenal 263
  therapy, exogenous 276
Hospital disasters, classification of 436
Human herpesvirus 205, 216
Human immunodeficiency virus 473
Hume fracture 396
Humeral head 371
Hutchinson fracture 397
Hydrochlorothiazide 477
Hydrocortisone 31, 61, 264, 429
Hydrogen ion 16
Hydroxycobalamin 142
Hydroxyurea 246
Hydroxyzine 430
Hymenoptera sting removal, technique of 133*f*
Hyoscine 302, 430
Hyperacute T waves 174*f*
Hyperaldosteronism 62
Hypercalcemia 60, 227
  causes of 60*t*
Hypercapnic respiratory failure 45
Hyperemesis gravidarum 278
  evaluation 278
  management 278
Hyperglycemia 33
  management of 39
Hyperhomocysteinemia 252
Hyperkalemia 16, 56, 57, 124, 244
  treatment of 58*t*
Hypermagnesemia 62
Hypernatremia 55
  causes of 55*t*
Hyperosmotic hyperglycemic nonketotic state 268
Hyperparathyroidism 62
Hyperphosphatemia 244
Hyperplasia 275
  endometrial 275
Hypertension 481
  gestational 282
  pregnancy induced 282
  pulmonary 32
  severe 154
  treatment of 283

Hypertensive
  crisis, acute 270
  disorders 282
  emergency 154, 155
Hyperthermia 56
  malignant 453
Hyperthyroidism 62
Hypertriglyceridemia 227
Hyperuricemia 244
Hypoalbuminemia 59
Hypocalcemia 59, 244
  chronic 60
  severe 60
  symptomatic 60
Hypoglycemia 80, 232, 261, 264, 265
  causes 265
  discharge recommendation 266
  management 265
  symptoms 265
Hypokalemia 16, 56, 232
Hypokalemic periodic paralysis 57, 206
Hypomagnesemia 62
  treatment of 63*t*
Hyponatremia 53, 261
  causes of 53*t*
  correction 54
  management of 53*t*
  symptoms of 53
Hypoparathyroidism 59
Hypoperfusion 32
Hypotension 14, 21, 23, 33, 113, 125, 407*t*
  orthostatic 134, 284
Hypothalamic disease 264
Hypothalamic-pituitary axis 261
Hypothermia 16, 56, 256, 261, 390, 510
Hypothyroidism
  primary 261
  secondary 261
Hypoventilation 261
Hypovolemia 16, 34, 232
Hypoxia 16, 232
  maternal 283

I

Ibuprofen 478
Ice pack application 452*f*
Idiopathic thrombocytopenic purpura
  250

Iliac fossa, right anterior 317
Imipenem 477
Immunization 102
Immunoglobulin E 29
Inactivated viral vaccines 89
Indian cobra 128
Indian krait 128
Infections 41, 232, 245, 256, 314, 498
  bacterial 314
  middle ear 216
  respiratory 420
  viral 251
Infectious diseases 69
Influenza 84
  A virus 84
  B virus 84
  complications of 84
  virus 85
Infusion pumps 497
Inhalation injuries 140
Inherited clotting disorders 252
Injuries
  abdominal 361
  electrical 457
  evaluation of 388
  grievous 441
  hepatic 514
  management of 388
  mechanism of 371
  needle-stick 473
  nongrievous 441
  penetrating 362
  submersion 462
  thermal 457
Inorganic rodenticides 121
Inotropes 32, 33*t*, 38
Insecticide poisoning 116
Inspiratory reserve volume 185
Inspiratory stridor 41
Insulin
  administration 267
    sliding scale for 269
  infusion 267, 269*t*
Intensive care, indications for 422
Internal jugular vein 199, 493
Intestinal obstruction 322
  causes of 322*t*
  examination 322
  history 322

investigations 322
  management 323
Intoxication, acute 135, 136
Intracellular fluid 52
Intracranial pressure 201, 204, 432
Intraosseous line 497
  complications 498
  procedure 497
Intraosseous needle insertion 497*f*
Intravenous fluids 187
  choice of 51
Intravenous thyroxine preparation
  method 262
Intubation 388
  protocol 509
Invasive mechanical ventilation 47, 87,
  88
Iritis 469
Iron 115
  deficiency anemia 238
  overload 256
Ischemia 33
  mesenteric 33, 324
Isoflurane 453
Isolated intracranial hypertension
  syndrome 199

J

Janus kinase inhibitor 89
Jaundice 80
Jaw thrust 6
Jefferson fracture 401
Jersey finger 398
Jones fracture 400
Jugular venous pressure 34

K

Kayexalatc 430
Kernig's sign 99
Kerosene poisoning 139
Ketamine 430, 478, 481, 509
Ketoacidosis, diabetic 266, 268
Ketosis 267
Kidneys 512
  disease, chronic 59, 512
  ultrasonography of 96

Kiesselbach's plexus 289*f*
King cobra 128
Klebsiella 297
Knee 398
Kocher's technique 372, 373*f*
Korsakoff's psychosis 465

L

Labetalol 155
Labyrinthine concussion 293
Labyrinthitis, bacterial 296
Lactate 65
  clearance 39
  dehydrogenase 87, 504
Larson's point 482*f*
Laryngeal mask airway 43
Laryngospasm 481
  notch 481, 482*f*
Le-Fort fractures 355, 402
Left ventricular hypertrophy 154
  diagnostic criteria 174
Leg 399
Leiomyomas 275
Leptomeningitis 98
Leptospira interrogans 73
Leptospirosis 73
Leukemia
  acute 241, 241*t*
    lymphoid 241, 243
    myeloid 241
  chronic myeloid 241, 242
Leukocyte esterase 96
Leukopenia 84
Levetiracetam 210, 430, 477
Levofloxacin 105, 476
Liberal sedation 102
Lidocaine 16, 290, 430, 491
Lignocaine 16, 17, 485, 491, 514
Limb ischemia, acute 335
Linezolid 104, 477
Lipid emulsion therapy 113, 492
Lisfranc fracture dislocations 400
Listeria monocytogenes 98
Lithium 115
Liver
  disease 251
  failure 465

function test 78, 84, 209, 228, 233, 318, 452, 512
injury 496
Local anesthetics
characteristics of 485*t*
infiltration 514
systemic toxicity of 491
toxicity, treatment of 491
Loop diuretics 61
Loratadine 477
Lorazepam 413, 430, 456
Losartan 477
Low flow priapism 308
Lower gastrointestinal bleeding 226
causes of 226
Lower motor neuron
facial nerve palsy 216
sudden-onset 216
Low-molecular weight heparin 201, 248, 249
Ludwig's angina 73, 298
Lumbar puncture 100
Lung
abscess 83
diseases, immunologic 191
injury, acute 256
Lyme disease 206, 216
Lymphocytic choriomeningitis virus 98
Lysergic acid diethylamide 136

M

Magnesium 62, 165
sulfate 16, 430
Magnetic resonance
angiography 219
imaging 154, 200, 213
venography 213
Maisonneuve fracture 400
Malabar pit viper 128
Malabsorption syndrome 62
Malaria 80, 81
complicated 81
prophylaxis of 81
severe 81
Malarial parasite test 80
Malgaigne's fracture 398
Malignancy 199, 337

Malignant hyperthermia 453
clinical presentation 453
diagnosis 453
management 454
Mallampati score 41
Mallet finger 398
Mammary duct ectasia 338
Mannitol 430
March fracture 401
Marijuana 134
Mass casualty 436
incidents 435
management protocol 437*fc*
Massive intra-abdominal bleed 362
Massive transfusion
complications of 347
protocol 346, 347, 347*fc*
Mastalgia 338
cyclical 338
Mastitis 338
acute 338
lactational 338
nonlactational 338
periductal 338
Mastodynia 338
Matsen's traction 373, 373*f*
Maxillary fractures, Le-Fort
classification of 355*f*
Maxillofacial trauma 41, 355
McBurney's point 318*f*
McBurney's sign 317
Mean arterial pressure 35, 36, 155
Mean corpuscular volume 237, 239
Mechanical ventilation 184
Median nerve block 487, 488*f*
Medicolegal cases 439, 441
death of 442
Mefenamic acid 279
Mefloquine 81
Melena 225
Ménière's disease 293, 296
Meningitis 98
bacterial 74
viral 98, 99
Meningoencephalitis 98, 99
Meropenem 73, 105, 325, 430, 477
Mesenteric arterial
embolism 324
thrombosis 324

Mesenteric artery, superior 324
Mesenteric ischemia 33, 324
  clinical features 324
  diagnosis 325
  management 325
  physical examination 324
Mesobuthus tamulus 131
Metered dose inhaler technique 184
Methanol 111
  metabolism of 138*f*
  poisoning 138, 467
Methemoglobinemia 142, 143
  acquired 142*t*
  induction of 141
Methergine 285
Methotrexate 478
Methyl alcohol poisoning 138
Methylene blue 143
Methylenedioxymethamphetamine 136
Metoclopramide 213, 218, 318, 455, 477
Metoprolol 160, 477
Metronidazole 106, 333, 431, 476, 517, 518
Midazolam 113, 413, 431, 481, 482, 509
Migraine 213, 214
  vestibular 293
Miller Fisher syndrome 205
Mineralocorticoids 263
Miosis 134
Mitral regurgitation, acute 169
Mitral stenosis 169, 170, 191
Moderna 89
Monoarthritis, acute 479
Monophasic defibrillators 12
Monosodium urate 480
Monteggia fracture 397
Moraxella catarrhalis 73
Morphine 431
Motor axonal neuropathy, acute 205
Mountain sickness, acute 158
Multifocal atrial tachycardia 164
Multiple organ dysfunction syndrome 46
Mumps 98, 227
Murphy's sign 321
Muscarinic receptors 116
Muscle
  damage 336
  relaxation 102

Musculoskeletal trauma 391
Myalgia 84
Mycoplasma pneumonia 82, 205, 245
Myelodysplastic syndrome 239, 241
Myelopathy, acute 206
Myocardial infarction 32, 147, 148, 161, 512
Myometritis 279
Myxedema coma 261
  clinical presentation 261
  diagnosis 262
  management 262

N

N-acetylcysteine 111
N-acetyl-P-aminophenol 111
Nail bed
  crush injury of 327
  emergencies 327
  injuries 327
Nail trephination 327, 328*f*
Naja naja 128
Naloxone 17, 111
  intravenous dose of 134
Naproxen 478
Nasal cannula 44, 88
Nasal decongestants 423, 477
Nasal fractures 356
Nasogastric tube 344
Nasopharyngeal airway 8, 8*f*
National Early Warning Score 2 36, 38*t*
National Emergency X-radiography Utilization Study Criteria 351
Native valve emergencies 169
Natural absorbable sutures 380
Nausea 53, 134, 278
Neck mobility 41
Necrotizing fasciitis 73, 313, 314
  investigations 314
  management 314
Needle
  cricothyroidotomy 499, 500*f*
  thoracostomy 189
Neisseria
  gonorrhoeae 279, 305, 479
  meningitidis 74, 98
Neoplasms 41
Nephrolithiasis 301

Nerve
  blocks 485
  conduction velocity 205
Nervous system disorder 101
Neuralgia, trigeminal 214
Neuritis, vestibular 293
Neuroleptic malignant syndrome 451, 455
  clinical manifestations 455
  diagnosis 455
  management 455
Neuropathy, peripheral 457
Neurotoxic bite 129
New York Heart Association 170
Nicotinic receptors 116
Nifedipine 114, 431, 477
Nightstick fracture 397
Nitrite test 96
Nitrofurantoin 106
Nonabsorbable suture materials 380
Noninvasive ventilation 45, 47, 88, 184
Nonpoliovirus enteroviruses 98
Non-rebreather mask 44, 88
Nonsteroidal anti-inflammatory drugs 213, 227, 302, 306, 315, 338, 479
  use of 225
Non-ST-segment elevation myocardial infarction 153*t*
  management of 152
Noradrenaline 33, 431
Norwalk virus 93
Nutcracker fracture 401
Nystagmus 198, 293

O

Obesity 40, 41, 337
Obstetric emergencies 271
Obstruction 40, 41
Obtundation 53
Occlusive mesenteric arterial disease 324
Oculomotor dysfunction 464
Oduvanthalai poisoning, management of 125*fc*
Olanzapine 455
Omeprazole 477

Ondansetron 477
Oophoritis 279
Opening airway, methods of 6*t*
Ophiophagus hannah 128
Ophthalmoplegia 205
Opioids 111, 134
  intoxication 134
Optic neuritis 467
Oral airway 388
Oral anaerobes 73, 83
Oral antibiotics 232
Oral anticoagulants 247
Oral contraceptive pills 199
  high-dose 277
Oral hydration 93
Oral iron therapy 239
Oral rehydration solution 93
Organ
  dysfunction 35
  ischemia 250
Organochlorides 120
  compounds 118
Organochlorine 118
Organophosphates 111, 120
Organophosphorus compounds 116
Organophosphorus poisoning
  clinical features of 116
  features of 116*t*
Orientia tsutsugamushi 74, 78
Orogenital ulcers 479
Oseltamivir 85
Osteomalacia 321
Osteomyelitis 73, 314
Otitis externa 423
Otitis media 293, 423
Ovarian cyst, ruptured 281
Ovarian torsion 280
  clinical presentation 280
  differential diagnosis 281
  investigations 280
  management 281
Oxcarbazepine 210
Oxygen 44
  flow rates 44
  saturation 36, 407
  therapy, dangers of 44
Oxymetazoline 290, 477

P

P mitrale 173
P pulmonale 173
P wave 171, 172
Packed cell volume 347, 365
Packed red cells 255
Paget's disease 321
Pain 336
    abdominal 315*t*, 317, 512
    control 228
    epigastric 282, 301
    lower abdominal 274
    relief 302, 460
        discharge plan for 514
    severity of 513
Painful crisis 245
Palamnaeus swammerdami 131
Pallor 336
Pamidronate 61
Pancreatic effusion 504
Pancreaticobiliary drainage, anatomy
    of 320*f*
Pancreatitis 278
    acute 227, 511
    biliary 228
    mild acute 227
    moderately severe acute 227
    severe acute 227
Pancuronium 431
Pantoprazole 278, 431, 477
Paracentesis 505
    therapeutic 505
Paracetamol 111, 302
Paradoxical chest wall movement 41
Paralysis 90, 336
    transient 457
Parametritis 279
Paraphimosis 307, 307*f*
    management 308
Paraquat poisoning 119
Parathyroid hormone 59
Paratrooper's fracture 400
Paresthesia 336
Paronychia 327, 328
    drainage 329, 329*f*
Parotid gland tumors 216
Paroxysmal supraventricular
    tachycardia 164, 164*f*
Parvovirus 245
Patellar dislocation 377
    reduction of 377*f*
Peak expiratory flow rate 182
Peaked T waves 174*f*
Pediatric
    basic life support 12*fc*
    cardiac arrest 25, 26*fc*
    emergencies 403
        drugs and dosages in 426
    resuscitative equipment 410*t*
    trauma 388
Pelvic
    compression test 368
    fractures 367
    inflammatory disease 279
        etiology 279
        management 279
Pelvis 398, 519
Penicillin 476
Penile
    emergencies 307
    fracture 308
Peptic ulcer disease 315
Pericardiocentesis 502, 502*f*
    complications 503
    emergency 502
    indications 502
    nonemergency 502
    technique 502
Pericarditis, constrictive 32
Peripheral capillary oxygen saturation
    183
Peritonitis 325, 362
    bacterial 72, 229, 231, 512
    secondary 72
Perphenazine 218
Pfizer 89
Pharyngitis, acute 73
Phenergan 218, 296, 477
Pheniramine maleate 431
Phenobarbitone 131, 210, 431, 477
Phenylephrine 309, 477
Phenytoin 210, 211, 477
    sodium 431
    therapeutic range 115
Pheochromocytoma 270
    laboratory investigations 270
    management 270

Phimosis 307, 307*f*
  management 307
Phosphorus compounds 122
Piedmont fracture 397
Piles 331
Pilon fracture 399
Piperacillin 72, 73, 103, 314, 316, 318,
    325, 431, 463, 476
Pituitary disease 264
Plant poisons 124
Plasmodium
  lactate dehydrogenase 80
  vivax 80
Plaster of Paris 378
Plastic surgery 461
Platelet 241, 255
  defects, acquired 250
  destruction 250
  disorders, congenital 250
  loss 251
  production 250
Pleural fluid analysis 504
Pneumatosis intestinalis 325
Pneumonia 420
  community-acquired 82, 83*t*
  necrotizing 83
Pneumothorax 188
  iatrogenic 188
  open 358, 359
  primary spontaneous 188
  secondary spontaneous 188
  traumatic 188
  types of 188
Poikilothermia 336
Poisonings 206, 511
Polyangiitis, microscopic 191
Polyarthritis 480
Polycystic ovarian syndrome 276
Polymicrobial 73
Polyps 275
Polyradiculoneuropathy, acute
    inflammatory demyelinating 205
Polytrauma 515
Pontine tumors 216
Porphyria, acute intermittent 206
Positive ascitic fluid bacterial culture 229

Posterior hip dislocations 374, 375
  reduction of 376
    Thompson and Epstein classification
      375*f*
Posterior tibial nerve block 490
Postexposure prophylaxis 90, 91, 473-
  475
Postpartum hemorrhage 284
  clinical features 284
  investigations 284
  management 284
Potassium 56
Pott's fracture 400
Pouteau fracture 396
Pralidoxime 111
Prazosin 131, 477
Prednisolone 61, 471
Preeclampsia 282
Pregnancy 84, 199, 252, 337
  drugs in 476
  ectopic 273, 278, 281
Preoxygenate 509
Preoxygenation 388
Pressure
  bag 497
  support 46
Priapism 245, 308
  management 308
Prilocaine 491
Prochlorperazine 218, 296
Progestogen therapy 276
Promethazine 218, 296, 455, 477
Prophylactic antibiotic protocol 517,
  517*t*
Prophylaxis 474*t*
Propranolol 431, 477
Prosthetic valve emergencies 170
Protein
  bound 59
  C 255
    deficiency 252
  S 255
    deficiency 252
Prothrombin
  gene mutation 252
  time 99, 233, 336, 347, 512

Protozoa 424
  infection 80
Pseudo Jones fracture 401
Pseudohyperkalemia 57
Pseudohyponatremia 53
Pseudomonas aeroginosa 216, 233, 240
Psoas sign 317
Psychosis 60
Puerperium 199
Pulmonary edema, high-altitude 158
Pulmonary function tests 183
Pulse
  check 11
  oximetry 407
  rate 36
Pulseless electrical activity 16
Pyelonephritis 95, 97, 278, 281
Pyogenic meningitis 98, 99
Pyrethroids 119, 120
Pyridoxine 278

Q

Q wave 173
QRS complex 171
Quinine 81

R

R wave 173
Rabies 90
  immunoglobulin 91
  vaccine 92
Radial nerve block 486, 487*f*
Raised intracranial pressure 213, 390
Ramsay Hunt syndrome 216
Ranitidine 432, 477
Rapid antigen test 86
Rapid blood borne virus screen 336
Rapid sequence induction 88, 509
  protocol 509, 509*t*
Rapid shallow breathing 41
Rash 479
Red blood
  cell 237, 239
    count 204
  distribution width 239
Red eye, acute 469

Regurgitant lesions 169
Regurgitation
  aortic 169
  paravalvular 170
Reiter syndrome 480
Renal calculi 281
Renal disease 251
Renal failure 80, 125, 282
Renal loss 56, 62
Renal replacement therapy 244
Renal tubular acidosis 62
Rescue breaths 8
Reservoir bag 44, 88
Resin casts 378
Respiratory arrest 53
Respiratory failure 44, 45, 47, 113
Respiratory rate 35, 36, 38
Respiratory system 29
Respiratory viruses 73
Resuscitation 341, 386
  cardiopulmonary 3, 4, 10, 11
  maternal 23
Reticulocyte count 237
Retina problems 466
Retinal detachment 467
Retropharyngeal abscess 297
  causes 297
  clinical features 297
  investigations 297
  management 297
Reverse transcription-polymerase chain
    reaction test 86
Rhinosinusitis, bacterial 73
Rifampicin 477
Right bundle branch block diagnostic
    criteria 175
Right upper quadrant pain 301
Ringer lactate 51
Risperidone 455
Rodenticides 121
  types of 121
Rolando fracture 397
Rotavirus 93
Rovsing's sign 317
Rubella 227
Rugby finger 398
Runner's fracture 399
Russell's viper 128

S

S wave 173
Saccular aneurysm 214
Salbutamol 432
  nebulization 31
Salmonella 480
  paratyphi 71
  typhi 71
Salpingitis 279
Saphenous nerve block 491
Sarcoidosis 216
Saw scaled viper 128
Scalp 517
  laceration 381
Scorpion sting 131
Scotoma 282
Scrotal pain, acute 304
Scrub typhus 74, 78, 99
  Eschar of 79*f*
Sea snakes 128
Seasonal influenza 84
Seatbelt fracture 401
Sedation, procedural 481
Segond fracture 398
Seizures 53, 62, 113, 131, 209, 512
  active 283
  complex febrile 412
  management of 209*t*
  new-onset 209
  simple febrile 412
  suppression 492
  withdrawal 464
Seldinger technique 494
Sensorimotor axonal neuropathy, acute 205
Sensorium, altered 14, 21, 36
Sepsis 35, 37, 37*fc*
Septic focus, control of 38
Septic shock 32, 35, 88, 325
  management of 37
Sequential organ failure assessment score 36*t*
Sequestration, hepatic 245
Serum beta-human chorionic gonadotropin 273
Sevoflurane 453

Sexually transmitted diseases 333
Sheehan's syndrome 284
Shenton's line 368, 368*f*
Shepherd fracture 400
Shigella 71, 480
Shock 32, 80
  anaphylactic 32
  cardiogenic 32
  classification of 32
  compensated 77
  distributive 32
  electric 457
  hemorrhagic 345, 345*t*
  hypovolemic 32, 284, 446
  management 34*t*
  mechanism of 33*fc*
  neurogenic 32
  obstructive 32
  overview of 32
  septic 32, 35, 88, 325
  signs of 14, 21
  stages of 32
  types of 32, 34
Shoulder
  dislocation 370
    types of 371*t*
  reduction, Kocher's technique for 373*f*
Sickle cell
  crisis 245
    clinical presentation of 245
  disease, acute complications of 245
Silver sulfadiazine 461
Sinoatrial nodal reentrant tachycardia 164
Sinus
  bradycardia 14, 17, 17*f*
  rhythm, normal 171
Skier's thumb 398
Skin
  and integumentary system 29
  hyperpigmentation 263
  infection 313
Smith fracture 396
Snakes 128*t*
  bites 128
Snoring 41

Sodium 53
bicarbonate 432
nitrite 142
polystyrene sulfonate 430
thiosulfate 142
valproate 210, 477
Soft tissue 354
infection 313
Sore throat 84
Sphincterotomy, endoscopic 234
Spider bites 133
Spinal cord injury 391
Spinal injuries, classification of 350
Spine 401
manual in-line stabilization of 342*f*
Spirometry 184
interpretation of 181*fc*
lung volumes on 185*f*
Spironolactone 432
Spleen injury 496
Splenic sequestration 245, 251
Splints 378
Sputnik 89
Staphylococcus
aureus 72, 82, 240, 290, 297, 328, 338, 479
epidermidis 240
organisms 93
Statins 478
Status asthmaticus 414
Status epilepticus 211, 212*fc*
management of 211
Steroids 31
Stevens–Johnson syndrome 472
Stieda fracture 398, 400
Stiff lungs 40
Stimson's technique 372, 372*f*
Stones, types of 301
Streptococcus
milleri 83
pneumonia 82, 83, 98, 245
pyogenes 72
viridans 240
Stridor 291, 417
acute 417
causes of 417*t*
classification of 418*t*
etiology 291
management 291

Stroke 165
hemorrhagic 196
ischemic 195, 196
Strychnine 126
ST-segment elevation myocardial infarction, management of 151
Subclavian line 493
Substance abuse 134
Succinylcholine 432, 453, 509
Sulbactam 103, 428
Sulfamethoxazole 306, 477
Sulfonamides 227
Sulfur donors 141
Superficial peroneal nerve block 490
Supratherapeutic international normalized ratio, management of 248*t*
Sural nerve block 491
Surgical cricothyroidotomy 500, 501*f*
complications of 501
Suture
materials 380
needles 380
Synovial fluid analysis 479
Synthetic braided sutures 380
Synthetic monofilament sutures 380
Systemic inflammatory response syndrome 35
Systemic lupus erythematosus 191
Systemic toxicity, management of 491

T

T wave 173
T2-weighted fluid-attenuated inversion recovery 219
Tachyarrhythmias 21, 33
classification of 21*t*
initial management of 21
Tachycardia 22*fc*, 33, 125, 259, 481
atrial 164
supraventricular 21, 168, 432
ventricular 21, 166, 167, 167*f*, 168, 432, 462
Tachypnea 125
Tardive
dyskinesia 218
dystonia 218
Tazobactam 72, 73, 103, 314, 316, 318, 325, 431, 463, 476

Temporary pacemaker insertion 19
Temporomandibular joint 356
   dislocation 356
Tennis elbow 397
Tense ascites 505
Tension pneumothorax 16, 32, 189*f*, 358, 359
Testicular cancer 304
Testicular torsion 304
Tetanus 101
   prophylaxis 90, 92, 102, 102*t*, 129, 379
Tetany 62
Tetracyclines 227
Tetralogy of Fallot 432
Thallium 121
Thiazides 227
Thioridazine 218
Third-degree atrioventricular block 14
Thompson and Epstein classification 375*f*
Thoracic injuries 358
Thorax 519
   examination of 343
Three-way occlusive dressing 360*f*
Thrombocytopenia 250
   heparin-induced 249
Thrombolysis in myocardial infarction score 153*t*
Thrombosis
   coronary 16
   pulmonary 16
Thrombotic thrombocytopenic purpura 250
Thrombus 335
Thyroid
   antibody titers 259
   gland, intrinsic dysfunction of 261
   hormone replacement 262
   stimulating hormone 259
   storm 259
      medical management of 260*t*
Thyrotoxic crisis 259
   clinical features 259
   investigations 259
   management 260
Tibia fractures 369
Tick borne paralysis 206

Tidal volume 185
Tigecycline 72
Tillaux fracture 400
Tinidazole 71
Tinnitus 296
Tissue factor pathway inhibitor 255
Tocilizumab 89
Toddler's fracture 399
Torsades de pointes 166, 167*f*
Torsion
   higher risk of 303
   testis 303
      clinical features 303
      management 303
Total lung capacity 185
Tourniquet test 76
Toxic epidermal necrolysis 472
Toxic shock syndrome 32, 290
Toxins 16
Tracheal tug 41
Tramadol 318, 432
Tranexamic acid 276, 285, 432
Transaminitis 84
Transcutaneous electrical nerve stimulation 217
Transcutaneous pacing 18, 19, 20*f*
Transfusion reaction 256
Transient ischemic attack 161, 165, 195
Transvenous pacing 18, 19
Trauma 216, 227, 283, 385, 515, 517
   abdominal 390
   early management of 341
Tremors 62
Tricyclic antidepressants 111-113
   overdose 112
Trifluoperazine 218
Triglycerides 504
Trihexyphenidyl 218
Triiodothyronine 259
Trimeresurus malabaricus 128
Trimethoprim 306, 477
Trousseau's sign 59
Tube thoracostomy 189*f*
Tuberculosis 190
Tubo-ovarian abscess 279, 281
Tumor lysis syndrome 243, 244

Tunica vaginalis 303
Typhoid fever 71

U

Ulnar nerve block 487, 488*f*
Ultrasonography 96, 188, 234, 393
Universal pain assessment tool 513*f*
Upper airway obstruction 45
Upper gastrointestinal
   bleeding 46, 225, 226*b*
      causes of 225
   surgery 45
Urea 84, 336
Ureaplasma urealyticum 279
Ureters 512
Urinary catheter 344
Urinary tract infection 95
   antibiotics for 97*t*
   diagnosis of 95*fc*
   lower 95
   management of 95*fc*
   upper 95
Urine
   alkalinization of 244
   osmolality 54
   output 390
   precolor 318
   spot sodium 54
Urological emergencies 299
Ursodeoxycholic acid 432
Urticaria 471
Uterine
   bleeding, abnormal 275
   rupture 387
Uveitis 469

V

Vaginal bleeding, management of 276
Valacyclovir 73, 476
Valproate 227, 432
Valve regurgitation 170
Valvular emergencies 169
Valvular thrombus, acute 170
Vancomycin 99, 104, 432
Varicella zoster virus 73, 98, 216

Vascular diseases 191
Vasculitis, systemic 227
Vaso-occlusive
   crisis 245
   phenomena 245
Vasopressin 17
Vasopressors 32, 33*t*, 187
Vasospasm, prevention of 204
Vecuronium 432
Vena cava, inferior 385
Venous blood gas 65
   analysis 112
Ventilation 7, 389
Ventricle septal rupture 32
Venturi mask 44, 88
Verapamil 114, 160, 477
Vertigo 198, 292, 292*fc*
   benign paroxysmal positional 292,
      293, 295*f*
   causes of 293*t*
   medications for 296
   peripheral 294
   posterior canal benign paroxysmal
      positional 294
Vibrio cholerae 71, 93, 94
Vincent's angina 73
Viral infection, arthropod-borne 75
Viridans spirillum minus *Streptobacillus*
   74
Viruses 240, 424
Vision
   loss of 282
   painless loss of 466
   sudden painless loss of 467
Visual disturbances 282
Visual field defects 198, 282
Visual loss, sudden 466
Vital capacity 185
Vitamin
   D deficiency 59
   K1 432
Vomiting 32, 46, 53, 134
von Willebrand disease 253, 254
   clinical features 254
   diagnosis 254
   management 254

W

Warm sitz baths 331, 332
Watery diarrhea, acute 425*t*
Weakness 62
Web space block 486*f*
Wegener's granulomatosis 191
Wellens' syndrome 149, 150*f*
Wells scoring system, modified 186*t*
Wernicke's encephalopathy 464
White blood cell count 96
Whole blood clotting time 129
Wide complex tachycardia 16, 166
  characteristics of 166*t*
Wound
  care 90
  classification of 91*t*
  cleansing 381
  closure 381
  debridement 381
  management 379, 460
  wash 379

Wrist block 486

X

X-rays 365-369, 371, 376, 394, 395
  role of 369

Y

Yellow
  oleander 124
  phosphorus 121, 122
Yersinia 480
  enterocolitica 93

Z

Zika virus 245
Zinc
  phosphide 121, 122
  supplementation 424
Zoledronic acid 61
Zygomycetes 314